Marine Anti-inflammatory and Antioxidant Agents 2021

Marine Anti-inflammatory and Antioxidant Agents 2021

Editors

Donatella Degl'Innocenti
Marzia Vasarri

MDPI • Basel • Beijing • Wuhan • Barcelona • Belgrade • Manchester • Tokyo • Cluj • Tianjin

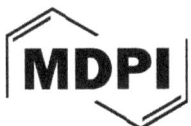

Editors
Donatella Degl'Innocenti Marzia Vasarri
Università degli Studi di Firenze Università degli Studi di Firenze
Italy Italy

Editorial Office
MDPI
St. Alban-Anlage 66
4052 Basel, Switzerland

This is a reprint of articles from the Special Issue published online in the open access journal *Marine Drugs* (ISSN 1660-3397) (available at: https://www.mdpi.com/journal/marinedrugs/special_issues/Anti_inflammatoryAntioxidantAgents).

For citation purposes, cite each article independently as indicated on the article page online and as indicated below:

LastName, A.A.; LastName, B.B.; LastName, C.C. Article Title. *Journal Name* **Year**, *Volume Number*, Page Range.

ISBN 978-3-0365-3373-5 (Hbk)
ISBN 978-3-0365-3374-2 (PDF)

© 2022 by the authors. Articles in this book are Open Access and distributed under the Creative Commons Attribution (CC BY) license, which allows users to download, copy and build upon published articles, as long as the author and publisher are properly credited, which ensures maximum dissemination and a wider impact of our publications.

The book as a whole is distributed by MDPI under the terms and conditions of the Creative Commons license CC BY-NC-ND.

Contents

About the Editors vii

Marzia Vasarri and Donatella Degl'Innocenti
Antioxidant and Anti-Inflammatory Agents from the Sea: A Molecular Treasure for New Potential Drugs
Reprinted from: *Mar. Drugs* **2022**, *20*, 132, doi:10.3390/md20020132 1

Xueyan Zhang, Zhilan Peng, Huina Zheng, Chaohua Zhang, Haisheng Lin and Xiaoming Qin
The Potential Protective Effect and Possible Mechanism of Peptides from Oyster (*Crassostrea hongkongensis*) Hydrolysate on Triptolide-Induced Testis Injury in Male Mice
Reprinted from: *Mar. Drugs* **2021**, *19*, 566, doi:10.3390/md19100566 7

Adrian S. Siregar, Marie Merci Nyiramana, Eun-Jin Kim, Soo Buem Cho, Min Seok Woo, Dong Kun Lee, Seong-Geun Hong, Jaehee Han, Sang Soo Kang, Deok Ryong Kim, Yeung Joon Choi and Dawon Kang
Oyster-Derived Tyr-Ala (YA) Peptide Prevents Lipopolysaccharide/D-Galactosamine-Induced Acute Liver Failure by Suppressing Inflammatory, Apoptotic, Ferroptotic, and Pyroptotic Signals
Reprinted from: *Mar. Drugs* **2021**, *19*, 614, doi:10.3390/md19110614 25

Indyaswan Tegar Suryaningtyas, Chang-Bum Ahn and Jae-Young Je
Cytoprotective Peptides from Blue Mussel Protein Hydrolysates: Identification and Mechanism Investigation in Human Umbilical Vein Endothelial Cells Injury
Reprinted from: *Mar. Drugs* **2021**, *19*, 609, doi:10.3390/md19110609 39

Vanessa Blas-Valdivia, Plácido Rojas-Franco, Jose Ivan Serrano-Contreras, Andrea Augusto Sfriso, Cristian Garcia-Hernandez, Margarita Franco-Colín and Edgar Cano-Europa
C-phycoerythrin from *Phormidium persicinum* Prevents Acute Kidney Injury by Attenuating Oxidative and Endoplasmic Reticulum Stress
Reprinted from: *Mar. Drugs* **2021**, *19*, 589, doi:10.3390/md19110589 53

Yinyan Yin, Nuo Xu, Yi Shi, Bangyue Zhou, Dongrui Sun, Bixia Ma, Zhengzhong Xu, Jin Yang and Chunmei Li
Astaxanthin Protects Dendritic Cells from Lipopolysaccharide- Induced Immune Dysfunction
Reprinted from: *Mar. Drugs* **2021**, *19*, 346, doi:10.3390/md19060346 73

Yinyan Yin, Nuo Xu, Tao Qin, Bangyue Zhou, Yi Shi, Xinyi Zhao, Bixia Ma, Zhengzhong Xu and Chunmei Li
Astaxanthin Provides Antioxidant Protection in LPS-Induced Dendritic Cells for Inflammatory Control
Reprinted from: *Mar. Drugs* **2021**, *19*, 534, doi:10.3390/md19100534 89

Elisabetta Bigagli, Mario D'Ambrosio, Lorenzo Cinci, Alberto Niccolai, Natascia Biondi, Liliana Rodolfi, Luana Beatriz Dos Santos Nascimiento, Mario R. Tredici and Cristina Luceri
A Comparative In Vitro Evaluation of the Anti-Inflammatory Effects of a *Tisochrysis lutea* Extract and Fucoxanthin
Reprinted from: *Mar. Drugs* **2021**, *19*, 334, doi:10.3390/md19060334 103

Qian Yang, Yanhui Jiang, Shan Fu, Zhaopeng Shen, Wenwen Zong, Zhongning Xia, Zhaoya Zhan and Xiaolu Jiang
Protective Effects of *Ulva lactuca* Polysaccharide Extract on Oxidative Stress and Kidney Injury Induced by D-Galactose in Mice
Reprinted from: *Mar. Drugs* **2021**, *19*, 539, doi:10.3390/md19100539 . . . . **117**

Muhammad Bilal, Leonardo Vieira Nunes, Marco Thúlio Saviatto Duarte, Luiz Fernando Romanholo Ferreira, Renato Nery Soriano and Hafiz M. N. Iqbal
Exploitation of Marine-Derived Robust Biological Molecules to Manage Inflammatory Bowel Disease
Reprinted from: *Mar. Drugs* **2021**, *19*, 196, doi:10.3390/md19040196 . . . . **129**

Vittoria Roncalli, Chiara Lauritano and Ylenia Carotenuto
First Report of OvoA Gene in Marine Arthropods: A New Candidate Stress Biomarker in Copepods
Reprinted from: *Mar. Drugs* **2021**, *19*, 647, doi:10.3390/md19110647 . . . . **149**

About the Editors

Donatella Degl'Innocenti Ph.D. Prof. Donatella Degl'Innocenti obtained a Ph.D. in Biochemistry, and she has been an Associate Professor of Biochemistry in the Department of Experimental and Clinical Biomedical Sciences "Mario Serio" (University of Florence, Italy) since 2001. During her scientific career, she built national and international scientific collaborations. She is an active researcher and the leader of her department laboratory (https://www.sbsc.unifi.it/vp-223-gruppo-degl-innocenti.html). She has strong, independent research experience, with an impact in the field, as demonstrated by several publications as a senior author in international, peer-reviewed journals. She is also a member of the Scientific Committee of the Interuniversity Center of Marine Biology and Applied Ecology (CIBM) of Livorno (Italy). In recent years, she has focused her research on the health role of natural and marine compounds. She studied the amyloid aggregation process and potential inhibitory mechanisms of natural compounds and the extract of Mediterranean red seaweed. Prof. Degl'Innocenti has also studied the biological properties of extracts obtained from the leaves of the *Posidonia oceanica* (L.) Delile marine plant, focusing on these extracts' role in pathophysiological cellular processes, such as inflammation and oxidative stress, as well as on cancer cell migration and protein glycation processes.

Marzia Vasarri Ph.D. Dr. Marzia Vasarri is a Post-Doc fellow at the Department of Experimental and Clinical Biomedical Sciences "Mario Serio" (University of Florence, Italy). She obtained a Bachelor's degree in Biotechnology in 2014 and a Master's degree in Medical and Pharmaceutical Biotechnology in 2016. During her studies, she acquired technical-scientific skills in biochemistry and molecular biology. Her research focuses on the bioactive properties of natural products, with particular reference to products of marine origin. Much of her research targets the marine plant *Posidonia oceanica* (L.) Delile, which has been investigated by Dr. Vasarri for a variety of pathophysiological cellular processes, from inflammation and oxidative stress to cancer cell migration, protein glycation processes, lipid accumulation in hepatic cells and its potential as an inducer of autophagy. Her research interest also includes the field of neurodegeneration and amyloid aggregation process, and the protective role of natural compounds against amyloid cytotoxicity. She has also conducted research on the biological properties of natural products delivered within nanoformulations that can improve the efficacy and bioavailability of the encapsulated compounds/phytocomplex to exploit their full potential.

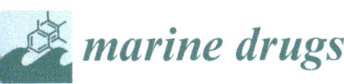

Editorial

Antioxidant and Anti-Inflammatory Agents from the Sea: A Molecular Treasure for New Potential Drugs

Marzia Vasarri * and Donatella Degl'Innocenti

Department of Experimental and Clinical Biomedical Sciences, University of Florence, Viale Morgagni 50, 50134 Florence, Italy; donatella.deglinnocenti@unifi.it
* Correspondence: marzia.vasarri@unifi.it

Nowadays, natural compounds are widely used worldwide for the treatment of human diseases and health disorders. Throughout history, plants have been the primary sources of many pharmaceutical agents. However, over the years, great attention has been paid to the incredible biodiversity of life in seas, which has proven to be an exceptional reservoir of novel bioactive molecules with disparate structural and chemical characteristics, and a source of inspiration for new drug discovery.

To date, several marine drugs have been pharmacologically approved for the treatment of various diseases, while many other compounds are in clinical trials. At the same time, the global preclinical marine pharmaceutical pipeline involves research with more than 1000 marine chemicals with diverse biological properties.

The treasures of the sea have provided fundamental contributions to modern medicine, supplying important scientific discoveries for human health. Thus, in recent decades, marine bio-discovery has become "frontier" research for many scientists in academia and industry.

Today, it is well recognized that inflammation and oxidative stress are two closely related biological processes. The impact of inflammation and related oxidative stress is a huge issue in human health, as most chronic diseases and disorders are deeply linked to the interaction between these two biological phenomena.

In the relentless demand to discover new safe and effective agents with anti-inflammatory and antioxidant properties beneficial to human health, the marine environment has emerged as an unexplored molecular treasure trove.

The Special Issue "Marine Anti-Inflammatory and Antioxidants Agents 2021" collected the latest research, both in vitro and in vivo, on natural compounds from a variety of deep-sea organisms (including arthropods, oysters, mussels, algae, microalgae and cyanobacteria) with anti-inflammatory and/or antioxidant properties as potential candidates for new drug discovery, and in general for the field of marine biotechnology.

Among the natural occurring biomolecules, peptides are natural products present in many marine species. A large amount of scientific evidence reports that marine peptides have a high nutraceutical and medicinal power thanks to their wide spectrum of biological properties, as in the case of peptides from oyster hydrolysate (OPs). Oysters, the largest farmed shellfish in the world, are a good source of polypeptides, with antioxidant, immune, antimicrobial, antitumor, antifatigue and hepatoprotective properties. The work of Zhang et al. (2021) adds new insight to the benefits of peptides from oyster (*Crassostrea hongkongensis*) hydrolysate by describing their protective effect on testicular injury and disorders of spermatogenesis caused by tryptolide (TP) [1]. In mice with testicular injury, the ingestion of OPs for 4 weeks significantly improved the sperm count and motility of mice, and alleviated seminiferous tubule injury. OPs exerted antioxidant properties by upregulating the Nrf2 signaling pathway and thereby promoting the activity of antioxidant enzymes and the expression of antioxidant enzyme regulatory proteins in the testis. The activities of enzymes related to energy metabolism in the testis also improved after the

Citation: Vasarri, M.; Degl'Innocenti, D. Antioxidant and Anti-Inflammatory Agents from the Sea: A Molecular Treasure for New Potential Drugs. *Mar. Drugs* **2022**, *20*, 132. https://doi.org/10.3390/md20020132

Received: 24 January 2022
Accepted: 27 January 2022
Published: 10 February 2022

Publisher's Note: MDPI stays neutral with regard to jurisdictional claims in published maps and institutional affiliations.

Copyright: © 2022 by the authors. Licensee MDPI, Basel, Switzerland. This article is an open access article distributed under the terms and conditions of the Creative Commons Attribution (CC BY) license (https://creativecommons.org/licenses/by/4.0/).

ingestion of OPs, and serum hormone levels returned to normal. Severe testicular tissue damage improved due to the OP-induced inhibition of the JNK signaling pathway and Bcl-2/Bax-mediated apoptosis. For the first time, this study provides evidence on the potential improvement of male reproductive function by OPs, and discloses the experimental basis for the development of OPs in functional foods.

Siregar et al. (2021) also directed their research on the beneficial properties of OPs for human health [2]. Specifically, the authors explored the mechanism of hepatoprotective action of the peptide tyrosine-alanine (YA), identified as the main component of oyster (*Crassostrea gigas*) hydrolysate, in a mouse model with liver injury induced by intraperitoneal injection with lipopolysaccharide (LPS) and D-galactosamine (D-GalN). It has been demonstrated that the pre-administration of YA (50 mg/kg) significantly reduced inflammatory, apoptotic, ferroptotic and pyroptotic liver injury induced by the intraperitoneal injection of LPS/D-GalN showing hepatoprotective effects. This study provides clear evidence of YA as a potential hepatoprotective bioactive peptide in acute liver injury, such as acute or fulminant liver failure, and acute hepatitis.

The study of peptides as potential functional agents in human health was also undertaken by Suryaningtyas et al. (2021) [3]. Here, the authors demonstrated the cytoprotective activity of two peptides identified as FTVN and EPTF from the blue mussel (*Mytilus edulis*) and their role in preventing endothelial dysfunction (ED) mediated by oxidative stress induced by H_2O_2 exposure in human umbilical vein endothelial (HUVEC) cells. The investigation of the cytoprotective mechanism of these two peptides and their combination revealed that the peptides significantly reduced HUVEC death caused by H_2O_2 exposure through the enhancement of the antioxidant defense system via the upregulation of the cytoprotective enzyme heme oxygenase-1, and antinecrotic action. In light of these data, the authors suggest potential applications of peptides from the blue mussel as functional agents in protecting against ED-mediated oxidative stress.

Taken together, these briefly summarized works shed light on the possibility of using bioactive peptides and peptide-rich protein hydrolysates as an alternative to synthetic drugs for the prevention and treatment of acute and chronic diseases. However, further in vivo research will be required to develop a nutraceutical or pharmaceutical component based on these findings.

Among the marine-derived proteins studied over the years for their human health benefits, microalgae pigments (or phycobiliproteins) are well known. C-phycocyanin has been widely described as a phycobiliprotein with nephroprotective activity due to its antioxidant properties. Among others, C-phycoerythrin (C-PE), an oligomeric chromoprotein from cyanobacteria, is also already used in the food and cosmetic industries, as well as in diagnosis and research due to its nutraceutical properties, e.g., scavenging and antioxidant activity. Blas-Valdivia et al. (2021) contributed to the study of the biological properties of phycobiliproteins by revealing, for the first time, that the nephroprotective activity of C-PE (purified from *Phormidium persicinum*) is closely related to its antioxidant activity in the kidney of animal models of $HgCl_2$-induced acute kidney injury [4]. Specifically, C-PE has been shown to act by preventing the $HgCl_2$-induced increase in oxidative stress. In addition, C-PE prevents podocyte destruction and damage to glomerular and tubular cells by acting on intracellular signaling pathways involved in proteostasis.

As with terrestrial organisms, carotenoids represent the most common group of pigments in marine environments. Marine carotenoids exert strong antioxidant, restorative, antiproliferative and anti-inflammatory effects and can be used both as skin photoprotection to inhibit the negative effects of solar UV radiation and as nutraceutical/cosmeceutical ingredients to prevent oxidative stress-related diseases. In this regard, Yin et al. (2021) contributed with the publication of two research articles focused on the biological properties of astaxanthin, a naturally occurring red carotenoid pigment classified as xanthophyll native to marine organisms, such as microalgae and seafood, with known potent antioxidant properties [5,6]. The authors evaluated the anti-inflammatory and antioxidant capacity of astaxanthin on the immune functions of murine dendritic cells (DCs) in a sepsis model.

Astaxanthin was shown to protect DCs from LPS-induced immune dysfunction. Specifically, it reduced the expression of LPS-induced inflammatory cytokines and phenotypic markers of DCs. It promoted endocytosis in LPS-treated DCs and hindered LPS-induced DC migration and abrogated allogeneic T-cell proliferation. Astaxanthin inhibited the LPS-induced immune dysfunction of DCs through the activation of the HO-1/Nrf2 axis, and when administered orally, it increased the survival rate of LPS-affected mice in vivo [5]. Furthermore, the authors demonstrated that astaxanthin, again via the HO-1/Nrf2 axis, protected LPS-induced DCs and LPS-affected mice from oxidative stress to achieve overloaded inflammatory control [6]. These studies lend strength to astaxanthin as a potential drug candidate for applications in various inflammatory diseases.

Historically, whole plants or mixtures of plants were used in traditional medicine rather than isolated compounds. There is evidence that crude extracts often have greater bioactivity in vitro and/or in vivo than isolated constituents at an equivalent dose. This effect could be due to the positive interactions between the components of whole extracts, as opposed to the activity of the individual compound. In this regard, Bigagli et al. (2021) performed a comparative study between the in vitro anti-inflammatory properties of a methanolic extract of *Tosochrysis lutea* (*T. lutea*) F&M-M36, a marine microalga belonging to the Haptophyta, and the single xanthophyll fucoxanthin (FX), on RAW 264.7 macrophages stimulated by lipopolysaccharide (LPS) [7]. To date, the anti-inflammatory and antioxidant effects of *T. lutea* have been mostly attributed to FX, one of its major constituents. However, *T. lutea* is also a source of phenolic compounds with a large spectrum of biological activities, including antioxidant, antiaging and anti-inflammatory effects, so positive pharmacodynamic synergies among the various components, acting on different targets, cannot be ruled out. In this study, the authors showed that the methanolic extract of *T. lutea* F&M-M36 exerts promising anti-inflammatory activity against COX-2/PGE$_2$ and NLRP3/mir-223, even more pronounced than that of FX alone, which could be attributable to the known anti-inflammatory effects of the simple phenolic compounds found in the extract. These phenolic compounds could synergize with FX, and *T. lutea* F&M-M36 could serve as a source of anti-inflammatory compounds to be further evaluated in in vivo models of inflammation.

Among naturally occurring biomolecules, polysaccharides derived from algae and marine plants have received increasing attention among researchers. Indeed, marine polysaccharides possess numerous health benefits as well as raw materials for the pharmaceutical, nutrition and cosmetic industries. A wide variety of natural products with seaweed polysaccharides, with recognized antioxidant effects, are gradually entering people's line of sight.

In this context, Yang et al. (2021) revealed to the scientific community the ameliorative effects of polysaccharide extract of *Ulva lactuca* (UPE), a type of green alga from coastal areas of China, on D-galactose (D-gal)-induced oxidative stress renal damage [8]. The intragastric administration of UPE in mice subjected to subcutaneous injection decreases serum creatinine, blood urea nitrogen and serum cystatin C levels; increases the glomerular filtration rate; enhances antioxidant enzyme activities; and reduces biomacromolecule damage caused by oxidative damage. It also significantly reduces the levels of inflammatory cytokines caused by oxidative stress. In addition, UPE administration could prevent the D-gal-induced apoptosis of renal tubule cells. This study highlights the protective effects of UPE on renal injury caused by oxidative stress, providing a new theoretical basis for the treatment of oxidative damage diseases.

Overall, marine-derived bioproducts are attracting incredible interest and appear to be a revolutionary therapy for various inflammation-related diseases, due to their beneficial health properties, which are attributed to the presence of characteristic biologically active functional constituents. In this context, research is ongoing worldwide, and researchers have redirected or reclaimed their interests in exploiting natural biological entities/resources, such as the algal biome. In this regard, Bilal et al. (2021) compiled a review that presents some natural biological compounds derived from the algal biome for the efficient management of inflammatory bowel diseases (IBDs), a chronic inflammation of the gastrointestinal tract [9]. A large number of marine bioproducts have been purified and identified from marine sources and have shown antioxidant properties and anti-inflammatory effects. However, the need for further research efforts has emerged to inspect the bioavailability and efficiency of marine bioproducts in human and animal models in order to prevent and manage IBDs.

Marine biotechnology aims to discover bioactive molecules from marine organisms to reveal their functions and actions, but also to understand the genetics, biochemistry, physiology and ecology of the marine organism. In light of this, Roncalli et al. (2021) provided the first piece of evidence of the presence of the OvoA gene, a key player in the ovotiol biosynthetic pathway, in arthropods [10]. Ovotiol is one of the most potent antioxidants that acts in marine organisms as a defense against oxidative stress during development and in response to environmental cues. Through a transcriptomics analysis, a single OvoA gene was found in marine arthropods including copepods, decapods and amphipods. Additionally, in particular, changes in OvoA gene expression through development and under stress conditions suggest that ovotiol may play a role as a defensive compound in *C. finmarchicus*, thus proposing this gene as a novel biomarker of stress in holozooplanktonic species. This discovery sheds light on copepods as marine organisms capable of producing bioactive compounds, opening further possibilities both for drug discovery and in the field of marine biotechnology.

In conclusion, as summarized in Figure 1, the studies collected in this Special Issue confirm that deep-sea organisms represent an extraordinary source of bioactive molecules with antioxidant and anti-inflammatory activity that can direct research to the design of new drugs.

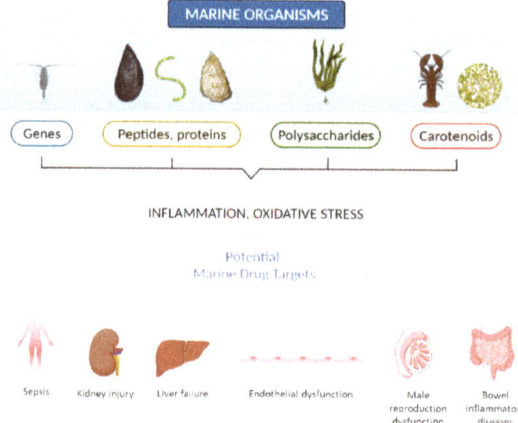

Figure 1. Schematic representation of the beneficial human health properties of biomolecules from marine organisms covered in the Special Issue "Marine Anti-inflammatory and Antioxidant Agents 2021", created with https://biorender.com/ (accessed on 5 January 2022).

Conflicts of Interest: The authors declare no conflict of interest.

References

1. Zhang, X.; Peng, Z.; Zheng, H.; Zhang, C.; Lin, H.; Qin, X. The Potential Protective Effect and Possible Mechanism of Peptides from Oyster (*Crassostrea hongkongensis*) Hydrolysate on Triptolide-Induced Testis Injury in Male Mice. *Mar. Drugs* **2021**, *19*, 566. [CrossRef] [PubMed]
2. Siregar, A.S.; Nyiramana, M.M.; Kim, E.-J.; Cho, S.B.; Woo, M.S.; Lee, D.K.; Hong, S.-G.; Han, J.; Kang, S.S.; Kim, D.R.; et al. Oyster-Derived Tyr-Ala (YA) Peptide Prevents Lipopolysaccharide/D-Galactosamine-Induced Acute Liver Failure by Suppressing Inflammatory, Apoptotic, Ferroptotic, and Pyroptotic Signals. *Mar. Drugs* **2021**, *19*, 614. [CrossRef] [PubMed]

3. Suryaningtyas, I.T.; Ahn, C.-B.; Je, J.-Y. Cytoprotective Peptides from Blue Mussel Protein Hydrolysates: Identification and Mechanism Investigation in Human Umbilical Vein Endothelial Cells Injury. *Mar. Drugs* **2021**, *19*, 609. [CrossRef] [PubMed]
4. Blas-Valdivia, V.; Rojas-Franco, P.; Serrano-Contreras, J.I.; Sfriso, A.A.; Garcia-Hernandez, C.; Franco-Colín, M.; Cano-Europa, E. C-phycoerythrin from *Phormidium persicinum* Prevents Acute Kidney Injury by Attenuating Oxidative and Endoplasmic Reticulum Stress. *Mar. Drugs* **2021**, *19*, 589. [CrossRef] [PubMed]
5. Yin, Y.; Xu, N.; Shi, Y.; Zhou, B.; Sun, D.; Ma, B.; Xu, Z.; Yang, J.; Li, C. Astaxanthin Protects Dendritic Cells from Lipopolysaccharide-Induced Immune Dysfunction. *Mar. Drugs* **2021**, *19*, 346. [CrossRef] [PubMed]
6. Yin, Y.; Xu, N.; Qin, T.; Zhou, B.; Shi, Y.; Zhao, X.; Ma, B.; Xu, Z.; Li, C. Astaxanthin Provides Antioxidant Protection in LPS-Induced Dendritic Cells for Inflammatory Control. *Mar. Drugs* **2021**, *19*, 534. [CrossRef] [PubMed]
7. Bigagli, E.; D'Ambrosio, M.; Cinci, L.; Niccolai, A.; Biondi, N.; Rodolfi, L.; Nascimiento, L.D.S.; Tredici, M.; Luceri, C. A Comparative In Vitro Evaluation of the Anti-Inflammatory Effects of a *Tisochrysis lutea* Extract and Fucoxanthin. *Mar. Drugs* **2021**, *19*, 334. [CrossRef] [PubMed]
8. Yang, Q.; Jiang, Y.; Fu, S.; Shen, Z.; Zong, W.; Xia, Z.; Zhan, Z.; Jiang, X. Protective Effects of *Ulva lactuca* Polysaccharide Extract on Oxidative Stress and Kidney Injury Induced by D-Galactose in Mice. *Mar. Drugs* **2021**, *19*, 539. [CrossRef] [PubMed]
9. Bilal, M.; Nunes, L.V.; Duarte, M.T.S.; Ferreira, L.F.R.; Soriano, R.N.; Iqbal, H.M.N. Exploitation of Marine-Derived Robust Biological Molecules to Manage Inflammatory Bowel Disease. *Mar. Drugs* **2021**, *19*, 196. [CrossRef] [PubMed]
10. Roncalli, V.; Lauritano, C.; Carotenuto, Y. First Report of OvoA Gene in Marine Arthropods: A New Candidate Stress Biomarker in Copepods. *Mar. Drugs* **2021**, *19*, 647. [CrossRef] [PubMed]

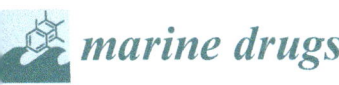

Article

The Potential Protective Effect and Possible Mechanism of Peptides from Oyster (*Crassostrea hongkongensis*) Hydrolysate on Triptolide-Induced Testis Injury in Male Mice

Xueyan Zhang [1], Zhilan Peng [1], Huina Zheng [1,2,3,4,5,6], Chaohua Zhang [1,2,3,4,5,6], Haisheng Lin [1,2,3,4,5,6] and Xiaoming Qin [1,2,3,4,5,6,*]

1. College of Food Science and Technology, Guangdong Ocean University, Zhanjiang 524088, China; xueyan@stu.gdou.edu.cn (X.Z.); pengzhilan@stu.gdou.edu.cn (Z.P.); zhenghn@gdou.edu.cn (H.Z.); zhangch@gdou.edu.cn (C.Z.); linhs@gdou.edu.cn (H.L.)
2. Guangdong Provincial Key Laboratory of Aquatic Product Processing and Safety, Zhanjiang 524088, China
3. National Research and Development Branch Center for Shellfish Processing (Zhanjiang), Zhanjiang 524088, China
4. Guangdong Province Engineering Laboratory for Marine Biological Products, Zhanjiang 524088, China
5. Guangdong Provincial Engineering Technology Research Center of Marine Food, Zhanjiang 524088, China
6. Collaborative Innovation Center of Seafood Deep Processing, Dalian Polytechnic University, Dalian 116034, China
* Correspondence: xiaoming0502@21cn.com; Tel.: +86-759-2396027

Abstract: Peptides from oyster hydrolysate (OPs) have a variety of biological activities. However, its protective effect and exact mechanism on testicular injury remain poorly understood. This study aimed to evaluate the protective effect of OPs on triptolide (TP)-induced testis damage and spermatogenesis dysfunction and investigate its underlying mechanism. In this work, the TP-induced testis injury model was created while OPs were gavaged in mice for 4 weeks. The results showed that OPs significantly improved the sperm count and motility of mice, and alleviated the seminiferous tubule injury. Further study showed that OPs decreased malonaldehyde (MDA) level and increased antioxidant enzyme (SOD and GPH-Px) activities, attenuating oxidative stress and thereby reducing the number of apoptotic cells in the testis. In addition, OPs improved the activities of enzymes (LDH, ALP and ACP) related to energy metabolism in the testis and restored the serum hormone level of mice to normal. Furthermore, OPs promoted the expression of Nrf2 protein, and then increased the expression of antioxidant enzyme regulatory protein (HO-1 and NQO1) in the testis. OPs inhibited JNK phosphorylation and Bcl-2/Bax-mediated apoptosis. In conclusion, OPs have a protective effect on testicular injury and spermatogenesis disorders caused by TP, suggesting the potential protection of OPs on male reproduction.

Keywords: oyster peptides; spermatogenesis; oxidative stress; apoptosis; hormone; testis

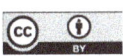

1. Introduction

Infertility is a universal and serious human health problem, reportedly affecting 8–12% of couples of childbearing age worldwide [1]. Male-related sterility accounts for around 50% of all infertility cases, with approximately 1 in 20 men of reproductive age suffering from infertility [2]. Infertility could be caused by a number of factors, including reproductive system injuries, endocrine disruption, environmental pollution, modern lifestyles, and drug side effects [3–7]. Spermatogenesis occurs in the seminiferous tubules and is strictly dependent on the structure of the testis. Therefore, the integrity of testicular morphological structure and the maintenance of physiological function play important roles in spermatogenesis [8]. Abnormal testicular tissue structure, changes in reproductive hormones, oxidative damage, and cell apoptosis may be the mechanisms of male reproductive dysfunction [9].

Triptolide (TP, $C_{20}H_{24}O_6$), as the main active ingredient of the pharmacological and toxic effects of *Tripterygium wilfordii multiglycoside* (GTW), has long been used in the treatment of inflammatory and immune diseases [10–12]. Among the toxic and side effects of TP, its reproductive toxicity leads to the highest incidence of reproductive dysfunction. Excessive triptolide intake interferes with testicular energy metabolism and normal reproductive function, resulting in reduced sperm quality and testicular atrophy, thereby leading to male reproductive dysfunction. Therefore, TP was used as a model drug in the animal models of male sterility to explore the pathogenesis of male sterility and the improvement effect of related drugs on this disease [13].

Oysters are the largest farmed shellfish in the world, rich in protein, glycogen, taurine, and trace elements [14]. In addition to rich nutrition, oyster meat can also affect a variety of physiological functions and has certain health care effects, thus it has been included in the medicine food homology list published by China's Ministry of Health [15]. As an aquatic product with high protein content, oysters are a good source of polypeptides. Several studies have focused on the health benefits of peptides from oyster hydrolysate (OPs) and have demonstrated their antioxidant [16], immunity-improving [17], antimicrobial [18], antitumor [19], anti-fatigue [20], and liver-protecting [21] properties. In previous studies, Li et al. reported that oyster polysaccharide administration could improve sperm quality and protect reproductive damage in cyclophosphamide-induced male mice [22]. However, the protective effects of OPs on reproductive damage have not been systematically reported. In addition, the study found that OPs may protect the ovary from D-galactose-induced female reproductive dysfunction by reducing oxidative stress, thereby preventing ovarian cell apoptosis [23]. Therefore, OPs have the potential to protect reproductive function against drug damage and deserve further study.

This study aimed to investigate the protective effect of peptides from the oyster hydrolysates on sperm parameters, testicular histopathology, sex hormone levels, activities of testicular marker enzymes, antioxidant level, and cell apoptosis in TP-induced ICR male mice. Furthermore, the activation of OPs on the nuclear factor-erythroid 2-related factor 2 (Nrf2) pathway and inhibition of OPs on the activation of the c-Jun N-terminal kinase (JNK) phosphorylation and Bcl-2/Bax-mediated apoptosis pathway was examined. Eventually, the correlation among the sperm analysis, morphological, biochemical indicators, cell apoptosis, and oxidative stress signaling pathway in the testis was established via the combination of experimental determination and statistical analysis. These findings not only deepen the understanding of OPs against TP-induced testis injury but also provide an experimental basis for the development of OPs as a functional agent.

2. Results

2.1. Molecular Weight and Main Peptide Sequences of OPs

The function and biological activity of peptides depends on their amino acid composition, sequence, and molecular mass. In this study, 89 peptides with molecular weight ranging from 662.41 to 1590.81 Da were identified by LC-MS/MS, and the peaks of OPs were mainly in the range of 300–800 m/z. As shown in Table 1, the scores for identifying peptide sequences were obtained, and 15 peptide sequences with higher scores were listed.

Table 1. Main peptide sequences of OPs.

No.	Peptide Sequence	Theoretical Mass (Mr)	Observed Mass (m/z)	Scores
1	LAGPQSIIGRTM	1242.68	622.34	56.04
2	IIDAPGHRDF	1139.57	380.87	62.28
3	YDNEFGYSFR	1296.55	649.28	56.59
4	RVPVPDVSVVDL	1293.73	647.87	48.44
5	AFRVPVPDVSVVDL	1511.84	756.93	37.93
6	GIVLDSGDGVSH	1154.56	578.28	57.46
7	LDLAGRDLTD	1087.56	544.78	36.34
8	PDGQVITI	841.46	421.73	35.7
9	KSYELPDGQVIT	1348.69	675.35	33.95
10	KSYELPDGQVITIG	1518.79	760.4	33.88
11	IAQDFKTDLR	1205.65	402.89	37.72
12	GLALLVP	681.45	341.73	32.1
13	LLQALD	671.39	336.7	35.92
14	GIVLDSGDGVTH	1168.58	585.3	42.1
15	LDLAGRDLTD	1087.55	544.78	36.34

2.2. Amino Acid Composition of OPs

Amino acid composition and content of OPs are presented in Table 2. The contents of total amino acids (TAA) in OPs were 54.75 g/100 g. The essential amino acid (EAA) cannot be synthesized by the body itself and must be obtained through the diet [24]. EAA content of OPs is 22.19 g per 100 g, accounted for 40.53% of TAA, which was highly sufficient to meet the minimum dietary intake of 35% recommended by the World Health Organization [25].

Table 2. The amino acids composition of OPs (g/100 g).

Amino Acid	Contents of OPs
Thr	2.81
Val	3.34
Met	1.41
Ile	3.02
Leu	4.56
Phe	2.27
Lys	4.78
His	1.03
Arg	4.23
Asp	5.56
Ser	2.88
Glu	8.41
Pro	2.30
Gly	3.25
Ala	2.69
Tyr	2.21
Cys	ND [e]
TAA [a]	54.75
EAA [b]	22.19
HAA [c]	17.29
BCAA [d]	10.92

[a] TAA: Total amino acids. [b] Essential amino acid (EAA): Thr, Val, Met, Ile, Leu, Phe, Lys. [c] Hydrophobic amino acids (HAA): Ala, Leu, Ile, Met, Phe, Pro, Tyr, and Val. [d] Branched-chain amino acids (BCAA) = Leu, Ile, and Val. [e] ND: not detected.

The composition, concentration, and sequence of amino acids have a great influence on the biological activity of proteolytic compounds [20]. The amino acid composition of spermatozoa was significantly changed by amino acid supplementation in the internal environment, which affected sperm motility [26]. Of the 17 amino acids contained in OPs, glutamic acid (8.41 g/100 g), aspartic acid (5.56 g/100 g), arginine (4.23 g/100 g), lysine (4.78 g/100 g), leucine (4.56 g/100 g), and valine (3.34 g/100 g) accounted for a higher proportion. Among them, a diet supplemented with amino acids (mainly lysine, valine, and threonine) improved sperm quality, changed amino acid composition in seminal plasma, and improved sperm motility [27]. Lysine, aspartic acid, and glutamic acid have the ability to chelate metal ions because of the amino or carboxyl groups in their side chains. Hydrophobic amino acids (HAA) accounted for 31.58% of TAA, and its high amounts in OPs offer properties that are able to promote lipid interactions, which enhance entry of the peptides into target organs via hydrophobic associations [28]. BCAAs accounted for 19.95% of TAA, which plays a strong role in maintaining energy supply, and Bahadorani et al. found that appropriate supplementation of BCAAs may have synergistic effects on sperm function and testosterone secretion [24].

2.3. Effects of OPs on Sperm Parameters of TP-Induced Mice

The model of TP-induced mice spermatogenesis dysfunction was established, and mice were treated for 4 weeks. The intervention of TP resulted in severe sperm distortion in mice, and the quantity and quality of sperm were significantly lower than those in the control group. It was even difficult to find an intact normal sperm. As shown in Figure 1A, the sperm morphology of TP-treated mice revealed an increase in acrosome abnormalities: fathead, bent neck, short tail, and coiled-in tail. The treatment of OPs significantly increased the number of normal sperms, elevated the sperm count, improved the sperm motility, and decreased the sperm deformity rate (Figure 1B–D). The effects of different doses of OPs showed a dose dependence, and high dose of OPs treatment significantly ameliorated sperm damage induced by TP ($p < 0.001$).

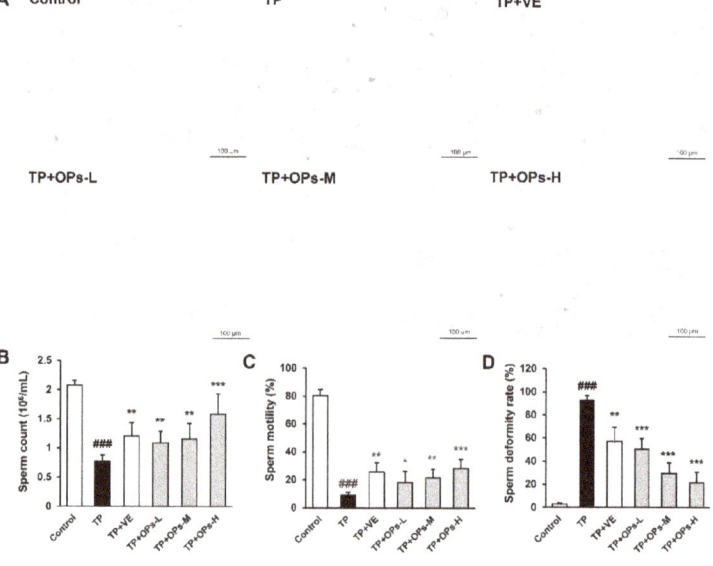

Figure 1. Effects of OPs on sperm quality of ICR mice induced by TP. (A) Sperm morphology was observed at 200× magnification; OPs -L, OPs -M, and OPs -H are the groups administrated with 100, 200, and 400 mg/kg OPs separately. (B), (C), and (D) indicate the sperm count, motility, and deformity rate of sperm, respectively. The data were expressed as mean ± SEM, n = 10. Compared with the control group, ### $p < 0.001$; compared with the TP group, * $p < 0.05$, ** $p < 0.01$ and *** $p < 0.001$.

In this research, VE was chosen as a positive control, based on the fact that its metabolite tocopheryl frequently applied for the promotion of reproductive hormone secretion, increasing sperm numbers and motility, preventing male infertility in the clinic. As shown in Figure 1, VE treatment significantly ameliorated sperm damage induced by TP ($p < 0.01$).

2.4. Effects of OPs on Testicular Injury of TP-Induced Mice

The results revealed that there was no significant difference in the bodyweight of mice among the groups (Figure 2B). As shown in Figure 2C, the testis index of the TP group was significantly lower than that in the control group ($p < 0.001$), while treatment of OPs ameliorated the testicular weight loss compared with the TP group. The structure of testicular tissue and the number of testicular cells play an important role in spermatogenesis and sperm quality. The testicular structures and cells play important roles during spermatogenesis, while an ample array of factors can influence its quality and quantity [29]. Histological analysis on the tissue sections of H&E staining showed that OPs treatment protected testis tissue against the damage caused by TP. As compared with controls, TP-induced mice showed severe vacuolation of germ cells, enlarged intercellular spaces, irregular shape, and atrophied seminiferous tubules with only a few Sertoli cells, spermatogonia, and primary spermatocytes (Figure 2A). VE and high-dose OPs (400 mg/kg) treatment restored morphological abnormalities compared with the TP group; vacuolation of germ cells and spermatocyte was decreased. The size of the seminiferous tubule, the layer of the spermatocytes, and the number of Sertoli cells were preserved by the treatment of VE and high-dose OPs (Figure 2A). The overall structures of the seminiferous tubule in testis were evaluated by Johnsen's scoring method. Compared with the TP group, the middle and high dose of OPs elevated Johnsen's score significantly ($p < 0.01$) (Figure 2D).

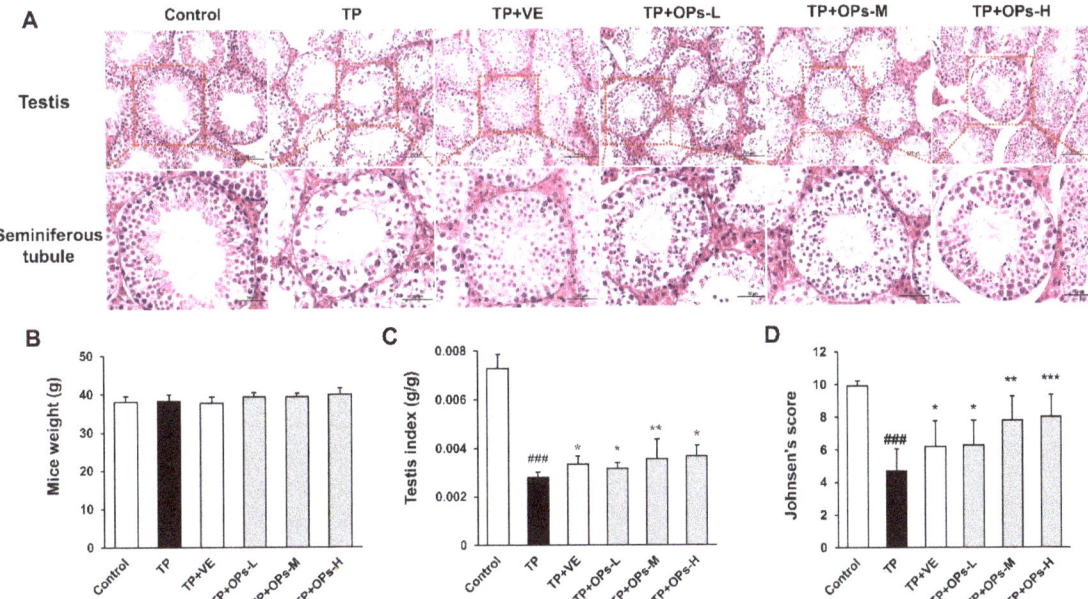

Figure 2. Effects of OPs on testicular injury of ICR mice induced by TP. (**A**) Histopathology with H&E staining (200× and 400×) of the testicular section in mice after treatment for 28 days; (**B**) body weight of mice was measured every 3 days; (**C**) testis index was measured by the ratio of testicular weight to body weight; (**D**) Johnsen's score in the testicular tissue was determined in each group. The data were expressed as mean ± SEM, n = 10. Compared with the control group, ### $p < 0.001$; compared with the TP group, * $p < 0.05$, ** $p < 0.01$ and *** $p < 0.001$.

2.5. Effects of OPs on TP-Induced Reproductive Hormone Level

Male reproductive hormones regulate the process of spermatogenesis. As shown in Figure 3, the concentration of serum testosterone and estradiol was significantly increased in the TP group, and the levels of follicle stimulating hormone (FSH) and luteinizing hormone (LH) were significantly decreased compared with the control group ($p < 0.01$). Obviously, it was shown that TP disturbed the serum hormone level of mice compared with the controls. As compared with the TP group, the treatment of OPs restored the serum testosterone and estradiol level of mice, which were close to the control group. Additionally, a significant increase in FSH and LH levels was seen in the TP+OPs-H group compared with the TP group ($p < 0.01$). VE as a positive control significantly restored the TP-induced serum reproductive hormone (testosterone, estradiol, and FSH) disorder in mice.

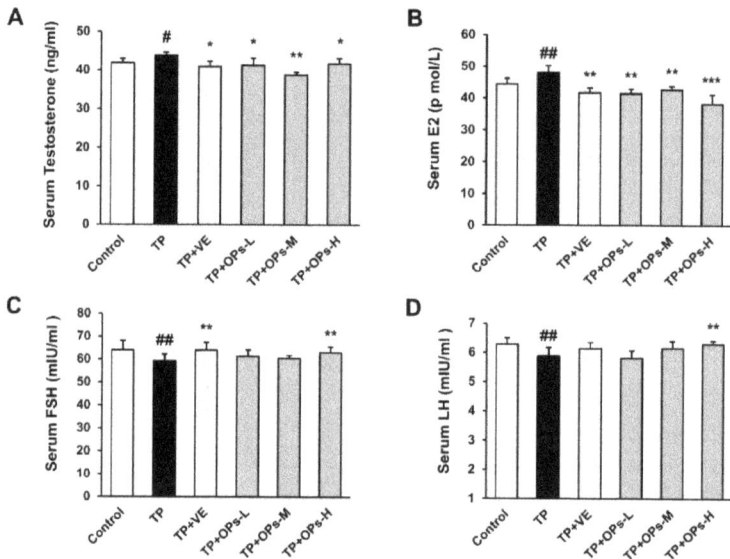

Figure 3. Effects of OPs on serum reproductive hormone level of ICR mice induced by TP. (**A**) Serum testosterone level, (**B**) serum estradiol (E2) level, (**C**) serum follicle stimulating hormone (FSH) level, (**D**) serum luteinizing hormone (LH) level. The data were expressed as mean ± SEM, n = 10. Compared with the control group, # $p < 0.05$ and ## $p < 0.01$; compared with the TP group, * $p < 0.05$, ** $p < 0.01$ and *** $p < 0.001$.

2.6. OPs Increased Testicular Marker Enzyme Activity and Reduced Oxidative Stress Induced by TP

Oxidative stress is a cause of testis injury which was also found in the TP-induced mice model (Figure 4A–C). TP raised the lipid peroxidation product malondialdehyde (MDA) and disrupted the antioxidative system of the testis, including the enzyme superoxide dismutase (SOD) and glutathione peroxidase (GSH-Px). OPs treatment reduced the level of MDA and increased the activity of SOD and GSH-Px, and especially the middle and high two-dose groups of OPs showed extremely significant changes ($p < 0.001$). Meanwhile, VE treatment as a positive control also significantly reduced oxidative stress in testicular tissue induced by TP.

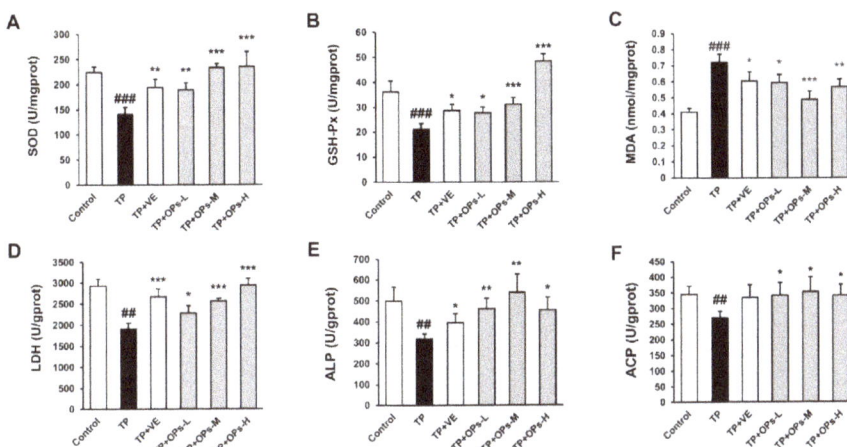

Figure 4. Effects of OPs on testicular marker enzymes and bio markers of oxidative stress in testes tissues of ICR mice induced by TP. (**A**) superoxide dismutase (SOD) level, (**B**) glutathione peroxidase (GSH-Px) level, (**C**) malondialdehyde (MDA) level, (**D**) lactate dehydrogenase (LDH) level, (**E**) alkaline phosphatase (ALP) level, (**F**) acid phosphatase (ACP) level. The data were expressed as mean ± SEM, n = 10. Compared with the control group, ## $p < 0.01$ and ### $p < 0.001$; compared with the TP group, * $p < 0.05$, ** $p < 0.01$ and *** $p < 0.001$.

Activities of testicular marker enzymes such as lactate dehydrogenase (LDH), acid phosphatase (ACP) level, and alkaline phosphatase (ALP) are considered as functional indicators of spermatogenesis and testicular development. The alterations of testicular marker enzyme activity could affect the energy metabolism pathway, thus interfering with the energy supply of spermatogenesis. As were shown in Figure 4D–F, TP significantly suppressed the level of testicular marker enzymes in testis tissue, including LDH, ALP, and ACP ($p < 0.01$). As compared with the TP group, middle and high doses of OPs significantly increased the activity of LDH ($p < 0.001$), and different dose of OPs ameliorated the activity of ALP and ACP. Meanwhile, VE treatment significantly increased the activity of testicular marker enzymes (LDH and ALP).

2.7. Effects of OPs on the Testicular Apoptotic Induced by TP

The results of terminal deoxynucleotidyl transferase dUTP nick-end labeling (TUNEL) staining of cell apoptosis were shown in Figure 5. There were few apoptotic cells in the testicular tissue of the control group, which is common during spermatogenesis. However, in the TP group, the proportion of the apoptotic cells was significantly increased despite the loss of total cells in seminiferous tubules (Figure 5B,C). VE and OPs treatment significantly ameliorated the decrease in the total number of cells in seminiferous tubules induced by TP (Figure 5B). Meanwhile, VE and high dose of OPs treatment reduced the number and proportion of the apoptotic cells (Figure 5C).

To further elucidate the testicular apoptotic events, the protein expression of Bcl2, Bax, caspase-3, and PARP reliable apoptotic markers were analyzed. As shown in Figure 6, TP stimulated the upregulation of Bax, caspase-3, cleaved caspase-3, and cleaved PARP, and inhibited the expression of Bcl-2. The upregulated Bax, caspase-3, cleaved caspase-3, and cleaved PARP were significantly inhibited by treatment of OPs at three doses. VE treatment downregulated the activation of cleaved caspase-3. The decrease in Bcl-2 expression was significantly upregulated by VE and high dose of OPs treatment. These findings suggested that OPs ameliorated TP-induced apoptosis in testicular tissue.

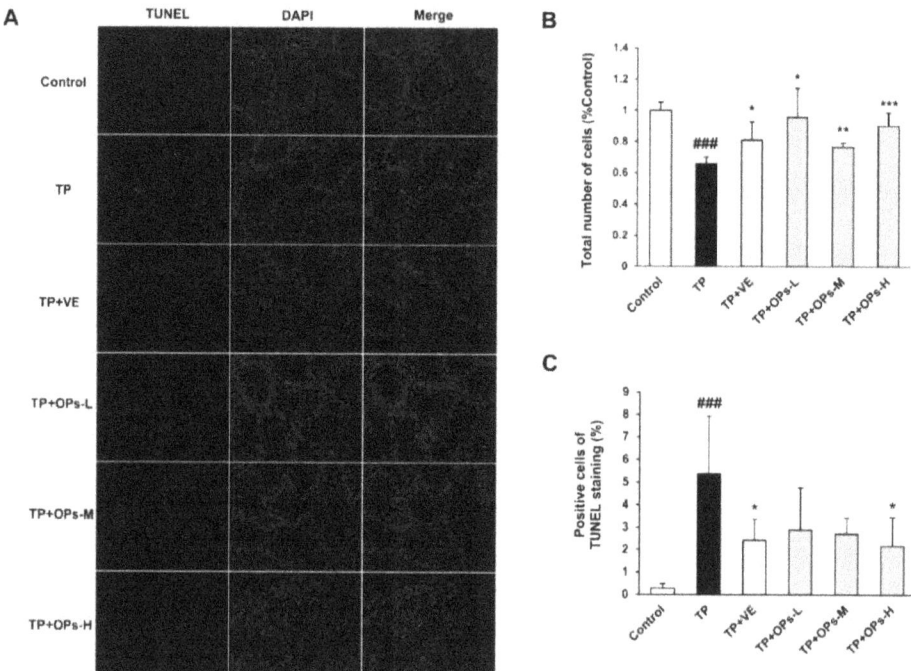

Figure 5. Effects of OPs on apoptotic index in testes tissues of ICR mice induced by TP. (**A**) Apoptotic cells in testicular tissue sections were detected by TUNEL assay (apoptotic cells: green fluorescence, cell nucleus: blue fluorescence). (**B**) The total number of cells in each group compared by Control group were shown. (**C**) The ratios of apoptotic cell were shown. The data were expressed as mean ± SEM, n = 3. Compared with the control group, ### $p < 0.001$; compared with the TP group, * $p < 0.05$, ** $p < 0.01$ and *** $p < 0.001$.

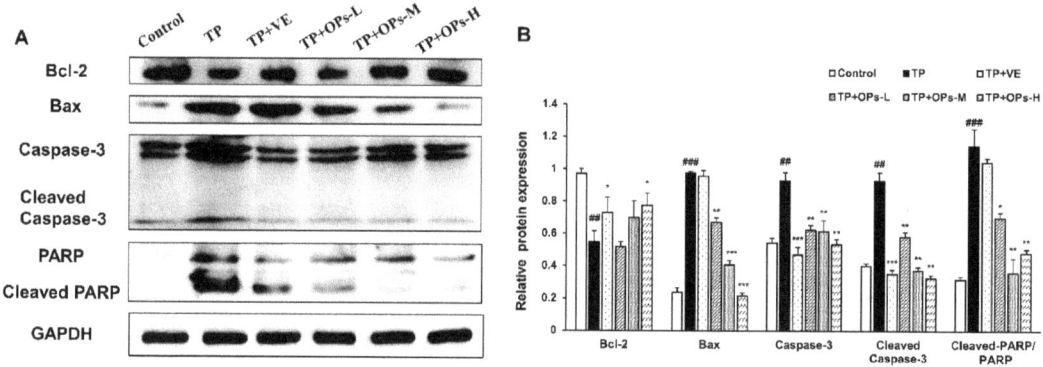

Figure 6. Effects of OPs on protein expression levels of markers of apoptosis in TP-induced testis tissues of male ICR mice. (**A**) Electrophoresis images of Bcl-2, Bax, Caspase-3, Cleaved Caspase-3, PARP, and GAPDH protein; (**B**) the quantitative densitometric analysis of Bcl-2, Bax, Caspase-3, Cleaved Caspase-3, and PARP proteins. The data were expressed as mean ± SEM, n = 3. Compared with the control group, ## $p < 0.01$ and ### $p < 0.001$; compared with the TP group, * $p < 0.05$, ** $p < 0.01$ and *** $p < 0.001$.

2.8. Effects of OPs on Related Proteins Expression in the Nrf2 and JNK Pathways

Detection of the levels of related protein factors in the testicular tissue via Western blot was illustrated in Figures 7 and 8. As displayed in Figure 7, administration of TP led to the downregulation of Nrf2, Keap1, HO-1, and NQO1 expression in mice testis tissues, concomitant with upregulated expressions of p-JNK and p-JNK/JNK, and total JNK protein expression was not affected by TP treatment, as shown in Figure 8. ImageJ software was used to obtain optical density values of the protein bands. The decrease in Nrf2, Keap1, HO1, and NQO1 protein expression were upregulated by treatment of OPs at middle and high doses. VE as a positive control upregulated the Nrf2, HO1, and NQO1 protein expression. The treatment with OPs downregulated the activation of p-JNK to a nearly normal level.

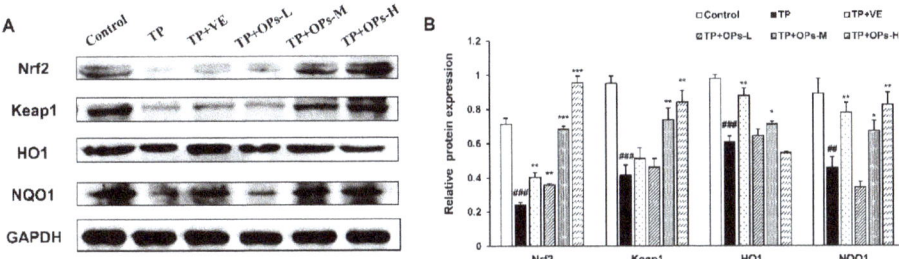

Figure 7. Effects of OPs on the Nrf2/Keap1 signaling pathway in TP-induced testis tissues of male ICR mice. (**A**) Electrophoresis images of Nrf2, Keap1, HO-1, NQO1, and GAPDH protein; (**B**) The quantitative densitometric analysis of Nrf2, Keap1, HO-1, and NQO1 proteins. The data were expressed as mean ± SEM, n = 3. Compared with the control group, ## $p < 0.01$ and ### $p < 0.001$; compared with the TP group, * $p < 0.05$, ** $p < 0.01$ and *** $p < 0.001$.

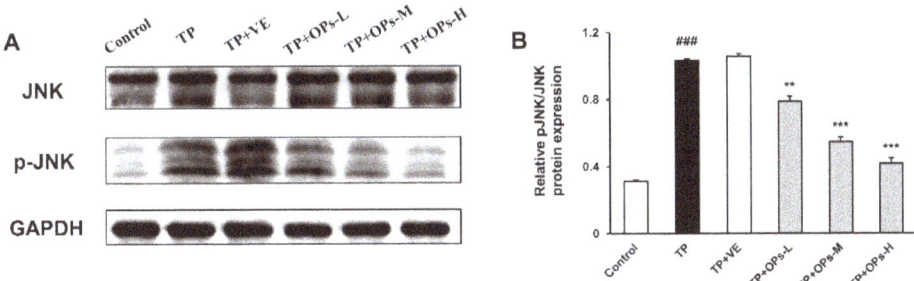

Figure 8. Effects of OPs on the JNK signaling pathway in TP-induced testis tissues of male ICR mice. (**A**) Electrophoresis images of JNK, p-JNK and GAPDH protein; (**B**) the quantitative densitometric analysis of p-JNK/JNK bands. The data were expressed as mean ± SEM, n = 3. Compared with the control group, ### $p < 0.001$; compared with the TP group, ** $p < 0.01$ and *** $p < 0.001$.

3. Discussion

In this study, male infertility disease model mice were successfully established by TP induction. In the model, the deteriorated sperm quality, altered testicle histomorphology, disordered hormone levels, the decreased activity of testicular marker enzyme, and the triggered testis oxidative stress and germ cells apoptosis were observed. The observed altered sperm quality and testicle histomorphology in this study is consistent with the previous reports [8,13,30]. Gastric administration of appropriate dose of OPs could reverse these abnormalities. The results showed that OPs treatment in TP-induced mice has beneficial effects on the testis index, sperm parameters, histological structure of testis, hormone level, testicular marker enzyme activity, and oxidative stress, as well as testicular apoptosis. The mechanism of the protective effects of OPs may be through inhibiting the oxidative stress by Nrf2 and JNK pathways, increasing the expression of Bcl2, and reducing the level of cell apoptosis by suppressing the expression of the apoptotic markers Bax, caspase-3, and PARP.

Oxidative stress due to toxic substances is considered to be closely related to male infertility [31]. Production of reactive oxygen species (ROS) and consequent oxidative damage have been established as mechanisms for TP toxicity [13]. It is well known that oxidative stress leads to sperm dysfunction by inducing peroxidation damage to the plasma membrane. In this study, TP-induced increased MDA levels and decreased GSH-Px and SOD levels in mice, suggesting oxidative stress, which was consistent with the reports of some researchers [8,13,32]. As spermatozoa are high in polyunsaturated fatty acids (PUFAs), it is more sensitive to oxidative damage than other cells [33]. Furthermore, the generation of ROS decreased the number of spermatogonia cells in the testis, and it is thought to be detrimental for spermatogenesis [34]. In this study, the sperm count and motility of mice were significantly decreased, and the sperm deformity rate was increased, induced by TP. The significant reduction in spermatogonia was also observed on histopathological assay. The severe impairment of sperm characteristics induced by TP is closely related to the obvious oxidant/antioxidant imbalance in testis. The treatment of OPs effectively reduced the deterioration of sperm quality, which may be related to the amelioration of oxidative stress in testicular microenvironment as manifested by decreasing in the level of MDA and increasing in the activity of SOD and GSH-Px. It suggested that OPs exert significant antioxidant effects in testicular tissue, including the increase in activities of antioxidant enzymes and decrease in lipid peroxidation. It has been reported that peptides (2-20 amino acids) can completely cross the intestinal barrier and perform biological functions in tissues, while peptides the size of 5–16 amino acids show potent antioxidant activity [28,35], which is manifested in its ability to carry out DPPH (2,2-diphenyl-1-picrylhydrazyl) free radical scavenging [16,20]. Combined with the results of animal experiments, the main peptides of OPs with 6–14 amino acid residues in length may also show antioxidant activity, suggesting that its alleviation of ROS-induced testicular injury may be related to its antioxidant function. In addition, compared with other hydrophilic amino acids, hydrophobic amino acids have higher antioxidant activity in peptides, and its high amounts in OPs may play an important role in reducing the oxidative damage of the testis caused by ROS [36].

Decreased activity of antioxidant enzymes could induce the accumulation of ROS and lead to oxidative stress. The expression of antioxidant enzymes including HO-1, NQO1, and SOD were mainly mediated by the Nrf2 pathway. Under normal conditions, Nrf2 is mainly regulated by the repressor protein Keap1 in the cell cytoplasm. The disturbance of interaction between Nrf2 and Keap1 or degradation of Keap1 affect the further activation of downstream antioxidant enzyme expression by Nrf2 [37]. Recent studies have shown that the regulation of endogenous antioxidant system through the Nrf2 pathway significantly reduces oxidative stress-induced apoptosis of Sertoli cells and testicular injury [32]. In this study, TP-induced decrease the expression of NQO1 and HO-1 protein by decreasing Nrf2 and Keap1 expression was consistent with the results of the previous study [8]. Pretreatment with OPs may inhibit the decrease in antioxidant enzyme expression by activating Nrf2 expression. This finding suggests that the protective effect of OPs on testicular injury might be related to the upregulation of Nrf2 expression.

Previous studies showed that TP could promote the production of ROS in Sertoli cells, thus further activating the JNK pathway, which triggered the mitochondrial-mediated apoptosis pathway [13]. In vivo results showed that TP reduced testicular weight, destroyed the microstructure of the testis, disrupted the enzyme activity, increased MDA levels, activated JNK phosphorylation, and promoted testicular tissue apoptosis. In this study, treatment of OPs significantly reduced the activation of JNK phosphorylation, which indicated that OPs may protect testis against oxidative stress by mediating the JNK pathway.

Mitochondria are responsible for cells energy metabolism and are the main targets of ROS production and regulation of apoptosis. In our study, it was found that OPs may reduce the excessive apoptosis of testicular cells mediated by the mitochondrial apoptosis pathway, as shown in the results of TUNEL assay and the Western blotting of apoptosis-related proteins (Bax, Bcl-2, caspase-3, and PARP). Both the anti-apoptotic protein Bcl-2 and the pro-apoptotic protein Bax regulate apoptosis by controlling the permeability of the mitochondrial membrane. OPs treatment significantly upregulated the expression of Bcl-2, downregulated the expression of Bax, thereby regulating cell permeability, further inhibiting the activation of Caspase-3 and reducing the Caspase cascade reaction. Several studies have shown that increased ROS accumulation may lead to increased permeability of the mitochondrial outer membrane and then activate mitochondria-dependent apoptosis signaling pathway to induce cell apoptosis. At present, few studies have shown that OPs play a direct role in the inhibition of cell apoptosis, while in the activation of the apoptosis process, it is believed that oxidative stress-induced damage can trigger apoptotic signaling procedures, leading to cell death. Therefore, it indicated that OPs may mediate mitochondria-dependent apoptosis signaling pathways to reduce cell apoptosis and tissue damage by reducing oxidative damage of mitochondrial lipids caused by ROS. In our study, it was also showed that OPs reversed severe testicular tissue damage by ameliorating testicular apoptosis by assessing the testis histopathology.

Sertoli cells, as nursing cells, regulate the processes of spermatogenesis by providing nutritional support and a suitable situation for the survival and development of germ cells [38]. The altered testicular enzyme activities induced by TP may have resulted from the impairment of Sertoli cell function and disrupted metabolism in mice [39]. LDH enzyme is involved in the process of glycolysis and gluconeogenesis and controls the synthesis of the main energy source of germ cells. The ACP enzyme is mainly distributed in the cytoplasm of Sertoli cells, which is involved in protein synthesis and related to the phagocytosis of Sertoli cells. ALP is involved in the synthesis of nucleic acids, nucleoproteins, and phospholipids, such as in the cleavage of phosphate esters and in mobilizing carbohydrates and lipid metabolites to be used by spermatozoa [40]. In this study, TP inhibited the activities of LDH, ACP, and ALP, which not only interfered with the energy supply process of aerobic and anaerobic glycolysis but also disturbed the energy utilization of testis. OPs treatment improved the energy metabolism of testicular tissue and the energy supply of spermatogenesis by increasing the enzyme activity of LDH, ACP, and ALP. In addition, metabolic disorders may be due to the disintegration of mitochondrial membrane ultrastructure caused by mitochondrial lipid peroxidation. It has been found that lipid peroxidation induced by oxidative stress produces a strong cytotoxic effect in the testis, leading to the damage of nucleic acid, protein, carbohydrates, and lipids in cells. Spermatogenesis is reduced due to the resulting disturbances in energy metabolism, oxidative phosphorylation, tricarboxylic acid cycle, and glycolysis. Previous studies have shown that OPs could protect TM4 Sertoli cells from toxic damage induced by TP, including improving the cell viability of TM4 cells, reducing the production of intracellular ROS and lipid peroxidation, and enhancing the antioxidant activity of TM4 cells [41]. Combined with the results of this study, it was found that OPs ameliorated TP-induced metabolic disorders by inhibiting mitochondrial lipid peroxidation.

Spermatogenesis is a multistep process that could be disturbed by multifaceted factors. Expect for oxidative stress, hormone imbalance can affect the process of spermatogenesis [42]. Destructive endogenous hormone signaling might mediate the process of spermatogenesis and lead to low sperm count [43]. LH and FSH are considered to be key factors in the regulation of testis function. LH is related to produce testosterone by stimulating the Leydig cells and both FSH and testosterone in turn regulate Leydig cells activity and stimulate germ cell proliferation and differentiation by stimulating the Sertoli cells. Estradiol is converted from circulating testosterone by enzyme aromatase; therefore, its concentration is affected by the level of testosterone. However, dysregulation of circulating estradiol may lead to inhibition of LH production not beneficial for spermatogenesis [44].

In this study, TP increased the levels of serum testosterone and estradiol, and decreased serum LH and FSH levels in mice. The treatment of OPs restored the serum hormone level of mice to the normal, and reduced the disturbance of hormones on spermatogenesis in mice. Additionally, previous studies had found that oyster peptides improved the level of serum androgen induced by cyclophosphamide [45].

The identification of the active components of oyster peptides is of great interest in exploring new strategies for the treatment or prevention of testicular and sperm damage. Previous studies showed that some antioxidant peptides were identified from oysters, such as Pro-Val-Met-Gly-Asp, Glu-His-Gly-Val, and Leu-Lys-Gln-Glu-Leu-Glu-Asp-Leu-Leu-Glu-Lys-Gln-Glu [16,46]. These antioxidant peptides may play an important role in preventing oxidative damage in the testis, resulting in reduced sperm quality. However, other active ingredients still need to be identified by Sephadex gel chromatography, HPLC, mass spectrometry, and other purification methods.

In conclusion, the underlying mechanism of OPs in the potential protective effect on testis and sperm is attributed to the synergistic modulations, and these results deepen the understanding of the potential improvement of male reproductive function by OPs, thus demonstrating the potential application of OPs in functional foods (Figure 9).

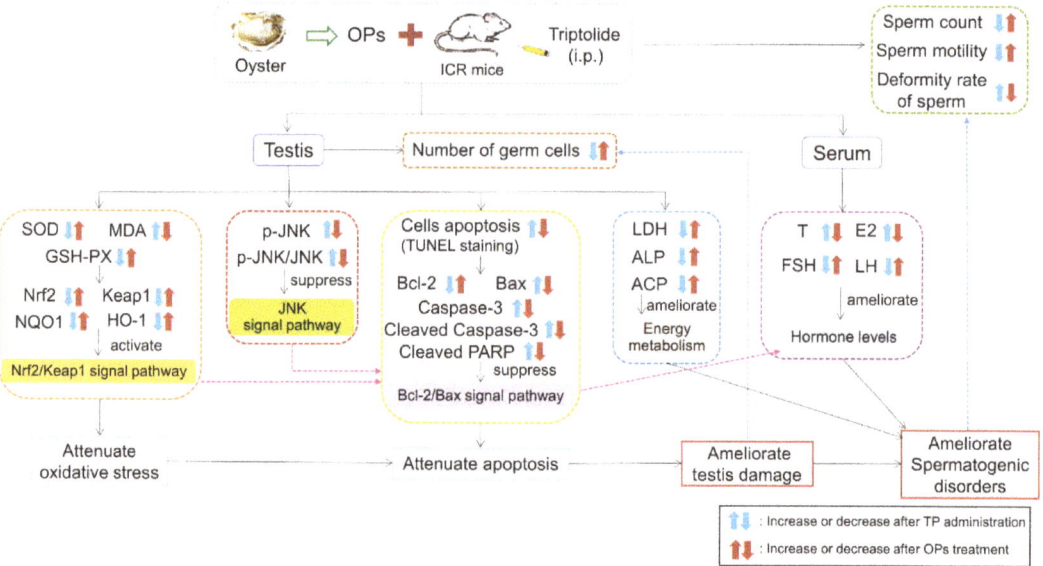

Figure 9. Possible mechanism underlying the protective effects of OPs intervention on TP-induced testicular damage in mice. By detecting MDA, antioxidant enzymes and related proteins in the testis, as well as sexual hormone levels in serum, the anti-effect of OPs was shown to be related to Nrf2/Keap1, JNK, and Bcl-2/Bax pathways.

4. Materials and Methods

4.1. Materials and Reagents

Fresh oysters (*Crassostrea hongkongensis*) were purchased from the local market in Zhanjiang, China (oysters were shelled at the market and immediately stored at −30 °C until use). Compound protease (4.5×10^5 U g^{-1}) was obtained from Pangbo Biotech (Nanjing, China). Triptolide (purity > 98%) were purchased from Meilun-Biotech Co., Ltd. (Dalian, China). Vitamin E (VE) (H44021026) was purchased from Baiyunshan Pharmaceutical Factory (Guangzhou, China). All chemicals and reagents used were of analytical grade and commercially available.

4.2. Preparation of OPs

OPs were prepared by enzymatic hydrolysis from the oyster meat according to the methods of Li et al., Peng et al., and Zhang et al. [17,41,47]. Briefly, three kilograms of oyster meat were ground into mince and then mixed with distilled water (1:3 w/v). The mixture was homogenized at 8000 rpm for 5 min by using a homogenizer. Homogenates were hydrolyzed at pH 7.0 with compound protease (enzyme concentration 1000 U g^{-1} of raw material). The hydrolysis reaction lasted for 5 h in a 53 °C water bath. Subsequently, the protease was inactivated at 100 °C for 10 min and the enzymatic hydrolysate was centrifuged at 15,000g at 4 °C for 20 min to obtain the supernatant. The supernatant was fractionated by an ultrafiltration device (XX42PMINI, Millipore, USA) and 10 kDa, 5 kDa, and 3 kDa ultrafiltration membranes (Mili Pellicon, Millipore, USA) to obtain the components used in this study (<3 kDa hydrolysate fraction). The samples were freeze-dried into powder for subsequent experiments (FD-551, EYELA, Tokyo, Japan).

4.3. OPs Characterization by LC-ESI/MS/MS

The molecular weight and amino acid sequences of the OPs were identified by liquid chromatography–electrospray ionization tandem mass spectrometry (LC-ESI/MS/MS). The sample (1 μL) was injected with an autosampler and subsequently separated by a C18 column and eluted with conditions of mobile phase A (H$_2$O, 0.1% formic acid) and mobile phase B (95% acetonitrile, 0.1% formic acid). Peptides were first eluted with a linear gradient from 2% to 35% of mobile phase B for 40 min, and then from 35% to 80% of mobile phase B for 10 min, running temperature of 25 °C at a flow rate of 0.3 μL/min. After chromatography, ESI-MS/MS was carried out using a Q-EXACTIVE mass spectrometer (Thermo Fisher Scientific, San Jose, CA) equipped with the electrospray ionization (ESI) source. The spectrometer worked in the positive ion mode, and the parameters of the ESI ionization interface were set as follows: capillary voltage 1.6 kV, Resolution 70,000, AGC target:1e5, NCE/stepped NCE: 27. Samples were analyzed with a full-scan MS mode in the range of 350–2000 m/z to obtain the total ion chromatogram. Then, the Mascot search engine was used to analyze the chromatographic peaks corresponding to the mass spectrometry of the custom oyster protein database. Only peptides identified with $p < 0.05$ significance were recorded.

4.4. Determination of Amino Acid Composition

The amino acid composition and content of OPs were determined by an amino acid autoanalyzer (L-8900, Hitachi, Tokyo, Japan). The sample and 6 mol/L HCl were added into a tube containing phenol for hydrolysis. After the tube was vacuumed, the mixture was washed with nitrogen and hydrolyzed at 110 °C for 22 h. After the filtrate had cooled, it was heated to 40–50 °C with a test tube concentrator and dried under reduced pressure until evaporated. Sodium citrate buffer solution was added to the dried test tube and dissolved. The solution was transferred to the injection flask of the instrument for determination by the amino acid analyzer [47]. According to the peak area in comparison with the standard, amino acid contents were calculated.

4.5. Animals and Treatment

The Laboratory Animal Committee of Guangdong Ocean University, China (no. GDOU-LAE-2020-014) approved all the animal protocols and experimental procedures for this study. Sixty adult ICR male mice (specific pathogen-free, approval no.11032201101487454) were purchased from the Huafukang Biotech Co., Ltd. (Beijing, China) and acclimatized for 7 days before the start of the experiments. All mice were housed at 4–5 mice per cage (23 cm × 32 cm × 15 cm) and randomly fed a normal diet in an environmentally controlled room (temperature was 25 ± 2 °C and relative humidity was 50–65%, with a 12 h light/dark cycle). Animals were randomly divided into six groups (n = 10). Control group: mice were given 0.9% NaCl orally and intraperitoneally, once a day; TP (model group): mice were pretreated with 0.9% NaCl and intraperitoneally injected with TP at a dose of 120 µg/kg; TP + VE (positive control group): mice were orally administered with VE at a dose of 7.5 mg/kg, and intraperitoneally injected with TP (120 µg/kg) after 1 h every day; TP + OPs: Mice were orally administered with OPs at the dose of 100 mg/kg (TP + OPs-L), 200 mg/kg (TP + OPs-M), 400 mg/kg (TP + OPs-H) and intraperitoneally injected with TP (120 µg/kg) after 1 h every day. Administration methods and doses of TP-induced testicular injury were conducted according to Wang et al., Ma et al., and Zhang et al. [8,13,32]. VE was determined as the positive control drug according to the study results of Li et al. and Hamza et al. [22,48]. After 28 days of continuous treatment, mice were sacrificed by enucleation of the eye and bled for the collection of blood, and all testes were removed and weighted to measure the testis index (testis weight/body weight). The right epididymis of mice was collected for sperm analysis, and the right testis of mice was stored at −80 °C for protein expression and other parameter detection. The left testis was fixed in 4% paraformaldehyde for further histological analysis.

4.6. Sperm Analysis

The entire right epididymis was placed in 1 mL of prewarmed saline and minced into small sections, incubating for 10 min (37 °C, 5% CO_2) to allow the spermatozoa to swim out from the epididymal tubules. The sperm suspension was dropped into a Neobar's hemocytometer, and the sperm count was estimated under a cover glass. The sperm motility was observed under a 400× light microscope (Olympus Corporation, Tokyo, Japan) and calculated and expressed as a percentage of motile sperm according to the World Health Organization manual criteria. The sperms were stained using the Quick sperm stain kit (Nanjing Jiancheng Bioengineering Institute, Nanjing, China) according to the manufacturer's instructions. Additionally, images of sperm after staining were observed under a light microscope and acquired by photographing using a Leica DMI4000B microscope with Leica DFd4500 imaging system (Leica Corporation, German). The rate of abnormal morphology of sperm was evaluated and calculated by observing sperm staining images. Sperm parameters of mice (count, motility, and morphology) were analyzed in each group according to the methods adopted by Qiu et al. and Oghbaei et al. [49,50].

4.7. Histopathological and Ultrastructural Assessment

The left testes of mice dehydrated in gradient concentrations of alcohol, and cleared with xylene, then embedded in paraffin at 65 °C. After cooling at −20 °C, the sections were cut at 4 µm and stained with hematoxylin and eosin (H&E). The sections of testis tissue were observed under a light microscope and photographed at magnifications of 200× and 400× using a Nikon Eclipse E100 microscope with Nikon DS-U3 imaging system (Nikon Corporation, Japan). The testicular structure of each animal was assessed, and Johnsen's score was assessed based on spermatogenic function and germ cell count from 1 (no spermatogenic epithelium) to 10 (normal spermatogenesis). All analyses were performed by an evaluator who was unaware of the treatment group.

4.8. Measurements of Enzyme and Hormone

The homogenates of right testis tissue were prepared to determine the levels of testicular superoxide dismutase (SOD), glutathione peroxidase (GSH-Px), malondialdehyde (MDA), and testicular marker enzymes containing lactate dehydrogenase (LDH), alkaline phosphatase (ALP), and acid phosphatase (ACP) according to the specific steps in the kit instructions (Nanjing Jiancheng Bioengineering Institute, Nanjing, China). The protein concentrations of testicular tissue homogenates were determined by the bicinchoninic acid (BCA) protein assay kit (Beyotime Biotechnology, Shanghai, China). Sex hormones of mice including testosterone (T), estradiol (E2), follicle-stimulating hormone (FSH), and luteinizing hormone (LH) in serum were measured by commercial enzyme-linked immunosorbent assay (ELISA) kits (Mmbio, Jiangsu, China) following the instructions.

4.9. TUNEL Apoptosis Assay

The embedded wax block sections were dewaxed in water and treated with proteinase K and rupturing cell membrane working solution at 37 °C for 22 min, then washed with PBS at pH 7.4 three times. The mixture of TDT and DUTP (1:5) was incubated at 37 °C for 2 h, followed by 4′,6-diamidino-2-phenylindole (DAPI) staining for 10 min after washing. The results were observed under a Nikon Eclipse C1 fluorescence microscope with Nikon DS-U3 imaging system (Nikon Corporation, Japan) and the images were collected. At a magnification of 200×, the positive cells of TUNEL staining were counted in 4 random fields on each section.

4.10. Western Blotting

Testicular tissues were homogenized over ice using a homogenizer with 1% protease inhibitor cocktail (Service bio). Then, after repeated mixing for 30 min in ice, the supernatant was collected after centrifugation at 12,000 g and 4 °C for 10 min. Total protein concentrations were determined by a BCA protein assay kit (Service bio) and adjusted to the same level. A total of 30 μg of protein extracts from testicular issues were separated by 5% SDS-polyacrylamide gel electrophoresis (SDS-PAGE) and transferred to polyvinylidene fluoride (PVDF) membranes (Millipore, USA), and followed by blocking with 5% skimmed milk at room temperature for 1 h. The primary antibodies were added into the membrane and then incubated overnight at 4 °C. Primary antibodies to the following proteins were used: Keap1 (sc-514914; 1:500), Heme Oxygenase 1 (sc-390991; 1:1000), NQO1 (sc-376023; 1:1000), Bax (sc-20067; 1:1000), JNK (sc-7345; 1:500), p-JNK (sc-6254; 1:500), cleaved PARP (sc-56196; 1:1000) (Santa Cruz, CA) and Nrf2(16396-1-AP; 1:1000), Bcl2 (26593-1-AP; 1:1000), Caspase-3 (19577-1-AP; 1:1000) (Proteintech, USA). After washing, the membranes were incubated with secondary antibodies at 1:2000 at room temperature for 2 h, and the marked proteins were illuminated using ECL Reagent Kit (Service bio). The bands were visualized by the scanner EPSON V300 (Seiko Epson Corporation, Japan) as well as its intensity was analyzed by ImageJ software and normalized to GAPDH levels.

4.11. Statistical Analysis

Results were expressed as the mean ± standard deviation (SD) and analyzed by SPSS version 17. All the experimental data were analyzed using One-way ANOVA. Differences at $p < 0.05$ was considered statistically significant.

Author Contributions: Conceptualization, X.Q. and X.Z.; methodology, X.Z. and Z.P.; formal analysis, X.Z.; investigation, X.Z.; resources, C.Z.; data curation, X.Z.; writing—original draft preparation, X.Z.; writing—review and editing, X.Z., Z.P., H.Z. and H.L.; supervision, X.Q.; project administration, X.Q.; funding acquisition, X.Q. All authors have read and agreed to the published version of the manuscript.

Funding: This research was financially supported by the China Agricultural Research System of MOF and MARA, High Value Aquatic Products Processing and Utilization Innovation Team of Higher Education Institutions of Guangdong Province (GDOU2016030503).

Institutional Review Board Statement: The study was conducted according to the guidelines of the Declaration of Helsinki, and approved by the Laboratory Animal Committee of Guangdong Ocean University, China (no. GDOU-LAE-2020-014).

Data Availability Statement: Data are available upon request.

Conflicts of Interest: The authors declare no conflict of interest.

References

1. Inhorn, M.C.; Patrizio, P. Infertility around the globe: New thinking on gender, reproductive technologies and global movements in the 21st century. *Hum. Reprod. Update* **2015**, *21*, 411–426. [CrossRef]
2. Jarow, J.P.; Sharlip, I.D.; Belker, A.M.; Lipshultz, L.I.; Sigman, M.; Thomas, A.J.; Schlegel, P.N.; Howards, S.S.; Nehra, A.; Damewood, M.D.; et al. Best practice policies for male infertility. *J. Urol.* **2002**, *167*, 2138–2144. [CrossRef]

3. Karna, K.K.; Choi, B.R.; Kim, M.-J.; Kim, H.K.; Park, J.K. The Effect of Schisandra chinensis Baillon on Cross-Talk between Oxidative Stress, Endoplasmic Reticulum Stress, and Mitochondrial Signaling Pathway in Testes of Varicocele-Induced SD Rat. *Int. J. Mol. Sci.* **2019**, *20*, 5785. [CrossRef]
4. Benoff, S.; Jacob, A.; Hurley, I.R. Male infertility and environmental exposure to lead and cadmium. *Hum. Reprod. Update* **2000**, *6*, 107–121. [CrossRef]
5. Clavijo, R.I.; Hsiao, W. Update on male reproductive endocrinology. *Transl. Androl. Urol.* **2018**, *7*, S367–S372. [CrossRef] [PubMed]
6. Ilacqua, A.; Izzo, G.; Emerenziani, G.P.; Baldari, C.; Aversa, A. Lifestyle and fertility: The influence of stress and quality of life on male fertility. *Reprod. Biol. Endocrinol.* **2018**, *16*, 115. [CrossRef] [PubMed]
7. Semet, M.; Paci, M.; Saïas-Magnan, J.; Metzler-Guillemain, C.; Boissier, R.; Lejeune, H.; Perrin, J. The impact of drugs on male fertility: A review. *Andrology* **2017**, *5*, 640–663. [CrossRef] [PubMed]
8. Ma, B.; Zhang, J.; Zhu, Z.; Bao, X.; Zhang, M.; Ren, C.; Zhang, Q. Aucubin, a natural iridoid glucoside, attenuates oxidative stress-induced testis injury by inhibiting JNK and CHOP activation via Nrf2 up-regulation. *Phytomedicine* **2019**, *64*, 153057. [CrossRef] [PubMed]
9. Liu, F.J.; Dong, W.Y.; Zhao, H.; Shi, X.H.; Zhang, Y.L. Effect of molybdenum on reproductive function of male mice treated with busulfan. *Theriogenology* **2019**, *126*, 49–54. [CrossRef] [PubMed]
10. Kupchan, S.M.; Court, W.A.; Dailey, R.G., Jr.; Gilmore, C.J.; Bryan, R.F. Triptolide and tripdiolide, novel antileukemic diterpenoid triepoxides from Tripterygium wilfordii. *J. Am. Chem. Soc.* **1972**, *94*, 7194–7195. [CrossRef] [PubMed]
11. Wang, B.; Ma, L.; Tao, X.; Lipsky, P.E. Triptolide, an active component of the Chinese herbal remedy Tripterygium wilfordii Hook F, Inhibits production of nitric oxide by decreasing inducible nitric oxide synthase gene transcription. *Arthritis Rheum.* **2004**, *50*, 2995–3003. [CrossRef] [PubMed]
12. Lu, Y.; Bao, X.; Sun, T.; Xu, J.; Zheng, W.; Shen, P. Triptolide attenuate the oxidative stress induced by LPS/D-GalN in mice. *J. Cell Biochem.* **2012**, *113*, 1022–1033. [CrossRef] [PubMed]
13. Wang, Y.; Guo, S.H.; Shang, X.J.; Yu, L.S.; Zhu, J.W.; Zhao, A.; Zhou, Y.F.; An, G.H.; Zhang, Q.; Ma, B. Triptolide induces Sertoli cell apoptosis in mice via ROS/JNK-dependent activation of the mitochondrial pathway and inhibition of Nrf2-mediated antioxidant response. *Acta Pharmacol. Sin.* **2018**, *39*, 311–327. [CrossRef] [PubMed]
14. Matsuda, Y.; Watanabe, T. Effects of oyster extract on the reproductive function of zinc-deficient mice: Bioavailability of zinc contained in oyster extract. *Congenit. Anom.* **2003**, *43*, 271–279. [CrossRef]
15. Zhang, X.; Qin, X.; Gao, J.; Lin, H.; Zhang, C.; Huang, Y. Optimization of enzymatic hydrolysis from Crassostrea gigas and effects of its enzymatic hydrolysate on TM3 Leydig cells. *J. Guangdong Ocean. Univ.* **2019**, *39*, 96–102.
16. Wang, Q.; Li, W.; He, Y.; Ren, D.; Kow, F.; Song, L.; Yu, X. Novel antioxidative peptides from the protein hydrolysate of oysters (Crassostrea talienwhanensis). *Food Chem.* **2014**, *145*, 991–996. [CrossRef]
17. Li, W.; Xu, C.; Zhang, C.H.; Cao, W.H.; Qin, X.M.; Gao, J.L.; Zheng, H.N. The purification and identification of immunoregulatory peptides from oyster (Crassostrea hongkongensis) enzymatic hydrolysate. *Rsc. Adv.* **2019**, *9*, 32854–32863. [CrossRef]
18. Liu, Z.Y.; Dong, S.Y.; Xu, J.; Zeng, M.Y.; Song, H.X.; Zhao, Y.H. Production of cysteine-rich antimicrobial peptide by digestion of oyster (Crassostrea gigas) with alcalase and bromelin. *Food Control* **2008**, *19*, 231–235. [CrossRef]
19. Umayaparvathi, S.; Arumugam, M.; Meenakshi, S.; Drager, G.; Kirschning, A.; Balasubramanian, T. Purification and Characterization of Antioxidant Peptides from Oyster (Saccostrea cucullata) Hydrolysate and the Anticancer Activity of Hydrolysate on Human Colon Cancer Cell Lines. *Int. J. Pept. Res. Ther.* **2014**, *20*, 231–243. [CrossRef]
20. Miao, J.; Liao, W.; Kang, M.; Jia, Y.; Wang, Q.; Duan, S.; Xiao, S.; Cao, Y.; Ji, H. Anti-fatigue and anti-oxidant activities of oyster (Ostrea rivularis) hydrolysate prepared by compound protease. *Food Funct.* **2018**, *9*, 6577–6585. [CrossRef]
21. Byun, J.H.; Choi, Y.J.; Choung, S.Y. Protective effect of Oyster hydrolysate peptide in alcohol induced alcoholic fatty liver in SD-rats. *Planta Med.* **2016**, *82*, 571. [CrossRef]
22. Li, S.J.; Song, Z.Y.; Liu, T.T.; Liang, J.; Yuan, J.; Xu, Z.C.; Sun, Z.H.; Lai, X.P.; Xiong, Q.P.; Zhang, D.Y. Polysaccharide from Ostrea rivularis attenuates reproductive oxidative stress damage via activating Keap1-Nrf2/ARE pathway. *Carbohyd. Polym.* **2018**, *186*, 321–331. [CrossRef]
23. Li, Y.; Qiu, W.; Zhang, Z.; Han, X.; Bu, G.; Meng, F.; Kong, F.; Cao, X.; Huang, A.; Feng, Z.; et al. Oral oyster polypeptides protect ovary against d-galactose-induced premature ovarian failure in C57BL/6 mice. *J. Sci. Food Agric.* **2020**, *100*, 92–101. [CrossRef]
24. Bahadorani, M.; Tavalaee, M.; Abedpoor, N.; Ghaedi, K.; Nazem, M.N.; Nasr-Esfahani, M.H. Effects of branched-chain amino acid supplementation and/or aerobic exercise on mouse sperm quality and testosterone production. *Andrologia* **2019**, *51*, e13183. [CrossRef]
25. Wu, G. Dietary protein intake and human health. *Food Funct.* **2016**, *7*, 1251–1265. [CrossRef] [PubMed]
26. Leahy, T.; Gadella, B.M. Sperm surface changes and physiological consequences induced by sperm handling and storage. *Reproduction* **2011**, *142*, 759–778. [CrossRef] [PubMed]
27. Dong, H.-J.; Wu, D.; Xu, S.-Y.; Li, Q.; Fang, Z.-F.; Che, L.-Q.; Wu, C.-M.; Xu, X.-Y.; Lin, Y. Effect of dietary supplementation with amino acids on boar sperm quality and fertility. *Anim. Reprod. Sci.* **2016**, *172*, 182–189. [CrossRef] [PubMed]
28. Sarmadi, B.H.; Ismail, A. Antioxidative peptides from food proteins: A review. *Peptides* **2010**, *31*, 1949–1956. [CrossRef]
29. Neto, F.T.; Bach, P.V.; Najari, B.B.; Li, P.S.; Goldstein, M. Spermatogenesis in humans and its affecting factors. *Semin. Cell Dev. Biol.* **2016**, *59*, 10–26. [CrossRef]

30. Huynh, P.N.; Hikim, A.P.; Wang, C.; Stefonovic, K.; Lue, Y.H.; Leung, A.; Atienza, V.; Baravarian, S.; Reutrakul, V.; Swerdloff, R.S. Long-term effects of triptolide on spermatogenesis, epididymal sperm function, and fertility in male rats. *J. Androl.* **2000**, *21*, 689–699.
31. Bisht, S.; Faiq, M.; Tolahunase, M.; Dada, R. Oxidative stress and male infertility. *Nat. Rev. Urol.* **2017**, *14*, 470–485. [CrossRef]
32. Zhang, J.; Bao, X.; Zhang, M.; Zhu, Z.; Zhou, L.; Chen, Q.; Zhang, Q.; Ma, B. MitoQ ameliorates testis injury from oxidative attack by repairing mitochondria and promoting the Keap1-Nrf2 pathway. *Toxicol. Appl. Pharmacol.* **2019**, *370*, 78–92. [CrossRef]
33. El-Demerdash, F.M.; Yousef, M.I.; Kedwany, F.S.; Baghdadi, H.H. Cadmium-induced changes in lipid peroxidation, blood hematology, biochemical parameters and semen quality of male rats: Protective role of vitamin E and beta-carotene. *Food Chem. Toxicol.* **2004**, *42*, 1563–1571. [CrossRef]
34. Morimoto, H.; Iwata, K.; Ogonuki, N.; Inoue, K.; Atsuo, O.; Kanatsu-Shinohara, M.; Morimoto, T.; Yabe-Nishimura, C.; Shinohara, T. ROS are required for mouse spermatogonial stem cell self-renewal. *Cell Stem. Cell* **2013**, *12*, 774–786. [CrossRef]
35. Zhou, C.; Hu, J.; Ma, H.; Yagoub, A.E.; Yu, X.; Owusu, J.; Ma, H.; Qin, X. Antioxidant peptides from corn gluten meal: Orthogonal design evaluation. *Food Chem.* **2015**, *187*, 270–278. [CrossRef] [PubMed]
36. Zou, T.B.; He, T.P.; Li, H.B.; Tang, H.W.; Xia, E.Q. The Structure-Activity Relationship of the Antioxidant Peptides from Natural Proteins. *Molecules* **2016**, *21*, 72. [CrossRef] [PubMed]
37. Wajda, A.; Lapczuk, J.; Grabowska, M.; Slojewski, M.; Laszczynska, M.; Urasinska, E.; Drozdzik, M. Nuclear factor E2-related factor-2 (Nrf2) expression and regulation in male reproductive tract. *Pharmacol. Rep.* **2016**, *68*, 101–108. [CrossRef] [PubMed]
38. Griswold, M.D. The central role of Sertoli cells in spermatogenesis. *Semin. Cell Dev. Biol.* **1998**, *9*, 411–416. [CrossRef] [PubMed]
39. Geng, X.; Shao, H.; Zhang, Z.H.; Ng, J.C.; Peng, C. Malathion-induced testicular toxicity is associated with spermatogenic apoptosis and alterations in testicular enzymes and hormone levels in male Wistar rats. *Environ. Toxicol. Phar.* **2015**, *39*, 659–667. [CrossRef]
40. Sadik, N.A. Effects of diallyl sulfide and zinc on testicular steroidogenesis in cadmium-treated male rats. *J. Biochem. Mol. Toxicol.* **2008**, *22*, 345–353. [CrossRef] [PubMed]
41. Zhang, X.Y.; Qin, X.M.; Lin, H.S.; Cao, W.H.; Zheng, H.N.; Gao, J.L.; Zhang, C.H. Protective effect of hydrolyzed ultrafiltration fractions from the Oyster (Crassostrea hongkongensis) on oxidative damage of TM4 Sertoli cells. *South China Fish. Sci.* **2021**, *17*, 118–125.
42. Jiang, X.; Zhu, C.; Li, X.; Sun, J.; Tian, L.; Bai, W. Cyanidin-3-O-glucoside at Low Doses Protected against 3-Chloro-1,2-propanediol Induced Testis Injury and Improved Spermatogenesis in Male Rats. *J. Agric. Food Chem.* **2018**, *66*, 12675–12684. [CrossRef] [PubMed]
43. Bonde, J.P.; Flachs, E.M.; Rimborg, S.; Glazer, C.H.; Giwercman, A.; Ramlau-Hansen, C.H.; Hougaard, K.S.; Hoyer, B.B.; Haervig, K.K.; Petersen, S.B.; et al. The epidemiologic evidence linking prenatal and postnatal exposure to endocrine disrupting chemicals with male reproductive disorders: A systematic review and meta-analysis. *Hum. Reprod Update* **2016**, *23*, 104–125. [CrossRef] [PubMed]
44. Pitteloud, N.; Dwyer, A.A.; DeCruz, S.; Lee, H.; Boepple, P.A.; Crowley, W.F.; Hayes, F.J. Inhibition of luteinizing hormone secretion by testosterone in men requires aromatization for its pituitary but not its hypothalamic effects: Evidence from the tandem study of normal and gonadotropin-releasing hormone-deficient men. *J. Clin. Endocr. Metab.* **2008**, *93*, 784–791. [CrossRef] [PubMed]
45. Li, M.; Zhou, M.; Wei, Y.; Jia, F.; Yan, Y.; Zhang, R.; Cai, M.; Gu, R. The beneficial effect of oyster peptides and oyster powder on cyclophosphamide-induced reproductive impairment in male rats: A comparative study. *J. Food Biochem.* **2020**, *44*, e13468. [CrossRef]
46. Qian, Z.J.; Jung, W.K.; Byun, H.G.; Kim, S.K. Protective effect of an antioxidative peptide purified from gastrointestinal digests of oyster, Crassostrea gigas against free radical induced DNA damage. *Bioresour. Technol.* **2008**, *99*, 3365–3371. [CrossRef] [PubMed]
47. Peng, Z.; Chen, B.; Zheng, Q.; Zhu, G.; Cao, W.; Qin, X.; Zhang, C. Ameliorative Effects of Peptides from the Oyster (Crassostrea hongkongensis) Protein Hydrolysates against UVB-Induced Skin Photodamage in Mice. *Mar. Drugs* **2020**, *18*, 288. [CrossRef]
48. Hamza, R.Z.; Al-Harbi, M.S.; El-Shenawy, N.S. Ameliorative effect of vitamin E and selenium against oxidative stress induced by sodium azide in liver, kidney, testis and heart of male mice. *Biomed. Pharm.* **2017**, *91*, 602–610. [CrossRef]
49. Qiu, C.; Cheng, Y. Effect of Astragalus membranaceus polysaccharide on the serum cytokine levels and spermatogenesis of mice. *Int. J. Biol. Macromol.* **2019**, *140*, 771–774. [CrossRef]
50. Oghbaei, H.; Hamidian, G.; Alipour, M.R.; Alipour, S.; Keyhanmanesh, R. The effect of prolonged dietary sodium nitrate treatment on the hypothalamus-pituitary-gonadal axis and testicular structure and function in streptozotocin-induced diabetic male rats. *Food Funct.* **2020**, *11*, 2451–2465. [CrossRef]

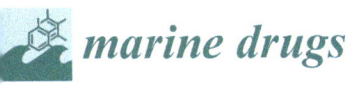

Article

Oyster-Derived Tyr-Ala (YA) Peptide Prevents Lipopolysaccharide/D-Galactosamine-Induced Acute Liver Failure by Suppressing Inflammatory, Apoptotic, Ferroptotic, and Pyroptotic Signals

Adrian S. Siregar [1,2,†], Marie Merci Nyiramana [1,2,†], Eun-Jin Kim [1], Soo Buem Cho [3], Min Seok Woo [1,2], Dong Kun Lee [1,2], Seong-Geun Hong [1], Jaehee Han [1], Sang Soo Kang [2,4], Deok Ryong Kim [2,5], Yeung Joon Choi [6] and Dawon Kang [1,2,*]

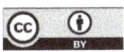

Citation: Siregar, A.S.; Nyiramana, M.M.; Kim, E.-J.; Cho, S.B.; Woo, M.S.; Lee, D.K.; Hong, S.-G.; Han, J.; Kang, S.S.; Kim, D.R.; et al. Oyster-Derived Tyr-Ala (YA) Peptide Prevents Lipopolysaccharide/D-Galactosamine-Induced Acute Liver Failure by Suppressing Inflammatory, Apoptotic, Ferroptotic, and Pyroptotic Signals. *Mar. Drugs* **2021**, *19*, 614. https://doi.org/10.3390/md19110614

Academic Editors: Donatella Degl'Innocenti and Marzia Vasarri

Received: 6 October 2021
Accepted: 26 October 2021
Published: 28 October 2021

Publisher's Note: MDPI stays neutral with regard to jurisdictional claims in published maps and institutional affiliations.

Copyright: © 2021 by the authors. Licensee MDPI, Basel, Switzerland. This article is an open access article distributed under the terms and conditions of the Creative Commons Attribution (CC BY) license (https://creativecommons.org/licenses/by/4.0/).

1. Department of Physiology and Institute of Health Sciences, College of Medicine, Gyeongsang National University, Jinju 52727, Korea; adriansiregar46@gmail.com (A.S.S.); mariemerci1994@naver.com (M.M.N.); eunjin1981@hanmail.net (E.-J.K.); whitewms@naver.com (M.S.W.); dklee@gnu.ac.kr (D.K.L.); hong149@gnu.ac.kr (S.-G.H.); jheehan@gnu.ac.kr (J.H.)
2. Department of Convergence Medical Science, Gyeongsang National University, Jinju 52727, Korea; kangss@gnu.ac.kr (S.S.K.); drkim@gnu.ac.kr (D.R.K.)
3. Department of Radiology, Ewha Womans University Seoul Hospital, Seoul 07804, Korea; kingnose80@gmail.com
4. Department of Anatomy and Institute of Health Sciences, College of Medicine, Gyeongsang National University, Jinju 52727, Korea
5. Department of Biochemistry, College of Medicine, Gyeongsang National University, Jinju 52727, Korea
6. Ocean-Pep, Jinju Bioindustry Foundation, Jinju 52839, Korea; yjchoi@gnu.ac.kr
* Correspondence: dawon@gnu.ac.kr
† These authors contributed equally to this work.

Abstract: Models created by the intraperitoneal injection of lipopolysaccharide (LPS) and D-galactosamine (D-GalN) have been widely used to study the pathogenesis of human acute liver failure (ALF) and drug development. Our previous study reported that oyster (*Crassostrea gigas*) hydrolysate (OH) had a hepatoprotective effect in LPS/D-GalN-injected mice. This study was performed to identify the hepatoprotective effect of the tyrosine-alanine (YA) peptide, the main component of OH, in a LPS/D-GalN-injected ALF mice model. We analyzed the effect of YA on previously known mechanisms of hepatocellular injury in the model. LPS/D-GalN-injected mice showed inflammatory, apoptotic, ferroptotic, and pyroptotic liver injury. The pre-administration of YA (10 mg/kg or 50 mg/kg) significantly reduced the liver damage factors. The hepatoprotective effect of YA was higher in the 50 mg/kg YA pre-administered group than in the 10 mg/kg YA pre-administered group. These results showed that YA had a hepatoprotective effect by reducing inflammation, apoptosis, ferroptosis, and pyroptosis in the LPS/D-GalN-injected ALF mouse model. We suggest that YA can be used as a functional peptide for the prevention of acute liver injury.

Keywords: acute liver injury; apoptosis; ferroptosis; inflammation; oyster; peptide; pyroptosis

1. Introduction

Acute liver failure (ALF) is the most common life-threatening disease in adults without pre-existing liver disease, and it mainly occurs in the 30s [1]. There are many causes of ALF that include hepatitis, acetaminophen overdose, toxins, autoimmune diseases, Wilson's disease, and unknown factors. Herbal supplements cannot be free from triggers of ALF [2]. Since there are few effective treatments for ALF other than liver transplantation, studies to find strategies for the treatment and prevention of ALF using experimental animal models are continuously being performed. In the early stages of ALF, the incidence of bacterial infection is high [3,4], which might aggravate the clinical condition and prognosis [5]. An uncontrolled inflammatory response not only impairs the liver's defenses but also causes massive cell death of hepatocytes, leading to acute liver damage and ultimately severe ALF [1,6].

A model made by the intraperitoneal injection of lipopolysaccharide (LPS) and D-galactosamine (D-GalN) has been widely used to study the pathogenesis of human ALF and drug development [7] because it shows clinically similar symptoms to ALF [8]. LPS, the major pathogenic component of Gram-negative bacteria, induces the secretion of large amounts of pro-inflammatory cytokines and ultimately causes liver injury [9–11]. D-GalN, a selective hepatotoxin, induces depletion of the intracellular uridine moiety, which in turn disrupts the hepatocyte RNA metabolism and results in liver injury [12,13]. D-GalN increases the sensitiveness of LPS and causes hepatotoxicity within a few hours. The LPS/D-GalN model shows typical hepatocellular death manifested by necrosis, apoptosis, autophagy, and inflammatory responses [14–16]. Although many studies have not been conducted, recent studies reported that cell death mechanisms by ferroptosis, pyroptosis, and necroptosis are involved in liver injury in the LPS/D-GalN model [17–19]. Substances that regulate signals related to the hepatocyte death mechanism are expected to be helpful in the prevention and treatment of LPS/D-GalN-induced liver injury.

Conventional drugs used to treat liver diseases, such as corticosteroids, antiviral drugs, and immunosuppressants, can cause serious adverse effects and even liver damage with long-term use [20]. A common strategy for preventing liver damage includes using substances with antioxidant and anti-inflammatory activity [21]. Natural products with antioxidant and anti-inflammatory activities, such as silymarin, were developed as hepatoprotectants [22]. However, since silymarin interacts with CYP2C9 inhibitors, caution is required when taking drugs related to CYP2C9 inhibitors [23]. It is necessary to broaden the choice of natural medicines suitable for individual patients by developing natural hepatoprotectants and therapeutic agents with fewer side effects than silymarin.

In our previous studies, oyster-derived hydrolysate (OH) showed hepatoprotective effects in a single ethanol binge model and a LPS/D-GalN-induced liver injury model [24,25]. In particular, the Tyrosine-Alanine (YA) peptide, the main component of OH, enhanced the ethanol metabolism and protected the liver from ethanol-induced toxicity [25]. YA has antioxidant and anti-inflammatory activities. Bioactive peptides affect various biological functions, and peptides have been used as therapeutic agents for various diseases for a long time [26]. Arg-Gly-Asp (RGD) peptide attenuates LPS-induced pulmonary inflammation [27] and hepatic fibrosis [28]. Currently, there are few studies on the hepatoprotective mechanism of YA against the LPS/D-GalN-induced liver injury model. Since the YA peptide is a food-derived substance, the preventive effect was first investigated before the therapeutic effect. This study was performed to determine the hepatoprotective effect of the YA peptide in the LPS/D-GalN-induced ALF model. We also compared the effects of two different concentrations of YA (10 and 50 mg/kg).

2. Results

2.1. Generation of Acute Liver Failure (ALF) Mouse Model

The method to produce an ALF mouse model and the experimental procedure to confirm the prophylactic effect of YA are summarized in Figure 1A. The ALF model was generated by the intraperitoneal injection of LPS (1 µg/kg) and D-galactosamine (400 mg/kg), and the mice were sacrificed 6 h after the LPS/D-GalN injection. The five experimental groups were divided into the vehicle, LPS/D-GalN, YA (10 or 50 mg/kg) + LPS/D-GalN, and silymarin (25 mg/kg) + LPS/D-GalN groups (each group with 10 mice). YA and silymarin were pre-administrated orally for 10 days. Saline was pre-administered instead of YA in the vehicle and LPS/D-GalN groups. Body weight was measured at the beginning and end of the experiment, and liver weight was measured immediately after sacrificing the mice. There was no significant change in body and liver weights among the experimental groups.

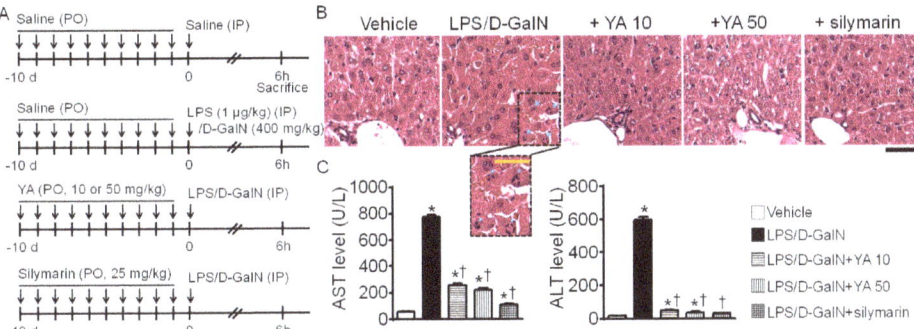

Figure 1. LPS/D-GalN-induced acute liver failure (ALF) mouse model. (**A**) Experimental design to determine the protective effect of YA in the ALF mouse model. Saline, YA, or silymarin was pre-administered daily for ten days by oral gavage before intraperitoneal injection of LPS/D-GalN. (**B**) LPS/D-GalN-induced pathological alterations in liver tissue attenuated by YA. The morphological changes were identified by H&E staining. The dotted rectangle representing the hemorrhage area is expanded to show. Blue arrowheads indicate nuclear fragmentation. Scale bar, 100 µm. (**C**) Effect of YA pre-administration on plasma ALT and AST levels in the LPS/D-GalN group. Data are shown as the mean ± SD (n = 10 in each group). * $p < 0.05$ compared to vehicle group. † $p < 0.05$ compared to the LPS/D-GalN group.

The morphological changes of the liver observed in the experimental groups were evaluated by hematoxylin and eosin (H&E) staining. The LPS/D-GalN group showed a remarkable increase in hemorrhage and nuclear fragmentation (dotted rectangle, Figure 1B). The morphological features of cell damage were reduced in the YA+LPS/D-GalN and silymarin+LPS/D-GalN groups. Comparing the effects of two different concentrations of YA, the cell damage was decreased more in the 50 mg/kg YA pre-administered group than in the 10 mg/kg YA pre-administered group. Silymarin (25 mg/kg), a positive control showing hepatoprotective effects, reduced the LPS/D-GalN-induced morphological features of cell damage (n = 3, Figure 1B). Alanine aminotransferase (ALT) and aspartate aminotransferase (AST) levels in the LPS/D-GalN group were significantly increased compared to the vehicle group ($p < 0.05$). In contrast, they were significantly decreased in the YA and silymarin pre-administered groups (Figure 1C, n = 10, $p < 0.05$).

2.2. YA Pre-Administration Attenuated Inflammatory Signals in ALF Model

YA significantly decreased the activity of the biosynthesis enzymes cyclooxygenase-2 (COX-2) and 5-lipoxygenase (5-LO), which are involved in the inflammatory process. The effect was dose-dependent (n = 4, $p < 0.05$, Figure 2A). The nuclear factor kappa-light-chain-enhancer of activated B cells (NF-κB), a key transcription factor for pro-inflammatory gene induction, was significantly activated in liver tissues obtained from the LPS/D-GalN groups compared to the vehicle group (Figure 2B, n = 4, $p < 0.05$). The NF-κB activation was significantly decreased in the 50 mg/kg YA + LPS/D-GalN and silymarin + LPS/D-GalN groups (Figure 2B, n = 4, $p < 0.05$). In the NF-κB activity, the 10 mg/kg YA + LPS/D-GalN group showed no significant difference from the vehicle and LPS/D-GalN groups.

Mitogen-activated protein kinase (MAPK) activation is related to LPS-induced inflammation [29]. Extracellular signal-regulated kinase 1/2 (ERK), c-Jun N-terminal kinases (JNK), and p38 MAPKs were significantly activated in the LPS/D-GalN group compared to the vehicle group (Figure 2B, $p < 0.05$, n = 4). ERK and JNK activation was significantly decreased in the 50 mg/kg YA + LPS/D-GalN group ($p < 0.05$), whereas p38 activation was significantly reduced in the 10 mg/kg and 50 mg/kg YA and silymarin pre-administered groups (Figure 2C, n = 4, $p < 0.05$), indicating that YA and silymarin may act through different mechanisms. Activation of NF-κB and MAPK is associated with the secretion of pro-inflammatory cytokines such as interleukin (IL)-1 β, IL-6, and tumor necrosis factor (TNF)-α [30,31]. High concentrations of IL-1β, IL-6, and TNF-α in the LPS/D-GalN group were significantly reduced in the YA + LPS/D-GalN group (Figure 2D, n = 4, $p < 0.05$). The secretion of IL-1β, IL-6, and TNF-α was more decreased in the 50 mg/kg YA pre-administered group than in the 10 mg/kg YA pre-administered group. The mRNA expression levels of IL-1β, IL-6, and TNF-α were also decreased in the YA + LPS/D-GalN groups (Figure 2D).

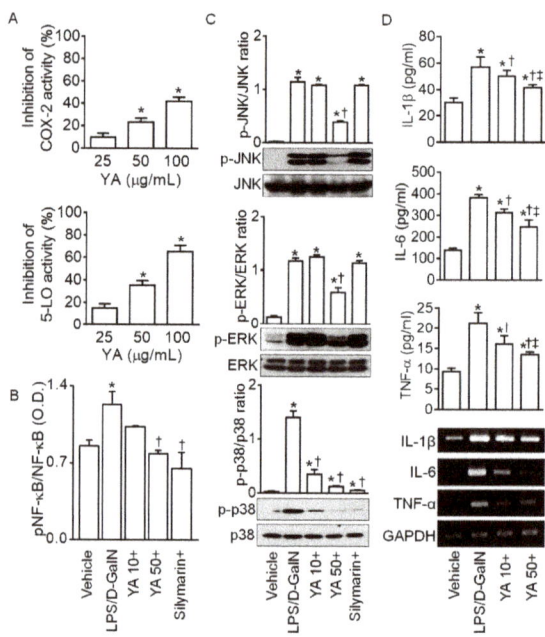

Figure 2. Anti-inflammatory effect of YA in LPS/D-GalN-induced ALF model. (**A**) Inhibition of cyclooxygenase-2 (COX-2) and 5-lipoxygenase (5-LO) activity by YA. * $p < 0.05$ compared to 25 μg/mL YA. (**B**) Changes in NF-κB activation. The NF-κB activity was measured using a phospho-NF-κB p65 (S536) ELISA kit. (**C**) Suppression of MAPK activation by YA. (**D**) Decrease in pro-inflammatory cytokines (IL-1β, IL-6, and TNF-α) by YA. Data are shown as the mean ± SD (n = 4 in each group). * $p < 0.05$ compared to vehicle group. † $p < 0.05$ compared to the LPS/D-GalN group. ‡ $p < 0.05$ compared to YA (10 mg/kg) + LPS/D-GalN group. The plus (+) sign, such as in YA10+, YA50+, and silymarin+, represents a combination of LPS/D-GalN and each substance.

2.3. YA Pre-Administration Attenuated Apoptotic Signals in ALF Model

Apoptotic signals were analyzed in liver tissues obtained from the LPS/D-GalN-injected mice. The number of apoptotic cells exhibiting green fluorescence was increased in the LPS/D-GalN group. In contrast, the number of these cells was decreased in the YA and silymarin pre-administered groups, according to terminal deoxynucleotidyl transferase dUTP nick end labeling (TUNEL) staining, a method detecting DNA fragmentation of apoptotic cells (Figure 3A). In the LPS/D-GalN group, the B-cell lymphoma protein 2 (Bcl-2)-associated X (Bax)/Bcl2 ratio was increased; poly ADP-ribose polymerase (PARP) and caspase 3 (Cas 3) were cleaved, and mitochondrial cytochrome C was secreted into the cytoplasm. In comparison to the LPS/D-GalN group, the apoptotic signals were significantly reduced in the YA and silymarin pre-administered groups (Figure 3B, $p < 0.05$, n = 4). The inhibitory effect on LPS/D-GalN-induced apoptotic signals was higher in the 50 mg/kg YA pre-administration group than in the 10 mg/kg YA pre-administration group.

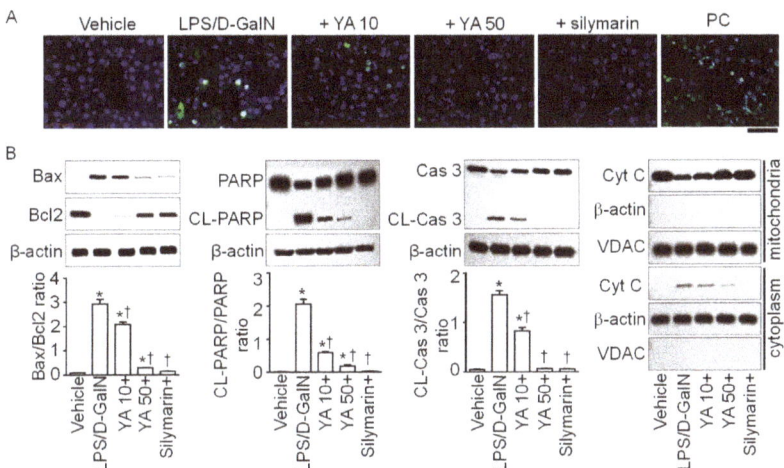

Figure 3. Anti-apoptotic effect of YA on liver tissues obtained from LPS/D-GalN-injected mice. (**A**) TUNEL staining. Representative fluorescence images of hepatocyte apoptosis in LPS/D-GalN group. Positive control (PC) treated with DNase I is displayed as a comparison. The cells showing green fluorescence in the nucleus are apoptotic. Scale bar, 200 μm. (**B**) Western blotting assay for detection of apoptotic signals. Pro-apoptotic Bax and anti-apoptotic Bcl2 expression levels, cleaved (CL) PARP and caspase 3 (Cas 3), and translocation of cytochrome C (Cyt C) into cytoplasm were analyzed. Data are shown as the mean ± SD (n = 4 in each group). * $p < 0.05$ compared to vehicle group. † $p < 0.05$ compared to the LPS/D-GalN group. The plus sign (+) represents a combination of LPS/D-GalN and each substance.

2.4. YA Pre-Administration Attenuated Endoplasmic Reticulum (ER) Stress and Ferroptosis and Pyroptosis Signals in ALF Model

ER stress is related to various cell death mechanisms. ER stress-related proteins such as GRP78, PERK, eIF2α, ATF4, ATF6, and CHOP were upregulated in the LPS/D-GalN group (Figure 4A). The upregulated ER stress markers were markedly decreased in the YA and silymarin pre-administered groups. SLC7A11, GPx4, and HO-1 suppression are linked to ferroptosis induction, while 4-HNE upregulation is related to lipid peroxidation during this process. SLC7A11, GPx4, and HO-1 protein expression levels were decreased in the LPS/D-GalN group, while the 4-HNE protein expression level was increased. The changes in the ferroptosis markers were significantly restored in the YA and silymarin pre-administered groups (Figure 4B, $p < 0.05$, n = 3).

Pyroptotic cell death was detected in the LPS/D-GalN group. The caspase-1 was cleaved, and the gasdermin D (GSDMD) was upregulated. In addition, the carboxy-terminal gasdermin-C domain cleaved in gasdermin D (CL-C-terminal GSDMD) was detected in the LPS/D-GalN group (Figure 4C). IL-1β was highly secreted in the LPS/D-GalN group (see Figure 2D). The pyroptotic signals were significantly reduced in the YA+LPS/D-GalN and silymarin+LPS/D-GalN groups (Figure 4C, $p < 0.05$, n = 3).

The mechanisms involved in liver injury in LPS/D-GalN-injected mice are summarized in Figure 5.

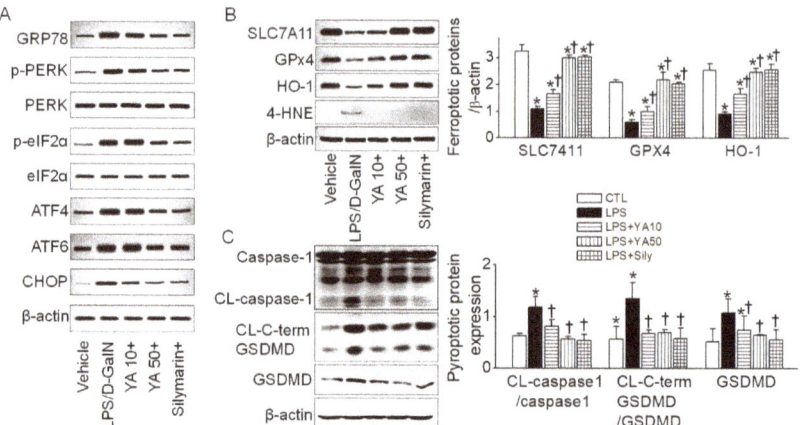

Figure 4. Ferroptotic and pyroptotic signals decreased by YA pre-administration. (**A**) Changes in ER stress markers. (**B**) Changes in ferroptosis markers. (**C**) Changes in pyroptosis markers. Data were shown as the mean ± SD (n = 3 in each group). (**B**,**C**) share a label representing each experimental group. * $p < 0.05$ compared to vehicle group. † $p < 0.05$ compared to the LPS/D-GalN group. The plus sign (+) means the combination of LPS/D-GalN and each substance.

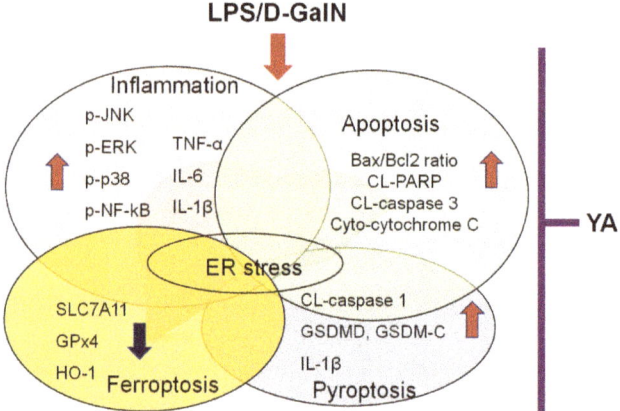

Figure 5. Various mechanisms were observed in liver tissues obtained from the LPS/D-GalN-induced ALF model. Pre-administration of YA reduced LPS/D-GalN-induced liver damage factors. The mechanisms are interconnected and can exacerbate liver damage.

3. Discussion

This study analyzed the effect of YA on previously known mechanisms of hepatocellular damage in a mouse model capable of mimicking ALF symptoms. LPS/D-GalN-injected mice used as an ALF model in this study are also referred to as models for fulminant liver failure (FLF), acute liver injury (ALI), and acute hepatitis. Previous studies reported that liver damage in LPS/D-GalN-injected mouse models is induced by multiple complex mechanisms, such as inflammation, apoptosis, necrosis, autophagy, pyroptosis, necroptosis, and ferroptosis [14–19]. However, most previous studies using LPS/D-GalN-injected mouse models analyzed one or two of the mechanisms mentioned above and reported that many hepatoprotectants proposed in those studies modulate the analyzed mechanisms. Since various factors and mechanisms cause ALF, substances that can control several mechanisms at once will be more helpful in treating ALF. Many hepatoprotective natural substances are more likely to exert their effects by regulating multiple mechanisms rather than specifically regulating a single mechanism. However, due to the lack of research, only some mechanisms of action of these substances are known. Even if the effects of these substances are excellent, it is challenging to develop new drugs or healthy functional foods if the mechanism of action is not sufficiently analyzed.

Here, we introduce a YA peptide that regulates many pathological mechanisms occurring in the LPS/D-GalN-induced ALF model. YA reduced inflammation, apoptosis, ER stress, ferroptosis, and pyroptosis in a LPS/D-GalN-injected mouse model, eventually reducing liver injury. Dipeptide YA used in this study has not been studied as much as other peptides. The mechanism of LPS/D-GalN-induced liver injury is also associated with increased autophagy [16]. However, in our study, autophagy-related signals did not show consistent results, so autophagy was excluded from the hepatoprotective mechanism of YA. Necrotic events were confirmed by H&E staining. Hepatocyte swelling along with shrinkage of the nucleus shown in the LPS/D-GalN-induced ALF model was reduced in the YA pre-administered group. Receptor-interacting protein kinase (RIPK) 1 and RIPK3, necroptosis markers, expression levels were also checked in the liver tissues obtained from the LPS/D-GalN-induced ALF model. There were no significant differences between the vehicle group and the LPS/D-GalN group. As a result, autophagy and necroptosis were excluded from YA-regulated mechanisms.

YA exerts an anti-inflammatory effect by reducing MAPK/NF-κB activity. Apoptosis plays a role in normal liver development. However, the over-activation of apoptosis may lead to hepatocellular damage [32,33]. YA exerts anti-apoptotic effects by decreasing the Bax/Bcl2 ratio, PARP and caspase 3 cleavages, and cytochrome C translocation from the mitochondria to the cytoplasm. ER stress plays a role during LPS/D-GalN-induced apoptosis in the ALF model [34–36]. YA decreased most of ER stress protein expression. ER stress is related to apoptosis, inflammation, and pyroptosis [37,38]. Ferroptosis agents cause ER stress responses, which play an essential role in the cross-talk between ferroptosis and other types of cell death [39]. ER stress appears to mediate many kinds of cell death. Dysregulation of ferroptosis has also been associated with various liver diseases [40]. Ferroptosis occurs mainly due to downregulated system x_c activity, inhibited glutathione peroxidase 4 (GPX4), and increased lipid ROS [41]. Functional subunit solute carrier family member 11 of system x_c (SLC7A11), GPx4, and HO-1 protein expression are reduced in the LPS/D-GalN-induced liver injury model [19,42]. YA pre-administration reversed ferroptotic signals in the LPS/D-GalN-induced ALF model. Apoptosis, necroptosis, and pyroptosis can be switched by some molecules. GSDMD is a pore-forming protein that promotes pyroptosis and the release of pro-inflammatory cytokines [43]. GSDMD-mediated hepatocyte pyroptosis extends the inflammatory response to ALF by upregulating monocyte chemotactic protein 1/CC chemokine receptor-2 to recruit macrophages [17,18]. YA pre-administration also decreased the upregulation of GSDMD, caspase 1 activation, C-terminal of GSDMD cleavage in the LPS/D-GalN induced ALF model. These signals are intricately intertwined in the ALF model and will act in complex ways. In addition, the analyzed mechanism may not be perfect. Other mechanisms will work. YA regulates various mechanisms, which can occur in the LPS/D-GalN-induced ALF model. Involvement in multiple mechanisms can be either an advantage or a disadvantage. The advantage is that it can be effective because it can block numerous pathways that can act as mechanisms of liver damage in the ALF model at once. The disadvantage is that since it blocks several pathways, the probability of side effects can be high, and YA may not work specifically for the ALF model. However, in terms of side effects, since YA is a peptide derived from natural products, it is considered that the possibility of side effects is low.

YA was used as a standard material for OH. Although several peptides have been suggested as standard materials in the OH, YA has advantages over other peptides. YA is readily available to be used because YA is synthesized and sold by several companies, including Sigma-Aldrich (#T5128). Short peptides produced from proteins that have biological activity beyond their nutritional value are known as bioactive peptides. To achieve their "bioactive" roles, these peptides must be released by proteolysis (in vivo digestion, in vitro enzymatic hydrolysis, or bacterial fermentation) [44]. YA was released from oysters by enzymatic hydrolysis. Our previous studies demonstrated that OH produced by in vitro enzymatic hydrolysis of oysters contained various bioactive peptides such as TAY, VK, KY, FYN, and YA and displayed antihypertensive, anti-inflammatory, antidiabetic, antioxidative, and hepatoprotective effects in in vitro and in vivo tests [24,25,45–47]. YA can be a bioactive peptide.

In the case of peptides, when administered orally, they are broken down into amino acids in the gastrointestinal tract, which may weaken their effectiveness. When comparing the effects of oral and intraperitoneal administrations in a preliminary study, the YA effect was slightly higher when injected intraperitoneally, indicating that the peptide may be digested into amino acids without being wholly absorbed when YA was administered orally. However, it is thought that this disadvantage can be overcome by intramuscular, subcutaneous, or intravenous injection. If YA is catabolized, tyrosine and alanine will be produced. Tyrosine and alanine are non-essential amino acids. Alanine is the most common amino acid catabolized by the liver in mammals, and it contributes the most to the gluconeogenesis of the 15 glucogenic amino acids [48,49]. To clear the N metabolites generated by amino acid catabolism, peripheral tissues such as skeletal muscle produce alanine and glutamine as nitrogen carriers in the blood, which are then taken up by the liver and gut and safely disposed of ureagenesis, resulting in glucose production from alanine [48,49]. Furthermore, the ALT expressed in the liver is responsible for the alanine-pyruvate interconversion [50]. When hepatocytes are damaged, ALT is released into the bloodstream, increasing serum ALT activity [51]. In an ALF rat model treated with D-GalN, alanine administration was found to lower plasma levels of ALT and total bilirubin dramatically [52]. In a CCl_4-induced hepatocyte necrotic rat model, alanine administration was shown to reduce the ALT rise and histological liver damage [53]. In addition, alanine treatment dramatically reduced lactate dehydrogenase levels in D-GalN-treated rat hepatocytes [53]. When dietary tyrosine levels are low, the liver can produce tyrosine by hydroxylating phenylalanine. Tyrosine can become an essential amino acid in conditions where the liver fails. Tyrosine shortage can cause net protein catabolism and muscle wasting, so it is important to get enough [54]. Furthermore, tyrosine that is overused is oxidized. Tyrosine is a ketogenic and glucogenic amino acid. Both glucose and fatty acids can be produced by tyrosine [54]. Blood tyrosine levels are supposed to rise as a result of all-cause liver disease [55]. However, the exact mechanism is not known, and there is little evidence that tyrosine has a direct influence on liver disease. The YA concentration in the gastrointestinal system did not vary significantly in the simulated digestion experiment, suggesting that YA can be absorbed into the blood without significant loss [45].

In addition, when comparing the hepatoprotective effect of YA between the group pre-administered with YA once a day for 10 days (10 days YA group) and the group pre-administered with YA once a day (1 day YA group), the hepatoprotective effect of YA was slightly lower in the 1 day YA group than the 10 day YA group, with a reduction in liver damage. At 10 and 50 mg/kg concentrations of YA, both concentrations effectively reduced liver damage in the LPS/D-GalN-induced ALF model, except for effects on ERK and JNK activation. The hepatoprotective effect was higher in the 50 mg/kg YA pre-administered group than in the 10 mg/kg YA pre-administered group. In addition, significant activation of ERK and JNK in the 50 mg/kg YA pre-administered group could act as a signaling pathway distinct from the silymarin pre-administered group. A single ethanol binge model with 50 mg/kg YA demonstrated a hepatoprotective effect [25]. Therefore, we compared the effect of low-dose (10 mg/kg) and high-dose (50 mg/kg) YA in the LPS/D-GalN-induced ALF model. It can become a more effective functional food and is more likely to be used as a pharmaceutical if it has an effect at a low concentration. Although less effective than 50 mg/kg YA, 10 mg/kg YA had a hepatoprotective effect, suggesting that it could be developed as a medication. YA did not cause hepatotoxicity at 50 mg/kg, and it may affect other mechanisms that were not fully explored in this study.

Food-derived bioactive peptides and peptide-rich protein hydrolysates could provide a safe alternative to synthetic pharmaceuticals for the prevention and treatment of acute and chronic diseases with fewer side effects. The positive effect of YA was confirmed in the acute inflammation models, but its effect should also be analyzed in the chronic models. The substances that modulate multiple mechanisms may be effective because they can control complex mechanisms that can coexist in a single disease. However, it will be necessary to investigate continuously the side effects of the substance on normal tissues. Our findings suggest that YA can be a hepatoprotectant in acute liver injury, such as ALF, FLF, and acute hepatitis as a bioactive peptide.

4. Materials and Methods

4.1. Preparation of YA Peptide

Crassostrea gigas specimens (length, 5.8 ± 0.4 cm; height, 3.2 ± 0.4 cm; body weight (BW), 9.8 ± 2.1 g) were harvested from a fish farm in Tongyeong (South Korea) in 2018–2019, frozen, and preserved for 1–2 years. The preparation of the oyster hydrolysate (OH) and YA was conducted according to a previous protocol [25]. The amino acid sequence of the purified peptide fragment in OH is determined using LC/MS/MS. The sequenced peptide YA was synthesized with a purity of 95% or higher to test their function. In addition, we validated histological changes in the liver and changes in liver enzymes (alanine aminotransferase, ALT; aspartate aminotransferase, AST) using synthetic YA purchased from Sigma-Aldrich (St. Louis, MI, USA).

4.2. Measurement of Cyclooxygenase-2 (COX-2) and 5-Lipoxygenase (5-LO) Inhibition Activity

The percentages of COX-2 inhibition and 5-LO inhibition of YA were measured according to the previous protocols [24]. Briefly, the assay mixture for COX-2 contained 450 µL of Tris-HCl buffer (pH 8.0, 100 mM), 100 µL of hematin (150 mM), 100 µL of ethylene-diamine-tetraacetic acid (EDTA, 30 µM), 200 µL of COX-2 (40 U/mL), and 100 µL of YA. The mixture was incubated for 15 min at room temperature. The reaction was initiated by adding 20 µL of arachidonic acid (20 mM) and 25 µL of N,N,N',N'-tetramethyl-p-phenylenediamine (TMPD, 10 mM) and evaluated after 5 min at 590 nm. To measure 5-LO activity, 200 µL of the enzyme solution (160 U/mL) were prepared in a 0.2 M boric acid buffer (pH 9.0), mixed with 50 µL of YA (1, 3, 5, and 100 mg/mL in boric acid buffer), and then incubated at room temperature for 3 min. The reaction was initiated by adding 250 µL of the substrate solution (100 µM of linoleic acid) and evaluated for 2 min at 234 nm using the VERSAmax microplate reader (Molecular Devices, San Jose, CA, USA).

4.3. LPS/D-GalN-Induced ALF Model

The animal experiments were carried out in compliance with the animal care and use committee guidelines at Gyeongsang National University (GNU-151208-M0068). Male C57BL/6 mice (7 weeks old) were purchased from Koatech Co. (Animal Breeding Center, Pyongtaek, Korea). Animals were kept on a 12 h light/dark cycle in a specific pathogen-free area with food and water freely available in the animal facility for 1 week before the experiment. All experimental animals were randomly separated into five groups as follows: Saline, LPS (1 µg/kg) + D-GalN (400 mg/kg), LPS/D-GalN + YA (10 mg/kg), LPS/D-GalN + YA (50 mg/kg), and LPS/D-GalN + silymarin (25 mg/kg). YA and silymarin were pre-administered for 10 days before LPS/D-GalN by oral gavage. LPS/D-GalN was injected intraperitoneally. Blood and tissues were collected 6 h after LPS/D-GalN injection. Liver tissues were quickly isolated and placed into a deep freezer at $-80\ °C$ or a 4% paraformaldehyde solution for further experimentation.

4.4. Measurement of Alanine Aminotransferase (ALT) and Aspartate Aminotransferase (AST) Levels

ALT and AST levels in the serum were measured by GC Labs (Yongin, Korea), which uses the International Federation of Clinical Chemistry standard method. ALT and AST levels were measured and analyzed according to previous methods [25].

4.5. Hematoxylin and Eosin (H&E) Staining

Histological changes in the liver tissue were analyzed by H&E staining (Sigma Aldrich., St Louis, MO, USA). Mice were perfused with a fixative solution containing 4% paraformaldehyde solution, and the liver was isolated and incubated in the same fixative solution overnight at 4 °C. The liver tissues were embedded in paraffin after washing three times. The paraffin blocks were sectioned to a thickness of 5 µm and air-dried on gelatin-coated slides. For H&E staining, the paraffin was removed from the liver tissue sections with xylene, and the tissue sections were rehydrated with graded alcohol series (100% to 70% EtOH). The liver tissue section was washed with tap water for 5 min, and the section slide was immersed in hematoxylin solution for 5 min. After checking the degree of hematoxylin staining, eosin staining was performed for 1 min. The sections were dehydrated through a graded series of EtOH (70% to 100% EtOH, each 3 min), removed from xylene, and mounted with mounting medium (Fisher Chemical, Geel, Belgium). The stained part was photographed using a BX61VS microscope (Olympus, Tokyo, Japan).

4.6. TUNEL Staining

The apoptotic signal in the testes was assessed using the DeadEnd Fluorometric TUNEL System (Promega, Madison, WI, USA) according to the manufacturer's protocol. The TUNEL staining was carried out as described previously [56]. Deparaffinized liver tissue sections were fixed in 4% paraformaldehyde in PBS for 15 min at room temperature, washed three times in PBS, and permeabilized with 20 µg/mL proteinase K solution for 10 min at room temperature. After three washes in PBS, the slides were refixed in 4% paraformaldehyde for 5 min at room temperature. The slides were washed in PBS for 5 min and equilibrated in an equilibration buffer for 10 min. The liver tissues on the slides were labeled with a TdT reaction mix for 60 min at 37 °C in a dark, humidified chamber. The reaction was stopped with a 2 × SSC solution, followed by washing three times in PBS. Counterstaining was carried out by incubating with 5 µg/mL PI for 10 min at room temperature in the dark. TUNEL-positive cells were observed using a confocal laser scanning microscope (Olympus).

4.7. RT-PCR

Total RNA isolated from liver tissues was used to synthesize first-strand cDNA using a reverse transcriptase kit (DiaStartTM RT kit; SolGent, Daejeon, Korea) for RT-PCR and real-time PCR. As previously mentioned, the procedure for RT-PCR was performed [57]. Table 1 shows the primer sequences used to detect mRNA of IL-1β, IL-6, TNF-α, and glyceraldehyde-3-phosphate dehydrogenase (GAPDH). GAPDH was used as a loading control. The PCR conditions included an initial denaturation at 94 °C for 5 min, followed by 30 cycles of 94 °C for 30 s, 58 °C for 30 s, and 72 °C for 30 s, and a final extension step at 72 °C for 10 min.

Table 1. Primer sequences used for PCR.

Gene Name	GenBank Acc. No.	Primer Sequences (5′–3′)	Expected Size (bp)
IL1b	NM_008361.4	Sense: GTTGACGGACCCCAAAAGAT Antisense: TCGTTGCTTGGTTCTCCTTG	440
IL6	NM_031168	Sense: CTTCACAAGTCCGGAGAGGAG Antisense: TGGTCTTGGTCCTTAGCCACT	489
Tnf	D84199	Sense: CAGCCTCTTCTCATTCCTGCT Antisense: TGTCCCTTGAAGAGAACCTGG	339
GAPDH	NM_017008.4	Sense: CTA AAG GGC ATC CTG GGC Antisense: TTA CTC CTT GGA GGC CAT	201

4.8. Western Blot Analysis

A Western blot analysis of total, cytoplasmic, and mitochondrial proteins was performed as described previously [25]. The total protein was isolated from liver tissue using the RIPA buffer (25 mM Tris-HCl (pH 7.4), 150 mM NaCl, 1% NP-40, 1% deoxycholate, 0.1% sodium dodecyl sulfate (SDS); Thermo Fisher Scientific, Carlsbad, CA, USA) containing a 1× protease inhibitor cocktail (Roche Diagnostics, Indianapolis, IN, USA). According to the manufacturer's protocol, mitochondrial and cytosolic fractions were isolated using a mitochondria isolation kit for the tissue (Thermo Fisher Scientific). Equal amounts (30 μg) of protein were analyzed among experimental groups. Equal volumes of the proteins and 2× SDS sample buffer were mixed, loaded on 10% SDS-polyacrylamide gel, and separated by electrophoresis for 120 min at 120 V. Then, the gel was transferred to a polyvinylidene difluoride membrane (Millipore, Billerica, MA, USA) for 1 h at 100 V using a wet transfer system (Bio-Rad, Hercules, CA, USA). The membranes blocked with 5% (w/v) fat-free dry milk in TBS with tween-20 at room temperature for 60 min were incubated with anti-Bax (1:200 dilution; Santa Cruz Biotechnology, Dallas, TX, USA), anti-Bcl-2 (1:200 dilution; Santa Cruz Biotechnology), anti-cytochrome C (1:1000; Cell Signaling, Danvers, MA, USA), anti-VDAC (1:1000; Cell Signaling, Danvers, MA, USA), anti-caspase-3 (1:1000; Cell Signaling), anti-GRP78 (1:1000 dilution, Abcam., Cambridge, UK), anti-pERK (1:200 dilution; Santa Cruz Biotechnology), anti-p-pERK (1:200 dilution; Santa Cruz Biotechnology), anti-eIF2α (1:1000; Cell Signaling), anti-p-eIF2α (1:1000; Cell Signaling), anti-ATF4 (1:200 dilution; Santa Cruz Biotechnology), anti-ATF6 (1:1000; Cell Signaling), anti-CHOP (1:200 dilution; Santa Cruz Biotechnology), anti-HO-1 (1:200 dilution; Santa Cruz Biotechnology), anti-SLC7A11/xCT (1:1000, arigo Biolaboratories Corp., Hsinchu City, Taiwan), anti-GPx4 (1:1000, arigo Biolaboratories Corp), anti-4-HNE (1:1000, arigo Biolaboratories Corp), anti-caspase 1 (1:1000, Adipogen Corporation, San Diego, CA, USA), anti-GSDMD (1:1000, Abcam), anti-cleaved C-terminal GSDMD (1:1000, Abcam), and anti-β-actin antibody (1:5000 dilution; Thermo Fisher Scientific) at 4 °C overnight. After the primary antibody incubation, it was incubated with a secondary HRP-conjugated anti-rabbit or anti-mouse antibody at 1:10,000 (Assay Designs, Ann Arbor, MI, USA). Immuno-positive bands were enhanced with chemiluminescence (EzWestLumi plus; ATTO Gentaur, Tokyo, Japan) and visualized using the iBright CL1500 imaging system (Thermo Scientific Fisher/Life Technologies Holdings Pte Ltd., Singapore).

4.9. Measurement of IL-1β, IL-6, and TNF-α Concentrations in Liver Tissues

According to the manufacturer's protocol, the concentrations of the pro-inflammatory cytokines IL-1β, IL-6, and TNF-α in the liver tissues were quantified using an ELISA kit (R&D system, Minneapolis, MN, USA). The protocol was previously described [25]. The absorbance of the plates at 450 nm was read with a microplate reader (Molecular Devices).

4.10. Measurement of Total and Phospho-NF-kB p65 Protein

The semi-quantitative measurement of NF-κB p65 (pS536) and total NF-κB p65 protein was performed using an ELISA kit (NF-κB p65 (pS536 + Total), Abcam) according to the manufacturer's protocol. The 100 mg of liver tissues were homogenized in cold 1× Extraction Buffer PTR (Abcam). The homogenates were incubated in ice for 20 min and subjected to centrifugation at 18,000× g for 20 min at 4 °C (Eppendorf Centrifuge 5424R, Eppendorf AG). After centrifugation, the supernatant was transferred to a clean tube and provided as tissue lysates. The protein concentration of tissue lysate was quantified using the BCA assay kit. Then, the tissue lysates were diluted to the desired concentration using 1× Extraction Buffer PTR. The diluted tissue lysates (50 μL), antibody cocktail (the mixture of Capture Antibody NF-κB p65 (pS536) or NF-κB p65 total with Detector Antibody) were added to a 96-well plate. The plates were covered with an adhesive strip, incubated for 1 h at room temperature, and washed three times with 1× wash buffer PT. Then, 100 μL of TMB substrate were added and incubated at room temperature for 15 min in the dark on a plate shaker set to 400 rpm. The reaction was quenched by adding 100 μL stop solution, and the absorbance of the plates was read at 450 nm with a microplate reader (Molecular Devices, Sunnyvale, CA, USA).

4.11. Data Analysis and Statistics

The images of the Western blots and agarose gel were captured using an iBright CL1500 imaging system (Thermo Scientific Fisher/Life Technologies Holdings Pte Ltd.). The bands were quantified by ImageJ software (version 1.49, National Institutes of Health, Bethesda, MD, USA). Data are presented as the mean ± standard deviation (SD). The one-way ANOVA/Bonferroni test or the Kruskal–Wallis/Mann–Whitney test was selected after the normality test to analyze differences among groups (OriginPro2020, OriginLab Corp., Northampton, MA, USA). A $p < 0.05$ value was considered as the statistical significance criterion.

5. Conclusions

Our findings demonstrate that YA regulates a complex mechanism induced by LPS/D-GalN. YA has anti-inflammatory, anti-apoptotic, anti-pyroptotic, and anti-ferroptotic effects against LPS/D-GalN-induced hepatic inflammation and cell death. YA may be a potential marine anti-inflammatory and antioxidative agent for treating acute liver diseases such as ALF.

Author Contributions: Conceptualization, S.S.K., Y.J.C. and D.K.; Data curation, A.S.S., M.M.N. and D.K.; Formal analysis, A.S.S., M.M.N., E.-J.K. and D.K.; Funding acquisition, S.S.K., Y.J.C., D.R.K. and D.K.; Investigation, A.S.S., M.M.N., E.-J.K., M.S.W. and D.K.; Methodology, A.S.S., M.M.N.; Project administration, E.-J.K.; Resources, Y.J.C.; Supervision, S.-G.H., J.H.; Writing—original draft, A.S.S., S.B.C. and D.K.; Writing—review and editing, D.K.L., J.H., S.S.K., S.-G.H. and D.K. All authors have read and agreed to the published version of the manuscript.

Funding: This work was supported by the National Research Foundation of Korea (MSIT, NRF-2015R1A-5A-2008833 and 2021R1I1A3044128) and by the Ministry of Oceans and Fisheries (Korea, D11410119H480000110/#2014042).

Institutional Review Board Statement: The study was conducted according to the guidelines of the Declaration of Helsinki and approved by the animal care and use committee of Gyeongsang National University (GNU-151208-M0068).

Data Availability Statement: The study did not report any data.

Acknowledgments: This work was from Adrian Syawaluddin Siregar's thesis for the degree of Doctor of Philosophy ("Hepatoprotective effect of dipeptide tyrosine-alanine in ethanol and lipopolysaccharide-induced liver injury models", 2021, Department of Convergence Medical Science, Graduate School, Gyeongsang National University).

Conflicts of Interest: The authors declare no conflict of interest. The funding sponsors had no role in the design of the study; in the collection, analyses, or interpretation of the data; in the writing of the manuscript; or in the decision to publish the results.

References

1. Bernal, W.; Wendon, J. Acute liver failure. *N. Engl. J. Med.* **2013**, *369*, 2525–2534. [CrossRef] [PubMed]
2. Toma, D.; Lazar, O.; Bontas, E. *Acute Liver Failure*; Springer Nature Switzerland AG: Cham, Switzerland, 2020; p. 12.
3. Rolando, N.; Wade, J.; Davalos, M.; Wendon, J.; Philpott-Howard, J.; Williams, R. The systemic inflammatory response syndrome in acute liver failure. *Hepatology* **2000**, *32*, 734–739. [CrossRef]
4. Rolando, N.; Harvey, F.; Brahm, J.; Philpott-Howard, J.; Alexander, G.; Gimson, A.; Casewell, M.; Fagan, E.; Williams, R. Prospective study of bacterial infection in acute liver failure: An analysis of fifty patients. *Hepatology* **1990**, *11*, 49–53. [CrossRef]
5. Zhai, X.R.; Tong, J.J.; Wang, H.M.; Xu, X.; Mu, X.Y.; Chen, J.; Liu, Z.F.; Wang, Y.; Su, H.B.; Hu, J.H. Infection deteriorating hepatitis B virus related acute-on-chronic liver failure: A retrospective cohort study. *BMC Gastroenterol.* **2020**, *20*, 320. [CrossRef]
6. Yin, X.; Gong, X.; Zhang, L.; Jiang, R.; Kuang, G.; Wang, B.; Chen, X.; Wan, J. Glycyrrhetinic acid attenuates lipopolysaccharide-induced fulminant hepatic failure in D-galactosamine-sensitized mice by up-regulating expression of interleukin-1 receptor-associated kinase-M. *Toxicol. Appl. Pharmacol.* **2017**, *320*, 8–16. [CrossRef]

7. Seo, M.J.; Hong, J.M.; Kim, S.J.; Lee, S.M. Genipin protects D-galactosamine and lipopolysaccharide-induced hepatic injury through suppression of the necroptosis-mediated inflammasome signaling. *Eur. J. Pharmacol.* **2017**, *812*, 128–137. [CrossRef] [PubMed]
8. Kemelo, M.K.; Wojnarova, L.; Kutinova Canova, N.; Farghali, H. D-galactosamine/lipopolysaccharide-induced hepatotoxicity downregulates sirtuin 1 in rat liver: Role of sirtuin 1 modulation in hepatoprotection. *Physiol. Res.* **2014**, *63*, 615–623. [CrossRef]
9. Nowak, M.; Gaines, G.C.; Rosenberg, J.; Minter, R.; Bahjat, F.R.; Rectenwald, J.; MacKay, S.L.; Edwards, C.K., 3rd; Moldawer, L.L. LPS-induced liver injury in D-galactosamine-sensitized mice requires secreted TNF-alpha and the TNF-p55 receptor. *Am. J. Physiol. Regul. Integr. Comp. Physiol.* **2000**, *278*, R1202–R1209. [CrossRef] [PubMed]
10. Guha, M.; Mackman, N. LPS induction of gene expression in human monocytes. *Cell. Signal.* **2001**, *13*, 85–94. [CrossRef]
11. Martich, G.D.; Danner, R.L.; Ceska, M.; Suffredini, A.F. Detection of interleukin 8 and tumor necrosis factor in normal humans after intravenous endotoxin: The effect of antiinflammatory agents. *J. Exp. Med.* **1991**, *173*, 1021–1024. [CrossRef]
12. Wang, H.; Xu, D.-X.; Lv, J.-W.; Ning, H.; Wei, W. Melatonin attenuates lipopolysaccharide (LPS)-induced apoptotic liver damage in D-galactosamine-sensitized mice. *Toxicology* **2007**, *237*, 49–57. [CrossRef] [PubMed]
13. Newsome, P.N.; Plevris, J.N.; Nelson, L.J.; Hayes, P.C. Animal models of fulminant hepatic failure: A critical evaluation. *Liver Transplant.* **2000**, *6*, 21–31. [CrossRef]
14. Eipel, C.; Kidess, E.; Abshagen, K.; Leminh, K.; Menger, M.D.; Burkhardt, H.; Vollmar, B. Antileukoproteinase protects against hepatic inflammation, but not apoptosis in the response of D-galactosamine-sensitized mice to lipopolysaccharide. *Br. J. Pharmacol.* **2007**, *151*, 406–413. [CrossRef]
15. Li, J.; Zhong, L.; Zhu, H.; Wang, F. The Protective Effect of Cordycepin on D-Galactosamine/Lipopolysaccharide-Induced Acute Liver Injury. *Mediat. Inflamm.* **2017**, *2017*, 3946706. [CrossRef]
16. Li, L.; Yin, H.; Zhao, Y.; Zhang, X.; Duan, C.; Liu, J.; Huang, C.; Liu, S.; Yang, S.; Li, X. Protective role of puerarin on LPS/D-Gal induced acute liver injury via restoring autophagy. *Am. J. Transl. Res.* **2018**, *10*, 957–965.
17. Li, H.; Zhao, X.K.; Cheng, Y.J.; Zhang, Q.; Wu, J.; Lu, S.; Zhang, W.; Liu, Y.; Zhou, M.Y.; Wang, Y.; et al. Gasdermin D-mediated hepatocyte pyroptosis expands inflammatory responses that aggravate acute liver failure by upregulating monocyte chemotactic protein 1/CC chemokine receptor-2 to recruit macrophages. *World J. Gastroenterol.* **2019**, *25*, 6527–6540. [CrossRef] [PubMed]
18. Bai, L.; Kong, M.; Duan, Z.; Liu, S.; Zheng, S.; Chen, Y. M2-like macrophages exert hepatoprotection in acute-on-chronic liver failure through inhibiting necroptosis-S100A9-necroinflammation axis. *Cell Death Dis.* **2021**, *12*, 93. [CrossRef]
19. Wang, Y.; Chen, Q.; Shi, C.; Jiao, F.; Gong, Z. Mechanism of glycyrrhizin on ferroptosis during acute liver failure by inhibiting oxidative stress. *Mol. Med. Rep.* **2019**, *20*, 4081–4090. [CrossRef]
20. Padmanabhan, P.; Jangle, S. Hepatoprotective activity of herbal preparation (HP-4) against alcohol induced hepatotoxicity in mice. *Int. J. Appl. Sci. Biotechnol.* **2014**, *2*, 50–58. [CrossRef]
21. Yang, S.; Kuang, G.; Zhang, L.; Wu, S.; Zhao, Z.; Wang, B.; Yin, X.; Gong, X.; Wan, J. Mangiferin Attenuates LPS/D-GalN-Induced Acute Liver Injury by Promoting HO-1 in Kupffer Cells. *Front. Immunol.* **2020**, *11*, 285. [CrossRef] [PubMed]
22. Gillessen, A.; Schmidt, H.H. Silymarin as Supportive Treatment in Liver Diseases: A Narrative Review. *Adv. Ther.* **2020**, *37*, 1279–1301. [CrossRef]
23. Doehmer, J.; Tewes, B.; Klein, K.U.; Gritzko, K.; Muschick, H.; Mengs, U. Assessment of drug-drug interaction for silymarin. *Toxicol. Vitr. Int. J. Publ. Assoc. BIBRA* **2008**, *22*, 610–617. [CrossRef]
24. Ryu, J.H.; Kim, E.J.; Xie, C.; Nyiramana, M.M.; Siregar, A.S.; Park, S.H.; Cho, S.B.; Song, D.H.; Kim, N.G.; Choi, Y.J.; et al. Hepatoprotective Effects of Oyster Hydrolysate on Lipopolysaccharide/D-galactosamine-Induced Acute Liver Injury in Mice. *J. Korean Soc. Food Sci. Nutr.* **2017**, *46*, 659–670.
25. Siregar, A.S.; Nyiramana, M.M.; Kim, E.J.; Shin, E.J.; Woo, M.S.; Kim, J.M.; Kim, J.H.; Lee, D.K.; Hahm, J.R.; Kim, H.J.; et al. Dipeptide YA is Responsible for the Positive Effect of Oyster Hydrolysates on Alcohol Metabolism in Single Ethanol Binge Rodent Models. *Mar. Drugs* **2020**, *18*, 512. [CrossRef] [PubMed]
26. Baig, M.H.; Ahmad, K.; Saeed, M.; Alharbi, A.M.; Barreto, G.E.; Ashraf, G.M.; Choi, I. Peptide based therapeutics and their use for the treatment of neurodegenerative and other diseases. *Biomed. Pharm.* **2018**, *103*, 574–581. [CrossRef] [PubMed]
27. Moon, C.; Han, J.R.; Park, H.J.; Hah, J.S.; Kang, J.L. Synthetic RGDS peptide attenuates lipopolysaccharide-induced pulmonary inflammation by inhibiting integrin signaled MAP kinase pathways. *Respir. Res.* **2009**, *10*, 18. [CrossRef]
28. Schon, H.T.; Bartneck, M.; Borkham-Kamphorst, E.; Nattermann, J.; Lammers, T.; Tacke, F.; Weiskirchen, R. Pharmacological Intervention in Hepatic Stellate Cell Activation and Hepatic Fibrosis. *Front. Pharmacol.* **2016**, *7*, 33. [CrossRef]
29. Yu, H.; Lin, L.; Zhang, Z.; Zhang, H.; Hu, H. Targeting NF-kappaB pathway for the therapy of diseases: Mechanism and clinical study. *Signal Transduct. Target. Ther.* **2020**, *5*, 209. [CrossRef]
30. Xiao, K.; Liu, C.; Tu, Z.; Xu, Q.; Chen, S.; Zhang, Y.; Wang, X.; Zhang, J.; Hu, C.A.; Liu, Y. Activation of the NF-kappaB and MAPK Signaling Pathways Contributes to the Inflammatory Responses, but Not Cell Injury, in IPEC-1 Cells Challenged with Hydrogen Peroxide. *Oxid. Med. Cell. Longev.* **2020**, *2020*, 5803269. [CrossRef]
31. Liu, T.; Zhang, L.; Joo, D.; Sun, S.C. NF-kappaB signaling in inflammation. *Signal Transduct. Target. Ther.* **2017**, *2*, 1–9. [CrossRef]
32. Wu, Y.H.; Hu, S.Q.; Liu, J.; Cao, H.C.; Xu, W.; Li, Y.J.; Li, L.J. Nature and mechanisms of hepatocyte apoptosis induced by D-galactosamine/lipopolysaccharide challenge in mice. *Int. J. Mol. Med.* **2014**, *33*, 1498–1506. [CrossRef]
33. Li, M.; Song, K.; Huang, X.; Fu, S.; Zeng, Q. GDF-15 prevents LPS and D-galactosamine-induced inflammation and acute liver injury in mice. *Int. J. Mol. Med.* **2018**, *42*, 1756–1764. [CrossRef]

34. Ren, F.; Yang, B.; Zhang, X.; Wen, T.; Wang, X.; Yin, J.; Piao, Z.; Zheng, S.; Zhang, J.; Chen, Y.; et al. Role of endoplasmic reticulum stress in D-GalN/LPS-induced acute liver failure. *Zhonghua Gan Zang Bing Za Zhi Chin. J. Hepatol. Abs* **2014**, *22*, 364–368. [CrossRef]
35. Wang, H.; Chen, L.; Zhang, X.; Xu, L.; Xie, B.; Shi, H.; Duan, Z.; Zhang, H.; Ren, F. Kaempferol protects mice from D-GalN/LPS-induced acute liver failure by regulating the ER stress-Grp78-CHOP signaling pathway. *Biomed. Pharmacother.* **2019**, *111*, 468–475. [CrossRef]
36. Chen, L.; Ren, F.; Zhang, H.; Wen, T.; Piao, Z.; Zhou, L.; Zheng, S.; Zhang, J.; Chen, Y.; Han, Y.; et al. Inhibition of glycogen synthase kinase 3beta ameliorates D-GalN/LPS-induced liver injury by reducing endoplasmic reticulum stress-triggered apoptosis. *PLoS ONE* **2012**, *7*, 45202. [CrossRef]
37. Zhang, K.; Kaufman, R.J. From endoplasmic-reticulum stress to the inflammatory response. *Nature* **2008**, *454*, 455–462. [CrossRef] [PubMed]
38. Lebeaupin, C.; Proics, E.; de Bieville, C.H.; Rousseau, D.; Bonnafous, S.; Patouraux, S.; Adam, G.; Lavallard, V.J.; Rovere, C.; Le Thuc, O.; et al. ER stress induces NLRP3 inflammasome activation and hepatocyte death. *Cell Death Dis.* **2015**, *6*, 1879. [CrossRef]
39. Lee, Y.S.; Lee, D.H.; Choudry, H.A.; Bartlett, D.L.; Lee, Y.J. Ferroptosis-Induced Endoplasmic Reticulum Stress: Cross-Talk between Ferroptosis and Apoptosis. *Mol. Cancer Res. MCR* **2018**, *16*, 1073–1076. [CrossRef]
40. Mao, L.; Zhao, T.; Song, Y.; Lin, L.; Fan, X.; Cui, B.; Feng, H.; Wang, X.; Yu, Q.; Zhang, J.; et al. The emerging role of ferroptosis in non-cancer liver diseases: Hype or increasing hope? *Cell Death Dis.* **2020**, *11*, 518. [CrossRef] [PubMed]
41. Xie, Y.; Hou, W.; Song, X.; Yu, Y.; Huang, J.; Sun, X.; Kang, R.; Tang, D. Ferroptosis: Process and function. *Cell Death Differ.* **2016**, *23*, 369–379. [CrossRef]
42. Ji, Y.; Si, W.; Zeng, J.; Huang, L.; Huang, Z.; Zhao, L.; Liu, J.; Zhu, M.; Kuang, W. Niujiaodihuang Detoxify Decoction Inhibits Ferroptosis by Enhancing Glutathione Synthesis in Acute Liver Failure Models. *J. Ethnopharmacol.* **2021**, *279*, 114305. [CrossRef] [PubMed]
43. Demarco, B.; Chen, K.W.; Broz, P. Cross talk between intracellular pathogens and cell death. *Immunol. Rev.* **2020**, *297*, 174–193. [CrossRef] [PubMed]
44. Chakrabarti, S.; Jahandideh, F.; Wu, J. Food-derived bioactive peptides on inflammation and oxidative stress. *BioMed. Res. Int.* **2014**, *2014*, 608979. [CrossRef]
45. Xie, C.L.; Kang, S.S.; Lu, C.; Choi, Y.J. Quantification of Multifunctional Dipeptide YA from Oyster Hydrolysate for Quality Control and Efficacy Evaluation. *BioMed. Res. Int.* **2018**, *2018*, 8437379. [CrossRef]
46. Xie, C.L.; Kim, J.S.; Ha, J.M.; Choung, S.Y.; Choi, Y.J. Angiotensin I-converting enzyme inhibitor derived from cross-linked oyster protein. *BioMed. Res. Int.* **2014**, *2014*, 379234. [CrossRef]
47. Byun, J.-H.; Shin, J.E.; Choi, Y.-J.; Choung, S.-Y. Oyster hydrolysate ameliorates ethanol diet–induced alcoholic fatty liver by regulating lipid metabolism in rats. *Int. J. Food Sci. Technol.* **2021**, *56*, 11. [CrossRef]
48. Felig, P. The glucose-alanine cycle. *Metab. Clin. Exp.* **1973**, *22*, 179–207. [CrossRef]
49. Okun, J.G.; Rusu, P.M.; Chan, A.Y.; Wu, Y.; Yap, Y.W.; Sharkie, T.; Schumacher, J.; Schmidt, K.V.; Roberts-Thomson, K.M.; Russell, R.D.; et al. Liver alanine catabolism promotes skeletal muscle atrophy and hyperglycaemia in type 2 diabetes. *Nat. Metab.* **2021**, *3*, 394–409. [CrossRef]
50. McCommis, K.S.; Chen, Z.; Fu, X.; McDonald, W.G.; Colca, J.R.; Kletzien, R.F.; Burgess, S.C.; Finck, B.N. Loss of Mitochondrial Pyruvate Carrier 2 in the Liver Leads to Defects in Gluconeogenesis and Compensation via Pyruvate-Alanine Cycling. *Cell Metab.* **2015**, *22*, 682–694. [CrossRef]
51. Kim, W.R.; Flamm, S.L.; di Bisceglie, A.M.; Bodenheimer, H.C.; Public Policy Committee of the American Association for the Study of Liver, D. Serum Activity of Alanine Aminotransferase (ALT) as an Indicator of Health and Disease. *Hepatology* **2008**, *47*, 1363–1370. [CrossRef]
52. Maezono, K.; Mawatari, K.; Kajiwara, K.; Shinkai, A.; Maki, T. Effect of alanine on D-galactosamine-induced acute liver failure in rats. *Hepatology* **1996**, *24*, 1211–1216. [CrossRef]
53. Maezono, K.; Kajiwara, K.; Mawatari, K.; Shinkai, A.; Torii, K.; Maki, T. Alanine protects liver from injury caused by F-galactosamine and CCl4. *Hepatology* **1996**, *24*, 185–191. [CrossRef] [PubMed]
54. Litwack, G. Metabolism of Amino Acids. In *Human Biochemistry*; Academic Press: Cambridge, MA, USA, 2018. [CrossRef]
55. Levine, R.J.; Conn, H.O. Tyrosine metabolism in patients with liver disease. *J. Clin. Investig.* **1967**, *46*, 2012–2020. [CrossRef]
56. Siregar, A.S.; Nyiramana, M.M.; Kim, E.-J.; Shin, E.-J.; Kim, C.-W.; Lee, D.; Hong, S.-G.; Han, J.; Kang, D. TRPV1 Is Associated with Testicular Apoptosis in Mice. *J. Anim. Reprod. Biotechnol.* **2019**, *34*, 7. [CrossRef]
57. Yang, J.H.; Siregar, A.S.; Kim, E.J.; Nyiramana, M.M.; Shin, E.J.; Han, J.; Sohn, J.T.; Kim, J.W.; Kang, D. Involvement of TREK-1 Channel in Cell Viability of H9c2 Rat Cardiomyoblasts Affected by Bupivacaine and Lipid Emulsion. *Cells* **2019**, *8*, 454. [CrossRef] [PubMed]

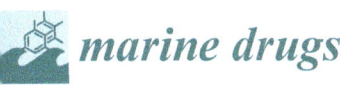

Article

Cytoprotective Peptides from Blue Mussel Protein Hydrolysates: Identification and Mechanism Investigation in Human Umbilical Vein Endothelial Cells Injury

Indyaswan Tegar Suryaningtyas [1,†], Chang-Bum Ahn [2,†] and Jae-Young Je [3,*]

1. Department of Food and Life Science, Pukyong National University, Busan 48513, Korea; indyaswantegar@gmail.com
2. Division of Food and Nutrition, Chonnam National University, Gwangju 61186, Korea; a321@jnu.ac.kr
3. Department of Marine-Bio Convergence Science, Pukyong National University, Busan 48547, Korea
* Correspondence: jjy1915@pknu.ac.kr
† These authors contributed equally to this work.

Citation: Suryaningtyas, I.T.; Ahn, C.-B.; Je, J.-Y. Cytoprotective Peptides from Blue Mussel Protein Hydrolysates: Identification and Mechanism Investigation in Human Umbilical Vein Endothelial Cells Injury. *Mar. Drugs* 2021, 19, 609. https://doi.org/10.3390/md19110609

Academic Editors: Donatella Degl'Innocenti and Marzia Vasarri

Received: 9 October 2021
Accepted: 26 October 2021
Published: 27 October 2021

Publisher's Note: MDPI stays neutral with regard to jurisdictional claims in published maps and institutional affiliations.

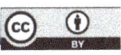

Copyright: © 2021 by the authors. Licensee MDPI, Basel, Switzerland. This article is an open access article distributed under the terms and conditions of the Creative Commons Attribution (CC BY) license (https://creativecommons.org/licenses/by/4.0/).

Abstract: Cardiovascular disease represents a leading cause of mortality and is often characterized by the emergence of endothelial dysfunction (ED), a physiologic condition that takes place in the early progress of atherosclerosis. In this study, two cytoprotective peptides derived from blue mussel chymotrypsin hydrolysates with the sequence of EPTF and FTVN were purified and identified. Molecular mechanisms underlying the cytoprotective effects against oxidative stress which lead to human umbilical vein endothelial cells (HUVEC) injury were investigated. The results showed that pretreatment of EPTF, FTVN and their combination (1:1) in 0.1 mg/mL significantly reduced HUVEC death due to H_2O_2 exposure. The cytoprotective mechanism of these peptides involves an improvement in the cellular antioxidant defense system, as indicated by the suppression of the intracellular ROS generation through upregulation of the cytoprotective enzyme heme oxygenase-1. In addition, H_2O_2 exposure triggers HUVEC damage through the apoptosis process, as evidenced by increased cytochrome C release, Bax protein expression, and the elevated amount of activated caspase-3, however in HUVEC pretreated with peptides and their combination, the presence of those apoptotic stimuli was significantly decreased. Each peptide showed similar cytoprotective effect but no synergistic effect. Taken together, these peptides may be especially important in protecting against oxidative stress-mediated ED.

Keywords: bioactive peptide; cytoprotective; oxidative stress; endothelial dysfunction; blue mussel

1. Introduction

The imbalance between the antioxidant defense mechanism and reactive oxygen species (ROS) generation in a physiological system leads to oxidative stress and associated disease consequences. Regulated ROS generation is critical for the activation of protective signaling pathways, but when in excess amount it induces oxidative stress. Oxidative stress induces depolarization of the mitochondrial membrane. When the mitochondrial membrane potential is reduced, a series of signaling proteins is activated, which leads to the activation of several stress-responsive genes, such as p53, Bax, Bcl-2, and caspase-3 [1]. This results in enhanced reactive oxygen species generation, severe cell damage, and apoptosis-induced cell death [2,3]. These risk factors can induce endothelial dysfunction (ED) through a variety of processes [4,5]. The endothelium, particularly the terminal arteries, is damaged by too much ROS, which disrupts the intracellular reduction-oxidation balance. Hence, ED is considered as an early indicator in the progression of cardiovascular disease (CVD) [6,7]. Since oxidative stress is defined as a possible cause of cardiovascular disease, treatment with antioxidants is a good strategy to prevent CVD-causing endothelial vein damage.

Recently, marine-derived food proteins have attracted much attention because of their wide range of bioactivity. Seafood consumption is thought to lower the risk of various diseases, as peptides derived from marine-food protein have an anti-inflammatory, antihypertensive, antidiabetic, anticancer, antioxidant, and anti-obesity potential [8–14]. Some identified antioxidant peptides or protein hydrolysates are important subjects of interest, due to their specific properties as therapeutic agents to protect the body from diseases related to oxidative damage [8,15,16]. Blue mussel (*Mytilus edulis*) is one of the prominent protein-rich marine food sources that can be converted into bioactive peptides (BAPs) through enzymatic hydrolysis to optimize their health benefits, such as anti-inflammation, antioxidant, and anti-obesity [17–19]. Fermented blue mussel sauce, a popular Asian-style culinary condiment, has also been associated with CVD risk by producing BAPs with antihypertensive activity [20,21]. An effective strategy to prevent CVD is to protect the venous endothelial cells, which are damaged by oxidative stress. In a previous study, α-chymotrypsin-assisted protein hydrolysate of blue mussel showed cytoprotective activity in protecting HUVECs from damage induced by H_2O_2-mediated oxidative stress [1]. However, there is insufficient information in previous reports about specific BAPs that play an important role in endothelial cell protection and certain mechanisms associated with ROS-mediated CVD that need to be understood. The purification of peptides is one of the procedures that needs to be carried out, in order to further expand the use of this compound as a pharmaceutical raw material or functional food source in the future. Therefore, the purpose of this study was to evaluate the capacity of purified peptides derived from blue mussel to protect HUVEC from oxidative stress caused by H_2O_2 exposure, as well as to understand the protective mechanism of these peptides.

2. Results

2.1. Purification and Identification of Cytoprotective Peptides

Cytoprotective peptides were purified from α-chymotrypsin-assisted protein hydrolysates of blue mussel by a cytoprotective activity-guided purification process. First, separation was performed by Sephadex G-25 gel filtration and four fractions (F1~4) were collected. After evaluating cytoprotective activity, the F3 fraction that showed the highest protective effect on HUVEC against H_2O_2-induced oxidative cell damage was selected and further purified by HPLC equipped with a C18 column (Figure 1). Six fractions were obtained by HPLC separation. After determination of cytoprotective activity, fractions H3 and H4 showed similar HUVEC protective activity and were analyzed by LC-MS/MS to identify the peptide sequence. Finally, two peptides of EPTF (calculated MW, 493 Da) and FTVN (calculated MW, 480 Da) were identified in H4 fraction (Figure 2). No peptides were identified in the H3 fraction. To evaluate more about their potential to protect HUVECs, these two peptides were chemically synthesized to further investigate their cytoprotective activity and underlying mechanism.

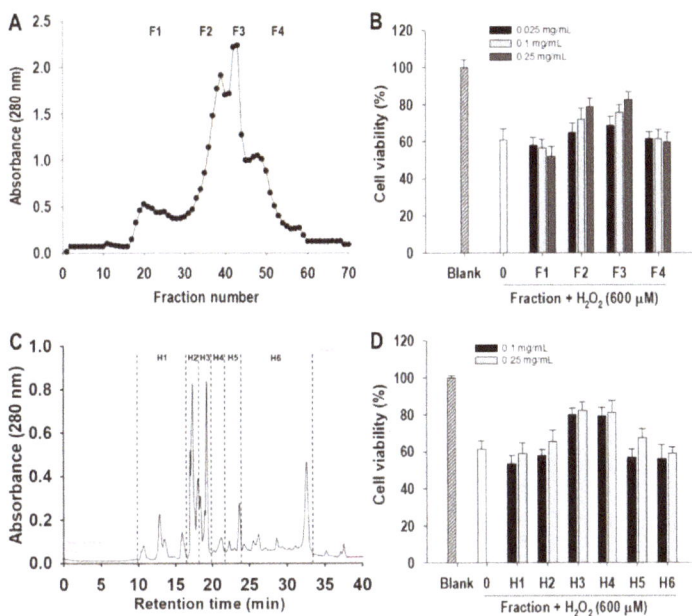

Figure 1. Peptide purification from α-chymotrypsin-assisted blue mussel hydrolysates. (**A**) Gel filtration chromatogram, (**B**) cytoprotective activity of gel filtration fraction, (**C**) HPLC chromatogram, and (**D**) cytoprotective activity of HPLC fraction. Detailed separation conditions are described in Section 2.1. Cells were treated with fraction for 2 h followed by the addition of 600 μM H_2O_2 and further incubation for 24 h.

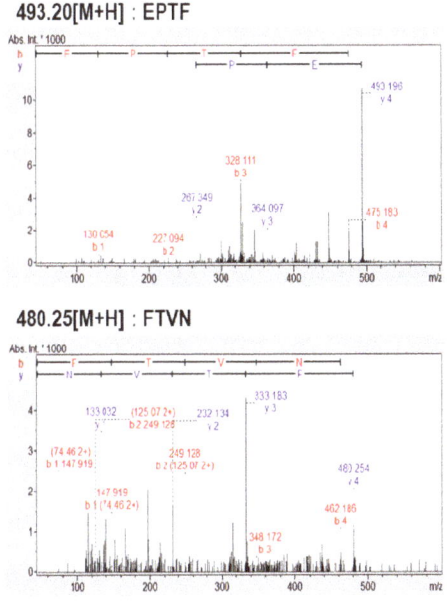

Figure 2. Identification of cytoprotective peptides from α-chymotrypsin-assisted protein hydrolysates of blue mussel by LC-MS/MS.

2.2. Cytoprotective Activity in H_2O_2-Mediated HUVECs Injury

Evaluation of cytoprotective activity was carried out on the identified peptides FTVN and EPTF, as well as their combination in the same proportion, to see if there was any synergy effect between the two peptides. Cell viability was evaluated using the MTT assay after cultured HUVECs were treated with sample peptides and subsequently challenged with 600 μM of H_2O_2, a concentration which was determined to significantly decrease cell viability in a previous report [22]. Compared with untreated cells that were not exposed to peptides or H_2O_2 (control), the addition of H_2O_2 significantly decreased the cell viability of HUVEC by 65.43%. Meanwhile, HUVECs pretreated with 100 μg/mL peptide samples showed remarkably increased cell viability of 85.46%, 83.11%, and 86.58% for FTVN, EPTF, and their combination (1:1), respectively. The results indicate the cytoprotective effect of FTVN, EPTF, and their combination. On the other hand, no significant difference was shown in improving HUVECs cell viability between the peptide samples or the combination of FTVN and EPTF. However, the concentration of the samples had a significant effect on cell viability (Figure 3A). Similar results were found in fluorescence microscopy with Calcein-AM/PI double staining analysis, where H_2O_2 treatment significantly reduced the green fluorescence of live cells, but pretreatment with FTVN, EPTF, and their combination reversed this effect. Moreover, in H_2O_2 treatment, more cells are stained with PI, while the peptides and their combination reduce the cells stained with PI, indicating a cytoprotective effect (Figure 3B).

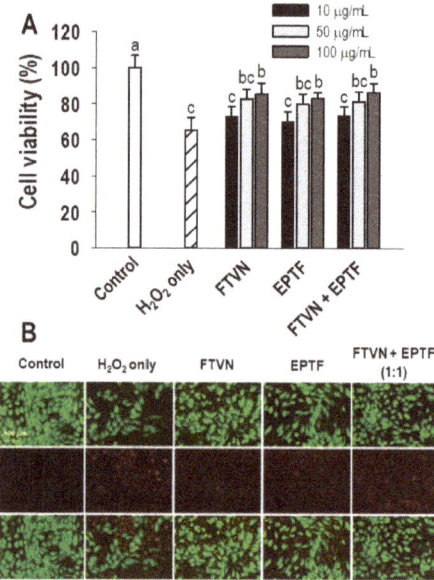

Figure 3. (**A**) The cell viability of HUVECs after BAPs pretreatment at different concentrations. (**B**) Calcein-AM/PI staining assay on EPTF, FTVN, and their combination pretreatment at 0.1 mg/mL. HUVECs were incubated with samples for 2 h before being challenged with 600 μM H_2O_2 for 24 h. The data are provided as means ± SD (n = 4). $^{a–c}$ Different letters show significance difference at $p < 0.05$.

2.3. Inhibition of Intracellular ROS Generation

It is hypothesized that ROS in cells is one of the causes of H_2O_2-induced HUVEC damage. Therefore, we also investigated the presence of ROS in the cells. The DCFH-DA fluorescent probe revealed the amount of intracellular ROS was significantly higher in HUVECs exposed to H_2O_2 alone compared to the control group. This is indicated by the visibility of the DCF fluorescence signal. The DCF fluorescence signal was decreased in HUVECs with pretreatment of FTVN and EPTF or their combination in H_2O_2-induced HUVEC injury (Figure 4A). Quantitatively, ROS generation in the cells significantly increased as a result of H_2O_2 exposure to HUVECs, whereas pretreatment of FTVN, EPTF, and the combination of both significantly reduced the intracellular ROS generation by approximately 40% (Figure 4B).

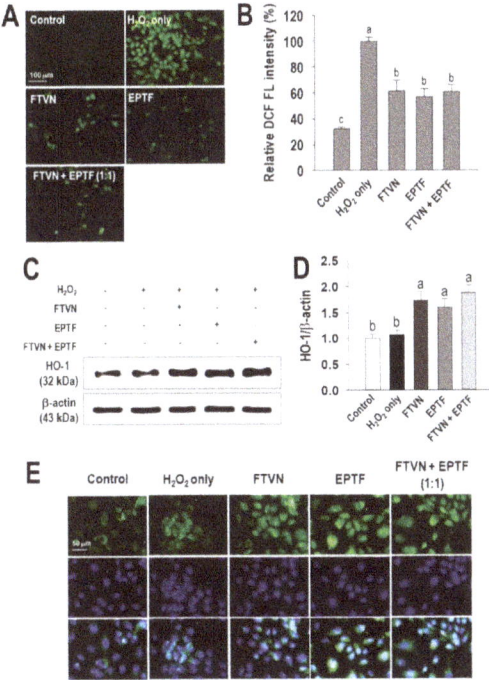

Figure 4. ROS generation in cells and the defense mechanism against it. (A) Visualization and (B) fluorescence intensity quantification on ROS existence. (C) Western blot analysis and (D) HO-1 expression value. (E) Nrf2 nuclear accumulation immunofluorescence stained HUVECs were incubated with 0.1 mg/mL of peptides for 2 h before being challenged with 600 µM H_2O_2 for 24 h (ROS generation and HO-1 analysis) or within 2 h for Nrf2 analysis. The data are provided as means ± SD (n = 4). $^{a-c}$ (ROS generation) and ± SD (n = 3). $^{a-c}$ (HO-1 and Nrf2 analysis). Different letters show significance difference at $p < 0.05$.

2.4. HO-1/Nrf2 Pathway Activation by Cytoprotective Peptides

HO-1 is one of the phase II detoxifying enzymes. In a ROS detoxifying mechanism, this enzyme must be induced by activation of a transcription factor such as Nrf2. This event is regarded as one of the most important cellular defense mechanisms [23]. As shown in Figure 4C,D, HO-1 expression slightly increased in the presence of H_2O_2 treatment alone, indicating spontaneous reaction for cytoprotection, and this finding is similar to a previous report [1]. However, the amount of HO-1 induction in the presence of H_2O_2 treatment alone is not enough to protect HUVECs, but we demonstrated that peptide treatment can increase the induction of HO-1, indicating the cytoprotective effect against exogenous stimuli. The induction of HO-1 is further confirmed by evidence of the translocation of Nrf2 into the nucleus, which regulates the expression of HO-1. As shown in Figure 4E, Nrf2 was detectable in the cytoplasm in the non-treated and H_2O_2 treated cells, whereas Nrf2 was slightly detectable in the nucleus in the H_2O_2 treated cells. Compared with the cells treated with H_2O_2 alone, treatment with FTVN and EPTF or their combination resulted in upregulation of Nrf2 expression in both the cytoplasm and nucleus of HUVECs, indicating activation of Nrf2 followed by induction of HO-1.

2.5. Anti-Apoptotic Activity against H_2O_2-Induced HUVECs Damage

A high dose exposure of powerful oxidants such H_2O_2 causes severe damage to macromolecules, which leads to cell death through apoptosis and/or necrosis mechanisms [24]. The cytoprotective activity of EPTF, FTVN, as well as their combination was evaluated by measuring the anti-apoptotic activity. Annexin V-FITC/PI and Hoechst 33342 staining was performed after the peptide treatments.

The results revealed that 94.1% of HUVECs were located in the lower left quadrant in the non-treated cells (control), which decreased to 60.8% in the H_2O_2 group. There was a high percentage of necrotic cell (28.5%) compared to apoptotic cell (10.72%) in the presence of H_2O_2 treatment alone. Pretreatment of HUVECs with EPTF, FTVN, and their combination significantly reduced the total percentage of dead cells compared to the H_2O_2 treatment group (Figure 5A). This indicates that our model treatment leads to apoptosis first, followed by necrosis. However, peptide treatment decreased predominantly the necrosis rate (Figure 5B). Figure 6 confirmed that peptide treatment modulated the protein expression related to apoptosis, indicating that cell survival by peptide treatment is attributed to downregulation of apoptotic protein expression.

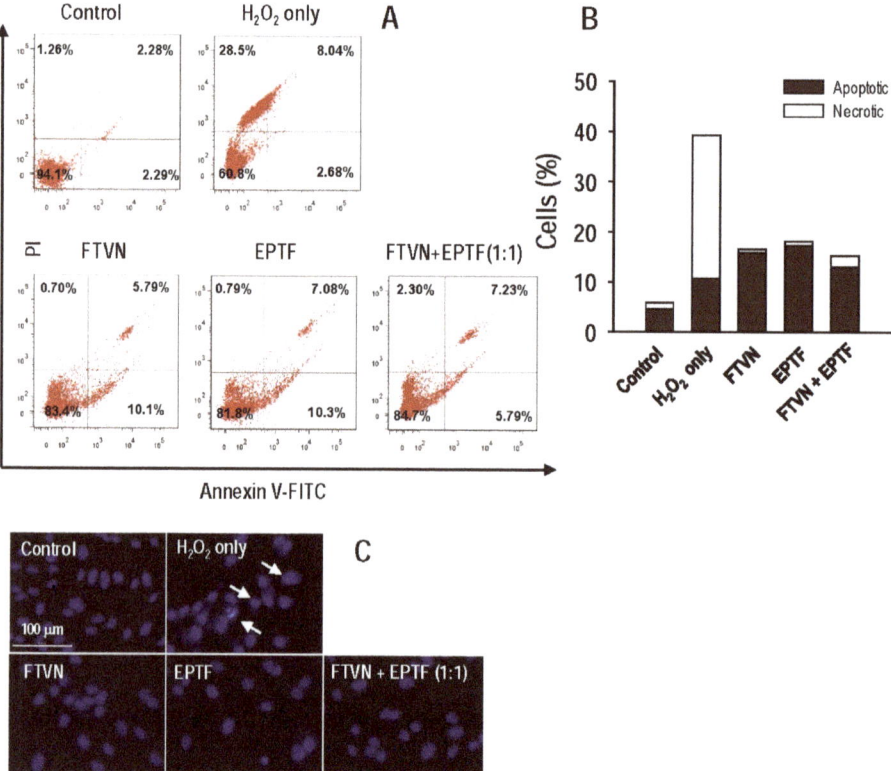

Figure 5. The effect of EPTF, FTVN, and combination in inhibiting HUVEC apoptosis. (**A**) Quadrant dot analysis showing live–dead cells, and (**B**) apoptotic and necrotic ratio using flow cytometer analysis using Annexin V-FITC/PI staining assay. (**C**) Morphological changes under fluorescence microscope with Hoechst 33342 staining assay (white arrows showed apoptosis occurrence). HUVECs were pretreated with 0.1 mg/mL of peptides for 2 h before being challenged with 600 μM H_2O_2 for 24 h. All treatment was carried out in triplicate.

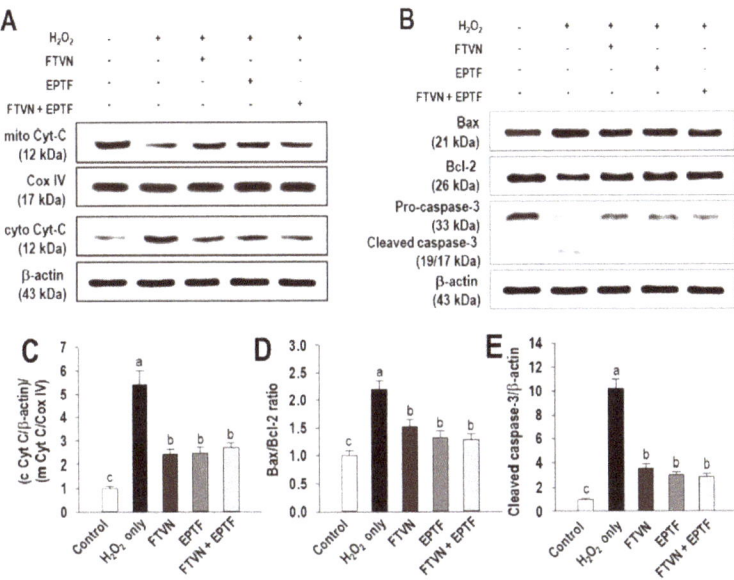

Figure 6. Western blot analysis of (**A**) released mitochondrial cytochrome C (Cyt-C) found in cytosol, and (**B**) Bax, Bcl-2, and activated caspase-3 (procaspase-3/cleaved caspase-3) expression. As protein loading control, Cox IV and β-actin were used. Expression level of (**C**) released Cyt C within mitochondria and cytoplasm, (**D**) ratio of Bax/Bcl-2 expression, and (**E**) cleaved caspase-3/β-actin for caspase-3 activation. HUVECs were incubated with 0.1 mg/mL of peptides for 2 h before being challenged with 600 µM H_2O_2 for 24 h. All treatment was carried out in triplicate. The data are provided as means ± SD (n = 3). Different letters show significance difference at $p < 0.05$.

Observation of nuclear morphology with a fluorescence microscope shows that H_2O_2 treatment leads to morphological changes, especially nuclear shrinkage, segregation, and chromatin condensation (Figure 5C). HUVECs in the peptides-pretreated group were comparable to those in the non-treated cells (control), suggesting that EPTF, FTVN, and their combination protect the HUVECs from apoptotic cell death.

It is known that disruption of mitochondrial membrane integrity by H_2O_2 insult leads to the release of cytochrome C (Cyt C), which in turn causes apoptosis in cells [25]. Western blot analysis was performed to investigate the effect of EPTF, FTVN, and their combination on the released of Cyt C into the cytoplasm. As shown in Figure 6A, mitochondrial Cyt C was strongly detected in the non-treated cells, while cytosolic Cyt C was weakly detected. On the other hand, H_2O_2 treatment resulted in cytoplasmic release of Cyt C from mitochondria into the cytoplasm, and Cyt C was strongly detected in the cytoplasm, indicating activation of apoptosis mediated by the intrinsic pathway. However, the release of the Cyt C from mitochondria in the cytoplasm by H_2O_2 treatment was significantly reduced after pretreatment with EPTF, FTVN, and their combination (Figure 6A,C), indicating suppression of the intrinsic pathway by H_2O_2 exposure.

The expression ratio of Bcl-2 and Bax plays a crucial role in the apoptosis process by regulating mitochondrial membrane permeability, which is associated with the disruption of mitochondrial membrane integrity [26]. In this study, H_2O_2 exposure resulted in an increase in Bax expression but a decrease in Bcl-2 expression (Figure 6B). In the cells pretreated with EPTF, FTVN, and their combination, the Bax and Bcl-2 expression was reversed and the Bax/Bcl-2 ratio was also significantly reduced compared to the cells with H_2O_2 treatment (Figure 6B,D). Finally, this study examined the activation of caspase-3, which is known to be the execution caspase in apoptosis. High expression of procaspase-3 was detected in the untreated cells, whereas the cleaved caspase-3, the active form of caspase-3, was negligible (Figure 6B,E). On the other hand, procaspase-3 was converted to cleaved caspase-3 in the presence of H_2O_2 treatment, but this process was abolished by pretreatment with EPTF, FTVN, and their combination, suggesting that the anti-apoptotic effect of the peptides came from suppression of the caspase-3 pathway.

3. Discussion

Recent studies have shown that BAPs derived from marine dietary proteins by enzymatic hydrolysis have versatile health benefits, as they have antioxidant, antihypertensive, and antidiabetic effects. To date, many BAPs have been isolated and identified from marine dietary protein hydrolysates [27]. In addition, previous studies have identified specific BAPs in blue mussel protein hydrolysates that have been attributed antioxidant, antithrombotic, antihypertensive, osteogenic, and anti-osteoporotic effects [19,20,28–31]. Blue mussel protein hydrolysate produced by α-chymotrypsin has been previously identified as a potential cytoprotective agent [1]. However, there is limited information on specific BAPs with cytoprotective effects of blue mussel protein hydrolysates in alleviating HUVEC damage caused by oxidative stress. In this study, two cytoprotective peptides were isolated and identified as EPTF and FTVN, and their molecular mechanism underlying the cytoprotective activity was investigated.

The idea of using antioxidants with cryoprotective affects to treat CVD is based on the evidence that the excess amount of ROS generates oxidative stress, which then leads to endothelial cell damage and induces apoptosis [31]. Endothelial dysfunction (ED) a physiological condition that occurs in the early development of atherosclerosis, is often characterized by cell death, including the mechanism of apoptosis [32]. H_2O_2 is one of the most understood ROS, serving as a second messenger in a variety of critical cellular signaling pathways, but when it presents in high concentrations it has toxic consequences that can lead to cellular dysfunction or even cell death. Therefore, to evaluate the cytoprotective effects of EPTF and FTVN, an H_2O_2-mediated HUVEC injury model was used. Since these two peptides were identified in the same fraction (H4), we investigated the cytoprotective effect of each peptide as well as their combination (synergic effect). It was found that pretreatment with EPTF, FTVN and both combinations reversed the cell death induced by H_2O_2 treatment. Moreover, increased ROS generation by H_2O_2 treatment was remarkably quenched by pretreatment of EPTF, FTVN, and their combination. There was no significant difference in the cytoprotective effect between the peptides and their combination. Each peptide had a potent cytoprotective effect on its own. This indicates that the contribution of each peptide to cytoprotective is similar.

To uncover the mechanism underlying the cytoprotective activity, the effect of EPTF, FTVN, and their combination in the cellular antioxidant defense system was investigated. Nuclear factor erythroid 2-related factor 2 (Nrf2) is a regulator of species lifespan that regulates the expression of genes coding for detoxifying proteins, antioxidants, and anti-inflammatories [33]. In this study, H_2O_2 plays a role as an exogenous stimulus that induces the oxidative damage and triggers the activation of Nrf2. In this condition, the Nrf2-Keap1-Cullin3 complex was disrupted, which then allowed the translocation of Nrf2 from cytoplasm to nucleus [34]. From Figure 4E, we can see that Nrf2 was accumulated in nucleus as an indication of cytoprotective activity. One of the genes regulated through Nrf2 is HO-1, which is recognized as a cytoprotective enzyme through catalyzing heme protein into ferritin, biliverdin, and carbon monoxide [35]. In our study, H_2O_2 stimulated the production of HO-1 but only with insignificant concentration; this result is similar to another study using H_2O_2 as the stress model [36,37]. This might be due to the very high concentrations of exogenous stimuli that exceed the cell capacity to perform cytoprotective mechanisms, which also results in cellular damage. To eliminate damaged cells, the apoptosis process occurs. We demonstrated that pretreatment of EPTF, FTVN, and their combination upregulated HO-1 expression through Nrf2 activation in H_2O_2-mediated HUVEC injury.

Induction of HO-1 by peptide treatment may have influenced cell survival and the decrease in intracellular ROS generation. Mitochondria is a natural source of cellular ROS; their membranes contain certain key compounds involved in antioxidant responses and in stimulating apoptotic pathways [38]. When oxidative stress surpasses a cell's ability to balance it, mitochondrial dysfunction occurs, which then leads mitochondria to generate more ROS. Furthermore, oxidative stress promotes nuclear damage and triggers the cascade of apoptotic cell death. Apoptosis is a programmed cell death that is governed by two major pathways including the intrinsic mitochondria pathway and the extrinsic death receptor pathway [39]. Since H_2O_2 is known to induce apoptosis through the intrinsic mitochondria pathway, in this study the role of EPTF, FTVN, and their combination was investigated in the intrinsic mitochondria pathway [40]. A key event of this pathway is mitochondria Cyt C released into the cytoplasm through the relative ratio of Bax and Bcl-2 proteins expression, i.e., a high Bax/Bcl-2 ratio increased cell death probability through an intrinsic mitochondria pathway-mediated apoptosis [41]. The released Cyt C then binds to apoptotic protease-activating factor-1 and forms an apoptosome with procaspase-9. This activates caspase-3, an important trigger of apoptosis. In this study, H_2O_2 exposure increased Bax expression while decreasing Bcl-2 expression in HUVEC and showed a high ratio of Bax/Bcl-2, indicating the increase of mitochondrial membrane permeability. However, its value was decreased in HUVEC that received pretreatment with EPTF, FTVN, and their combination. In addition, our data clearly showed H_2O_2-mediated mitochondria dysfunction, which is proved by the accumulation of Cyt C in the cytoplasm, while pretreatment of EPTF, FTVN, and their combination inhibited this event in the cytoplasm.

Finally, H_2O_2-mediated activation of caspase-3 in HUVEC was inhibited by cascade activation via alteration of the Bax-Bcl-2 ratio and release of Cyt C by pretreatment of EPTF, FTVN, and their combination. This suggests that the intrinsic mitochondrial pathway is involved in the cytoprotective effect induced by EPTF, FTVN and their combination in H_2O_2-mediated HUVEC damage.

Similar results of BAPs from various food proteins, including edible seahorse, rice bran, and *Mytilus coruscus*, have been reported in H_2O_2-mediated HUVEC injury where these BAPs showed the cytoprotective effect through modulation of the intrinsic mitochondria pathway [24,42,43]. These findings suggest that BAPs may be useful for ameliorating oxidative stress-mediated ED and may be helpful for treating CVD.

4. Material and Methods

4.1. Materials

Blue mussel (*Mytilus edulis*) was purchased from Yeosu Fisheries Co. (Yeosu, Korea). Calcein AM solution, propidium iodide (PI), 2′7′-dichlorofluorescein diacetate (DCFH-DA), H_2O_2, Hoechst 33342, and 3-(4,5-dimethylthiazol-2-yl)-2,5-diphenyltetrazolium bromide (MTT) were purchased from Sigma-Aldrich Chemical Co. (St. Louis, MO, USA). Trypsin-EDTA solution and PBS were purchased from Hyclone (Logan, UT, USA). The HUVEC (PCS-100-010™) are produced by the American Type Culture Collection (Rockville, MD, USA). Endothelial Growth Medium-2 Bullet Kit (EGM™-2) was produced by Lonza, (Walkersville, MD, USA).

4.2. Blue Mussel Protein Hydrolysate by α-Chymotrypsin-Assisted Hydrolysis

Blue mussel was rinsed and lyophilized before being hydrolyzed by α-chymotrypsin (pH 8.0 and 37 °C), with 1:100 (enzyme to substrate ratio) and 8 h incubation [1]. Enzyme activity was stopped by 10 min boiling in 100 °C. The supernatants were collected by centrifugation (5000 rpm for 20 min, Labogene 1248R, Seoul, Korea), lyophilized and kept at −20 °C before use.

4.3. Purification and Identification of Cytoprotective Peptides

Blue mussel hydrolysates were eluted at 1.0 mL/min rate over Sephadex G-25 column (3.0 × 90 cm), then every 5 min the eluate was collected. Fractions with cytoprotective activity were separated using HPLC equipped with C_{18} column at 2.0 mL/min flow rate (Hypersil Gold, 250 × 10 mm, 5 µm, Thermo Scientific, Pittsburgh, PA, USA). A linear gradient elution was carried out using acetonitrile, as mentioned in a previous publication [24]. Q-TOF LC-MS/MS coupled with an ESI source (maXis-HD™, Bruker Daltonics, Bremen, Germany) was used to perform peptide identification, and subsequently MS/MS spectrometry was used in peptide sequencing (Biotools 3.2, Bruker Daltonics, Bremen, Germany) [18]. The synthesized peptides were ordered from Biostem (Ansan, Korea). HPLC-MS/MS was used to check the purity of the synthesized peptides (over 96% purity).

4.4. HUVECs Culture and Treatment

HUVECs were cultured in 37 °C and 5% CO_2 incubation, using EGM™-2 Medium Kit. The cells were subcultured and harvested using a 0.025% trypsin-EDTA solution. For experimental design, only HUVECs at passages 3–5 were used. They were then seeded in a 96- or 24-well plate, or 60 mm² dishes. Sample peptides were added for the pretreated group following 2 h incubation before being challenged with 600 µM H_2O_2 for 24 h. The control group was cells without peptides treatment and H_2O_2 exposure.

4.5. Cell Viability Assessment

Cytoprotective effect was evaluated by monitoring cell viability using MTT assay to HUVECs in a 96-well plate with 1×10^4 cells/well density. For further confirmation of the cytoprotective effect, live and dead cell assay was also performed. HUVECs were rinsed with warmed PBS in a 24-well plate with 2×10^4 cells/well, and then double stained using calcein-AM and PI 2.5 µM and 5 µM, respectively, following 30 min incubation at 37 °C. Stained cells were distinguished as live and dead cells under a fluorescence microscope (Leica DMI6000 B, Wetzlar, Germany).

4.6. Determination of Intracellular ROS

ROS generation in cells was detected in a 96-well black plate for quantification and a 24-well plate for microscopic observation. Pretreated cells were mixed with Hank's Balanced Salt Solution contained 20 µM DCFH-DA followed by 20 min incubation (37 °C). Fluorescence intensity was measured to determined intracellular ROS level at 485 and 528 nm (excitation and emission) (GENios, TECAN, Männedorf, Switzerland) and visually observed under fluorescence microscope (Leica DMI6000 B, Wetzlar, Germany).

4.7. Nrf2 Nuclear Translocation Assessment

To observe Nrf2 nuclear translocation, HUVECs culture was mixed with 3.7% paraformaldehyde in PBS for 15 min, and then permeabilized using 0.1% Triton X-100 dissolve with PBS (10 min), before being blocked in 2% bovine serum albumin with 30 min incubation. Later, anti-Nrf2 antibody with 1:200 dilution was added. After overnight incubation at 4 °C, the secondary antibody (Alexa Fluor® 488, Santa Cruz Biotechnology, Santa Cruz, CA, USA) was added (1:500 dilution with 1h incubation). To counterstain the nuclei, 2 µg/mL Hoechst 33342 was added following 10 min incubation. Visual observation was performed under fluorescence microscope (Leica DMI6000 B, Wetzlar, Germany).

4.8. Annexin V-FITC/PI for Apoptotic Cells

Treated cells were washed three times using PBS, harvested, and then resuspended with Annexin V-FITC and PI in binding buffer solution followed by 15 min incubation at room temperature. Apoptotic cells were then analyzed by a flow cytometry (FACSCalibur system, BD Biosciences, San Jose, CA, USA) using an Apoptosis Detection Kit (BD Pharmingen™, San Jose, CA, USA).

4.9. Hoechst 33342 Staining Analysis

Treated cells were then washed, harvested, and then fixated using ethanol. After incubation for 20 min, 10 µM Hoechst 33342 staining was added following another 20 min incubation in room temperature. Observation was perform using a fluorescence microscope (Leica DMI6000 B, Wetzlar, Germany).

4.10. Western Blot Analysis

Total proteins were extracted with a RIPA buffer (Sigma Chemical Co., St. Louis, MO, USA). The mitochondria and cytosol fractions were isolated using a Mitochondria Isolation Kit (Abcam, Cambridge, MA, USA) following the manufacturer's procedure. Western blotting was conducted as describe in our previous report [24]. Briefly, 25 µg of total extracted proteins were separated via 10–12% SDS-PAGE prior to nitrocellulose membranes transfer by electroblotting, which was then blocked with 5% skimmed milk for 1 h. Blots were then incubated with specific antibodies HO-1 (1:200), Bax (1:200), Bcl-2 (1:200), cytochrom C (1:200), β-actin (1:500), and Cox IV (1:500) (Santa Cruz Biotechnology, Santa Cruz, CA, USA) and caspase-3 (1:500) (Cell Signaling Technology, Beverly, MA, USA) overnight at 4 °C;. The horseradish peroxidase-conjugated antibodies were regarded as the secondary antibody. The bands were detected by chemiluminescence using the ECL Western blotting assay kit (Life Technologies, Seoul, Korea) and visualized by Davinch-Chemi Imager™ (CAS-400SM, Core Bio, Seoul, Korea).

4.11. Data Analysis

SigmaPlot® 12.0 (Systat Software Inc., San Jose, CA, USA) software was used to perform statistical analysis of the data. All experiments are expressed as mean ± standard deviation (SD). Student's *t*-test was performed, and statistical significance was assigned in accordance with $p < 0.05$.

5. Conclusions

The findings of this study demonstrated the cytoprotective activity of the BAPs identified as FTVN and EPTF from blue mussel protein and their role in preventing oxidative stress-mediated endothelial dysfunction (ED). Investigations of the cytoprotective mechanism of these two peptides and their combination in H_2O_2-mediated HUVEC injury revealed that BAPs alleviated HUVEC injury through enhancement of the antioxidant defense system and anti-necrotic action. As a result, BAPs derived from blue mussel protein might be an alternative approach in preventing CVD through protecting cardiovascular vein endothelial cells. Furthermore, to develop a nutraceutical or pharmaceutical component based on this result, more in vivo research is required.

Author Contributions: I.T.S. and C.-B.A. methodology, writing, conceptualization, data investigation and analysis. J.-Y.J. editing, supervising, designing, and directing the project: funding acquisition. All authors have read and agreed to the published version of the manuscript.

Funding: This study was supported by the Basic Science Research Program through the National Research Foundation of Korea (NRF) funded by the Ministry of Education (NRF-2021R1I1A3047702).

Data Availability Statement: The original contribution presented in this study are included in the article, further inquiries can be directed to the corresponding author.

Conflicts of Interest: The authors declare that there are no conflict of interest.

References

1. Oh, Y.; Ahn, C.-B.; Nam, K.-H.; Kim, Y.-K.; Yoon, N.Y.; Je, J.-Y. Amino acid composition, antioxidant, and cytoprotective effect of blue mussel (Mytilus edulis) hydrolysate through the inhibition of caspase-3 activation in oxidative stress-mediated endothelial cell injury. *Mar. Drugs* **2019**, *17*, 135. [CrossRef] [PubMed]
2. Wang, J.; Toan, S.; Zhou, H. New insights into the role of mitochondria in cardiac microvascular ischemia/reperfusion injury. *Angiogenesis* **2020**, *23*, 299–314. [CrossRef] [PubMed]

3. Paone, S.; Baxter, A.A.; Hulett, M.D.; Poon, I.K. Endothelial cell apoptosis and the role of endothelial cell-derived extracellular vesicles in the progression of atherosclerosis. *Cell. Mol. Life Sci.* **2019**, *76*, 1093–1106. [CrossRef]
4. Oh, Y.S.; Jun, H.-S. Effects of glucagon-like peptide-1 on oxidative stress and Nrf2 signaling. *Int. J. Mol. Sci.* **2018**, *19*, 26. [CrossRef]
5. Xu, F.; Zhang, J.; Wang, Z.; Yao, Y.; Atungulu, G.G.; Ju, X.; Wang, L. Absorption and metabolism of peptide WDHHAPQLR derived from rapeseed protein and inhibition of HUVEC apoptosis under oxidative stress. *J. Agric. Food Chem.* **2018**, *66*, 5178–5189. [CrossRef] [PubMed]
6. Togliatto, G.; Lombardo, G.; Brizzi, M.F. The future challenge of reactive oxygen species (ROS) in hypertension: From bench to bed side. *Int. J. Mol. Sci.* **2017**, *18*, 1988. [CrossRef] [PubMed]
7. Wang, K.; Dong, Y.; Liu, J.; Qian, L.; Wang, T.; Gao, X.; Wang, K.; Zhou, L. Effects of REDOX in regulating and treatment of metabolic and inflammatory cardiovascular diseases. *Oxidative Med. Cell. Longev.* **2020**, *2020*, 5860356. [CrossRef]
8. Jin, J.-E.; Ahn, C.-B.; Je, J.-Y. Purification and characterization of antioxidant peptides from enzymatically hydrolyzed ark shell (Scapharca subcrenata). *Process Biochem.* **2018**, *72*, 170–176. [CrossRef]
9. Hyung, J.-H.; Ahn, C.-B.; Kim, B.I.; Kim, K.; Je, J.-Y. Involvement of Nrf2-mediated heme oxygenase-1 expression in anti-inflammatory action of chitosan oligosaccharides through MAPK activation in murine macrophages. *Eur. J. Pharmacol.* **2016**, *793*, 43–48. [CrossRef] [PubMed]
10. Kim, Y.-S.; Ahn, C.-B.; Je, J.-Y. Anti-inflammatory action of high molecular weight Mytilus edulis hydrolysates fraction in LPS-induced RAW264. 7 macrophage via NF-κB and MAPK pathways. *Food Chem.* **2016**, *202*, 9–14. [CrossRef]
11. Je, J.-Y.; Park, S.Y.; Hwang, J.-Y.; Ahn, C.-B. Amino acid composition and in vitro antioxidant and cytoprotective activity of abalone viscera hydrolysate. *J. Funct. Foods* **2015**, *16*, 94–103. [CrossRef]
12. Ahn, C.-B.; Cho, Y.-S.; Je, J.-Y. Purification and anti-inflammatory action of tripeptide from salmon pectoral fin byproduct protein hydrolysate. *Food Chem.* **2015**, *168*, 151–156. [CrossRef] [PubMed]
13. Oh, Y.; Shim, K.-B.; Ahn, C.-B.; Kim, S.S.; Je, J.-Y. Sea squirt (Halocynthia roretzi) hydrolysates induce apoptosis in human colon cancer HT-29 cells through activation of reactive oxygen species. *Nutr. Cancer* **2019**, *71*, 118–127. [CrossRef]
14. Je, J.-Y.; Qian, Z.-J.; Lee, S.-H.; Byun, H.-G.; Kim, S.-K. Purification and antioxidant properties of bigeye tuna (Thunnus obesus) dark muscle peptide on free radical-mediated oxidative systems. *J. Med. Food* **2008**, *11*, 629–637. [CrossRef] [PubMed]
15. Fernando, I.P.S.; Park, S.Y.; Han, E.J.; Kim, H.-S.; Kang, D.-S.; Je, J.-Y.; Ahn, C.-B.; Ahn, G. Isolation of an antioxidant peptide from krill protein hydrolysates as a novel agent with potential hepatoprotective effects. *J. Funct. Foods* **2020**, *67*, 103889. [CrossRef]
16. Kim, S.S.; Ahn, C.-B.; Moon, S.W.; Je, J.-Y. Purification and antioxidant activities of peptides from sea squirt (Halocynthia roretzi) protein hydrolysates using pepsin hydrolysis. *Food Biosci.* **2018**, *25*, 128–133. [CrossRef]
17. Park, S.Y.; Ahn, C.B.; Je, J.Y. Antioxidant and anti-inflammatory activities of protein hydrolysates from Mytilus edulis and ultrafiltration membrane fractions. *J. Food Biochem.* **2014**, *38*, 460–468. [CrossRef]
18. Oh, Y.; Ahn, C.-B.; Je, J.-Y. Low molecular weight blue mussel hydrolysates inhibit adipogenesis in mouse mesenchymal stem cells through upregulating HO-1/Nrf2 pathway. *Food Res. Int.* **2020**, *136*, 109603. [CrossRef]
19. Park, S.Y.; Kim, Y.-S.; Ahn, C.-B.; Je, J.-Y. Partial purification and identification of three antioxidant peptides with hepatoprotective effects from blue mussel (Mytilus edulis) hydrolysate by peptic hydrolysis. *J. Funct. Foods* **2016**, *20*, 88–95. [CrossRef]
20. Je, J.-Y.; Park, P.-J.; Byun, H.-G.; Jung, W.-K.; Kim, S.-K. Angiotensin I converting enzyme (ACE) inhibitory peptide derived from the sauce of fermented blue mussel, Mytilus edulis. *Bioresour. Technol.* **2005**, *96*, 1624–1629. [CrossRef] [PubMed]
21. Magtaan, J.K.; Fitzpatrick, B.; Murphy, R. Elucidating the Biological Activity of Fish-Derived Collagen and Gelatine Hydrolysates using Animal Cell Culture-A Review. *Curr. Pharm. Des.* **2021**, *27*, 1365–1381. [CrossRef] [PubMed]
22. Oh, Y.; Ahn, C.-B.; Yoon, N.Y.; Nam, K.H.; Kim, Y.-K.; Je, J.-Y. Protective effect of enzymatic hydrolysates from seahorse (Hippocampus abdominalis) against H_2O_2-mediated human umbilical vein endothelial cell injury. *Biomed. Pharmacother.* **2018**, *108*, 103–110. [CrossRef] [PubMed]
23. Keum, Y.-S. Regulation of Nrf2-mediated phase II detoxification and anti-oxidant genes. *Biomol. Ther.* **2012**, *20*, 144. [CrossRef] [PubMed]
24. Oh, Y.; Ahn, C.-B.; Je, J.-Y. Cytoprotective Role of Edible Seahorse (Hippocampus abdominalis)-Derived Peptides in H_2O_2-Induced Oxidative Stress in Human Umbilical Vein Endothelial Cells. *Mar. Drugs* **2021**, *19*, 86. [CrossRef]
25. Garrido, C.; Galluzzi, L.; Brunet, M.; Puig, P.; Didelot, C.; Kroemer, G. Mechanisms of cytochrome c release from mitochondria. *Cell Death Differ.* **2006**, *13*, 1423–1433. [CrossRef] [PubMed]
26. Chen, Q.; Liu, X.-F.; Zheng, P.-S. Grape seed proanthocyanidins (GSPs) inhibit the growth of cervical cancer by inducing apoptosis mediated by the mitochondrial pathway. *PLoS ONE* **2014**, *9*, e107045. [CrossRef]
27. Admassu, H.; Gasmalla, M.A.A.; Yang, R.; Zhao, W. Bioactive peptides derived from seaweed protein and their health benefits: Antihypertensive, antioxidant, and antidiabetic properties. *J. Food Sci.* **2018**, *83*, 6–16. [CrossRef] [PubMed]
28. Qiao, M.; Tu, M.; Wang, Z.; Mao, F.; Chen, H.; Qin, L.; Du, M. Identification and antithrombotic activity of peptides from blue mussel (Mytilus edulis) protein. *Int. J. Mol. Sci.* **2018**, *19*, 138. [CrossRef] [PubMed]
29. Oh, Y.; Ahn, C.-B.; Je, J.-Y. Blue Mussel-Derived Peptides PIISVYWK and FSVVPSPK Trigger Wnt/β-Catenin Signaling-Mediated Osteogenesis in Human Bone Marrow Mesenchymal Stem Cells. *Mar. Drugs* **2020**, *18*, 510. [CrossRef] [PubMed]
30. Oh, Y.; Ahn, C.-B.; Cho, W.H.; Yoon, N.Y.; Je, J.-Y. Anti-Osteoporotic Effects of Antioxidant Peptides PIISVYWK and FSVVPSPK from Mytilus edulis on Ovariectomized Mice. *Antioxidants* **2020**, *9*, 866. [CrossRef] [PubMed]

31. Wang, B.; Li, L.; Chi, C.-F.; Ma, J.-H.; Luo, H.-Y.; Xu, Y.-f. Purification and characterisation of a novel antioxidant peptide derived from blue mussel (Mytilus edulis) protein hydrolysate. *Food Chem.* **2013**, *138*, 1713–1719. [CrossRef]
32. Shah, D.; Das, P.; Alam, M.A.; Mahajan, N.; Romero, F.; Shahid, M.; Singh, H.; Bhandari, V. MicroRNA-34a promotes endothelial dysfunction and mitochondrial-mediated apoptosis in murine models of acute lung injury. *Am. J. Respir. Cell Mol. Biol.* **2019**, *60*, 465–477. [CrossRef]
33. Loboda, A.; Damulewicz, M.; Pyza, E.; Jozkowicz, A.; Dulak, J. Role of Nrf2/HO-1 system in development, oxidative stress response and diseases: An evolutionarily conserved mechanism. *Cell. Mol. Life Sci.* **2016**, *73*, 3221–3247. [CrossRef] [PubMed]
34. da Costa, R.M.; Rodrigues, D.; Pereira, C.A.; Silva, J.F.; Alves, J.V.; Lobato, N.S.; Tostes, R.C. Nrf2 as a potential mediator of cardiovascular risk in metabolic diseases. *Front. Pharmacol.* **2019**, *10*, 382. [CrossRef]
35. Ryter, S.W.; Choi, A.M. Targeting heme oxygenase-1 and carbon monoxide for therapeutic modulation of inflammation. *Transl. Res.* **2016**, *167*, 7–34. [CrossRef] [PubMed]
36. Choi, Y.H. Activation of the Nrf2/HO-1 signaling pathway contributes to the protective effects of coptisine against oxidative stress-induced DNA damage and apoptosis in HaCaT keratinocytes. *Gen. Physiol. Biophys.* **2019**, *38*, 281–294. [CrossRef] [PubMed]
37. Yuan, J.; Lu, Y.; Wang, H.; Feng, Y.; Jiang, S.; Gao, X.-H.; Qi, R.; Wu, Y.; Chen, H.-D. Paeoniflorin resists H_2O_2-induced oxidative stress in melanocytes by JNK/Nrf2/HO-1 pathway. *Front. Pharmacol.* **2020**, *11*, 536. [CrossRef] [PubMed]
38. Calabrese, G.; Peker, E.; Amponsah, P.S.; Hoehne, M.N.; Riemer, T.; Mai, M.; Bienert, G.P.; Deponte, M.; Morgan, B.; Riemer, J. Hyperoxidation of mitochondrial peroxiredoxin limits H_2O_2-induced cell death in yeast. *Embo J.* **2019**, *38*, e101552. [CrossRef] [PubMed]
39. Yaoxian, W.; Hui, Y.; Yunyan, Z.; Yanqin, L.; Xin, G.; Xiaoke, W. Emodin induces apoptosis of human cervical cancer hela cells via intrinsic mitochondrial and extrinsic death receptor pathway. *Cancer Cell Int.* **2013**, *13*, 71. [CrossRef] [PubMed]
40. Di Marzo, N.; Chisci, E.; Giovannoni, R. The role of hydrogen peroxide in redox-dependent signaling: Homeostatic and pathological responses in mammalian cells. *Cells* **2018**, *7*, 156. [CrossRef] [PubMed]
41. Redza-Dutordoir, M.; Averill-Bates, D.A. Activation of apoptosis signalling pathways by reactive oxygen species. *Biochim. Biophys. Acta (Bba)-Mol. Cell Res.* **2016**, *1863*, 2977–2992. [CrossRef] [PubMed]
42. Liang, Y.; Lin, Q.; Huang, P.; Wang, Y.; Li, J.; Zhang, L.; Cao, J. Rice bioactive peptide binding with TLR4 to overcome H_2O_2-induced injury in human umbilical vein endothelial cells through NF-κB signaling. *J. Agric. Food Chem.* **2018**, *66*, 440–448. [CrossRef] [PubMed]
43. Zhang, Z.; Jiang, S.; Zeng, Y.; He, K.; Luo, Y.; Yu, F. Antioxidant peptides from Mytilus Coruscus on H_2O_2-induced human umbilical vein endothelial cell stress. *Food Biosci.* **2020**, *38*, 100762. [CrossRef]

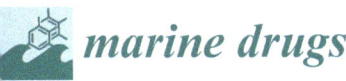

Article

C-phycoerythrin from *Phormidium persicinum* Prevents Acute Kidney Injury by Attenuating Oxidative and Endoplasmic Reticulum Stress

Vanessa Blas-Valdivia [1,†], Plácido Rojas-Franco [2,†], Jose Ivan Serrano-Contreras [3], Andrea Augusto Sfriso [4], Cristian Garcia-Hernandez [1,2], Margarita Franco-Colín [2,*] and Edgar Cano-Europa [2,*]

[1] Laboratorio de Neurobiología, Departamento de Fisiología, Escuela Nacional de Ciencias Biológicas, Instituto Politécnico Nacional, Ciudad de México 07738, Mexico; vblasv@ipn.mx (V.B.-V.); cgarciah1702@alumno.ipn.mx (C.G.-H.)

[2] Laboratorio de Metabolismo I, Departamento de Fisiología, Escuela Nacional de Ciencias Biológicas, Instituto Politécnico Nacional, Ciudad de México 07738, Mexico; projasf@ipn.mx

[3] Department of Metabolism, Digestion and Reproduction, Division of Systems Medicine, Section of Biomolecular Medicine, Faculty of Medicine, Imperial College London, South Kensington Campus, London SW7 2AZ, UK; j.serrano-contreras@imperial.ac.uk

[4] Department of Chemical and Pharmaceutical Sciences, University of Ferrara, 44121 Ferrara, Italy; sfrndr@unife.it

* Correspondence: mfrancoc@ipn.mx (M.F.-C.); ecanoe@ipn.mx (E.C.-E.); Tel./Fax: +52-55-57-29-60-00 (ext. 52351) (M.F.-C. & E.C.-E.)

† These authors contributed equally to this work.

Abstract: C-phycoerythrin (C-PE) is a phycobiliprotein that prevents oxidative stress and cell damage. The aim of this study was to evaluate whether C-PE also counteracts endoplasmic reticulum (ER) stress as a mechanism contributing to its nephroprotective activity. After C-PE was purified from *Phormidium persicinum* by using size exclusion chromatography, it was characterized by spectrometry and fluorimetry. A mouse model of $HgCl_2$-induced acute kidney injury (AKI) was used to assess the effect of C-PE treatment (at 25, 50, or 100 mg/kg of body weight) on oxidative stress, the redox environment, and renal damage. ER stress was examined with the same model and C-PE treatment at 100 mg/kg. C-PE diminished oxidative stress and cell damage in a dose-dependent manner by impeding the decrease in expression of nephrin and podocin normally caused by mercury intoxication. It reduced ER stress by preventing the activation of the inositol-requiring enzyme-1α (IRE1α) pathway and avoiding caspase-mediated cell death, while leaving the expression of protein kinase RNA-like ER kinase (PERK) and activating transcription factor 6α (ATF6α) pathways unmodified. Hence, C-PE exhibited a nephroprotective effect on $HgCl_2$-induced AKI by reducing oxidative stress and ER stress.

Keywords: C-phycoerythrin; *Phormidium persicinum*; acute kidney injury; mercury; oxidative stress; endoplasmic reticulum stress

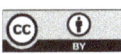

1. Introduction

Acute kidney injury (AKI), a syndrome engendered by sepsis, cardiorenal syndrome, urinary tract obstruction, and nephrotoxins, is known to increase the level of serum creatinine and/or decrease urine output. It is an important public health issue because of being a serious complication for 10–15% of hospitalized patients and ~50% of those in intensive care [1].

Animal models of AKI are induced by administering a drug or toxicant (e.g., $HgCl_2$) [2,3]. Mercury targets the kidney by binding to thiol-containing proteins in the tubular and glomerular nephron portion, disrupting the tubular transport mechanism related to Na^+/K^+-ATPase [4]. It also alters the intracellular calcium current and consequently the redox environment. The increase in oxidants is not counteracted by the antioxidant system and therefore leads to oxidative stress [5,6] and endoplasmic reticulum (ER) stress [3].

ER stress disrupts proteostasis in this organelle, causing the accumulation of unfolded and misfolded proteins. To maintain ER function, the unfolded protein response is activated through the protein kinase RNA-like ER kinase (PERK), activating transcription factor 6α (ATF6α), and inositol-requiring enzyme 1α (IRE1α) pathways.

The PERK pathway, crucial in regulating the unfolded protein response, reduces transcription through phosphorylation of the eukaryotic translation initiation factor-2α (eIF2α). If ER stress is controlled, protein folding can resume, and the phosphorylated eIF2α dephosphorylates. In the event that ER stress is sustained, the activating transcription factor 4 (ATF4)/growth arrest and DNA damage-inducible gene 153 (GADD153, also called CHOP) pathway activates the expression of genes that participate in redox homeostasis, autophagy, and/or apoptosis. The particular genes involved depend on the level of ER stress [7,8].

In parallel, the ATF6α pathway diminishes ER stress by regulating genes that encode ER chaperones and enzymes responsible for promoting folding, maturation, secretion, or degradation of misfolded proteins. When ER stress is sustained, the cell activates autophagy and apoptosis by upregulating the generation of reactive oxygen species (ROS) and activating ER membrane-associated caspase 12 through the ATF4/GADD153 pathway [7,8].

Additionally, IRE1α contributes to adaptation or apoptosis under chronic ER stress. The adaptation response of IRE1α is activated by selective cleavage of X-box binding protein 1 (XBP1) mRNA to produce spliced isoforms of XBP1, which enhance the transcription of chaperones, foldases, and components of the ER-associated protein degradation (ERAD) response to restore proteostasis. In case ER stress is still uncontrolled, IRE1α activates c-Jun N-terminal kinases 1 (JNK1) to promote the translocation of B-cell lymphoma 2 (Bcl-2)-associated X protein (Bax) into the mitochondrial membrane, which triggers the release of cytochrome c and the second mitochondrial-activated factor (Smac), leading to the activation of caspases 3 and 9 [9].

Some research groups have been developing eco-friendly therapeutic strategies for AKI from microalgae pigments such as phycobiliproteins, toroidal light-harvesting proteins in cyanobacteria, and the photosynthetic apparatus in algae. The most studied phycobiliprotein with nephroprotective activity is C-phycocyanin (C-PC). It impedes kidney failure by decreasing oxidative stress and ER stress in mice intoxicated with mercury [6,10,11]. Moreover, other phycobiliproteins, including C-phycoerythrin (C-PE), have nutraceutical activity against metabolic and toxic injury that affects certain organs (e.g., the liver) in animal models [12,13].

C-PE, an oligomeric chromoprotein of cyanobacteria, is composed of monomers αβ and prosthetic covalently linked open-chain tetrapyrrole moieties denominated C-phycoerythrobilin. In *Phormidium* sp., the monomer units oligomerize to form trimers $(\alpha\beta)_3$ and then stack as hexamers $[(\alpha\beta)_3]_2$ [14]. C-PE is widely used in the food and cosmetic industries, as well as in diagnosis and research. There are reports on its nutraceutical properties, which stem from scavenging and antioxidant activity [15]. Our research group demonstrated that a C-PE-rich protein extract from *Pseudanabaena tenuis* has nephroprotective activity [16], although its mechanism is still not completely understood. The aim of the current contribution was to determine whether the nephroprotective activity of C-PE (purified from *Phormidium persicinum*) is related to a reduction in oxidative stress and ER stress, and consequently an attenuation of the alterations in the levels of nephrin and podocin normally caused by $HgCl_2$-induced AKI.

2. Results

2.1. Characterization of C-PE from Phormidium persicinum

The absorbance spectra from various steps of purification (Figure 1) show an absorbance peak at 562 nm. The A_{562}/A_{280} ratio increased with each purification step, thus being the greatest (4.35) for the final product of purified C-PE.

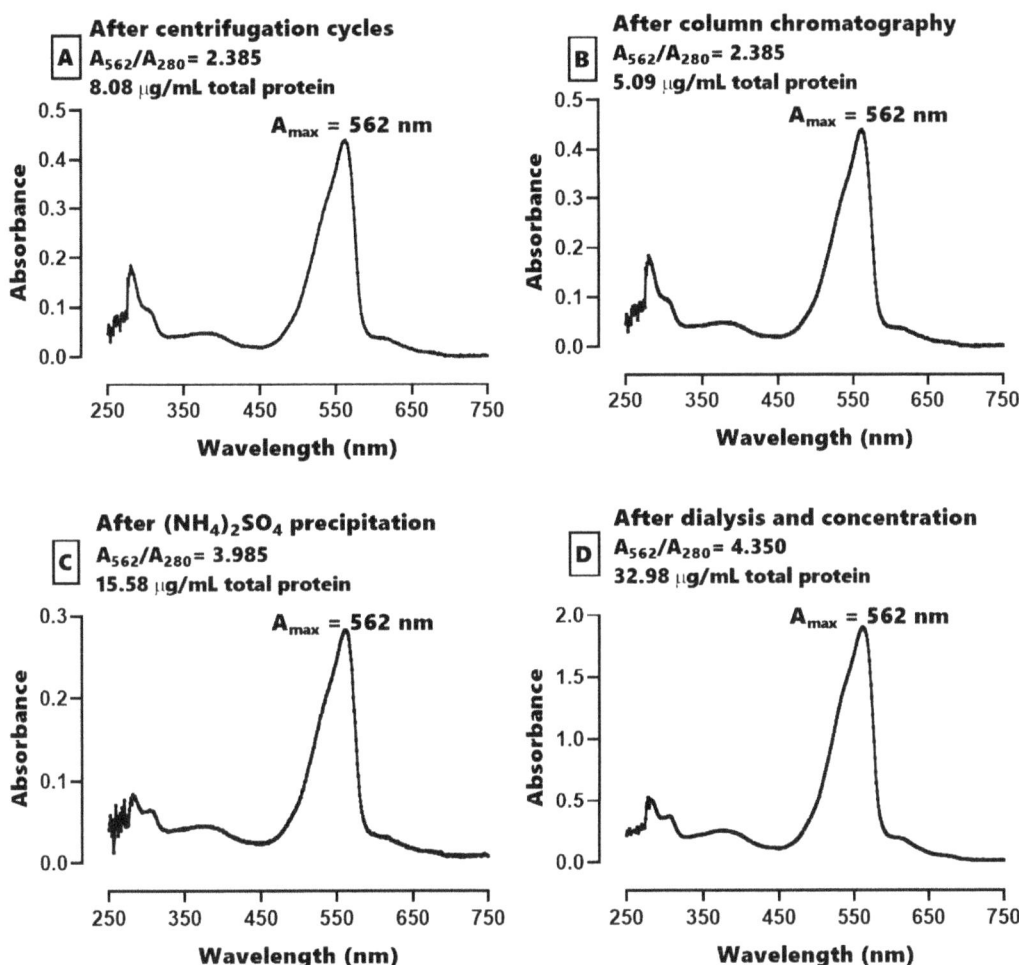

Figure 1. The absorbance spectra for the process of purification of C-phycoerythrin (C-PE) from *Phormidium persicinum* taken after the following events: the centrifugation cycles (**A**), Sephadex column chromatography (**B**), $(NH_4)_2SO_4$ precipitation (**C**), and dialysis and concentration (**D**).

The images of native- and SDS-PAGE at each step of the purification process show that the α and β C-PE subunits correspond to ~19 and ~21 KDa, respectively (Figure 2).

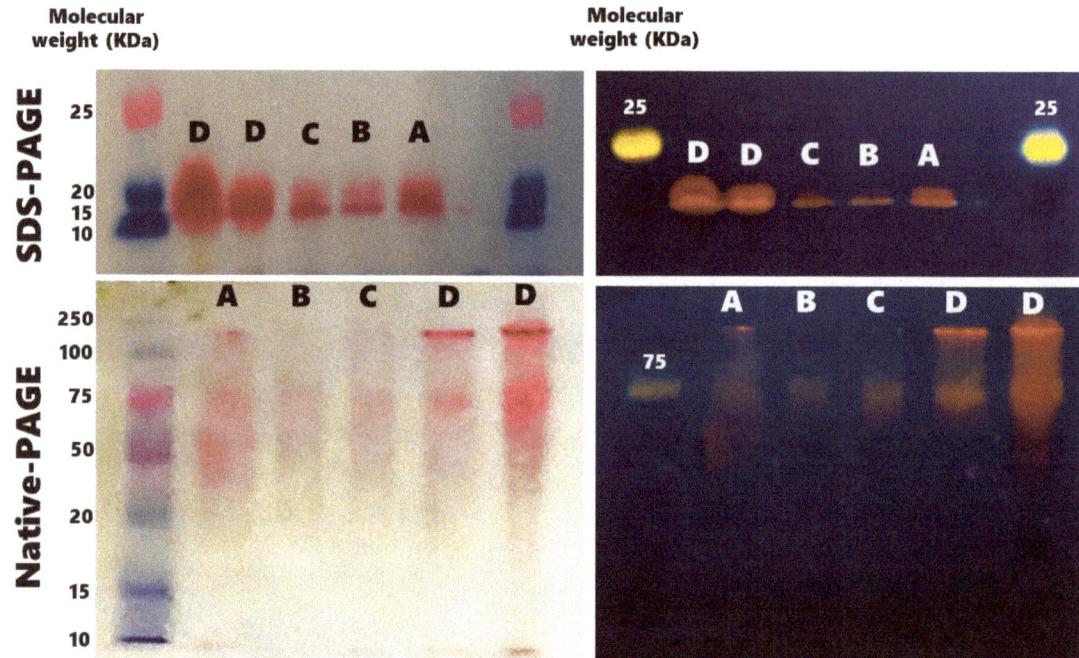

Figure 2. Representative native- and sodium dodecyl sulfate (SDS)-polyacrylamide gels (PAGE) during the process of purification of C-phycoerythrin (C-PE) from *Phormidium persicinum*, taken after the following events: the centrifugation cycles (A), Sephadex column chromatography (B), $(NH_4)_2SO_4$ precipitation (C), and dialysis and concentration (D).

The excitation-emission matrix (EEM) spectrum corresponding to the 3D fluorescence fingerprint of purified C-PE is shown in Figure 3 (panel A). The expansion of the same EEM displays the emission and excitation regions in the range of 555–595 and 510–570 nm, respectively (panel B). The fingerprint of C-PE exhibits a sharp fluorescence peak at E_{ex}/E_{em} 563/574 nm (corresponding to fluorochrome) next to Rayleigh-Tyndall's scattered light lines. The 3D spectrum of EEM features three principal Ex/Em peaks at 563/574, 545/574, and 530/574, and a small Ex/Em peak at 385/575. Two shoulders are present on the lower part of the main peak, the first at E_{ex}/E_{em} 545/574 nm and the second at E_{ex}/E_{em} 530/574 nm. Another weak peak can be observed at E_{ex}/E_{em} 385/575 nm.

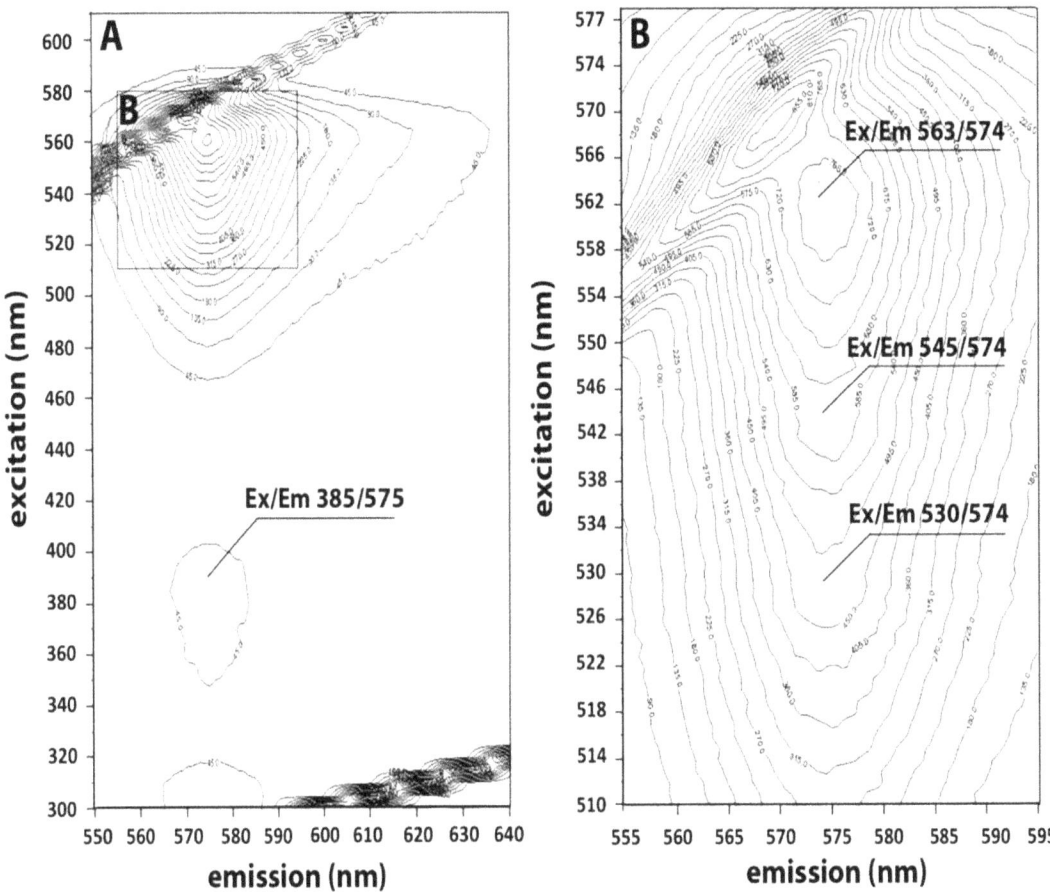

Figure 3. 3D spectrum of the excitation-emission matrix (EEM) of C-phycoerythrin (C-PE), with the emission and excitation regions in the range of 550–640 and 300–600 nm, respectively (**A**). Expansion of the EEM for emission (555–595 nm) and excitation (510–577 nm) (**B**).

2.2. Evaluation of Oxidative Stress, the Redox Environment, the Activity of Effector Caspases 3 and 9, the Expression of Nephrin and Podocin, and Renal Damage

The effect of C-PE on HgCl$_2$-induced oxidative stress and alterations in the redox environment is illustrated in Figure 4 (panels A–C and D–E, respectively). Animals intoxicated with HgCl$_2$ showed higher renal oxidative stress, indicated by the corresponding increase in lipid peroxidation (panel A, ~374%), ROS (panel B, ~211%), and nitrites (panel C, ~171%). Mercury intoxication also caused a lower GSH^2/GSSG ratio (panel F, ~66%) and greater GSSG content (panel E, ~269%). On the other hand, all doses of C-PE treatment prevented the HgCl$_2$-induced increase in lipid peroxidation, ROS, and GSSG, and the alteration in the GSH^2/GSSG ratio, while ameliorating the elevated level of nitrites (from 171% to 139%).

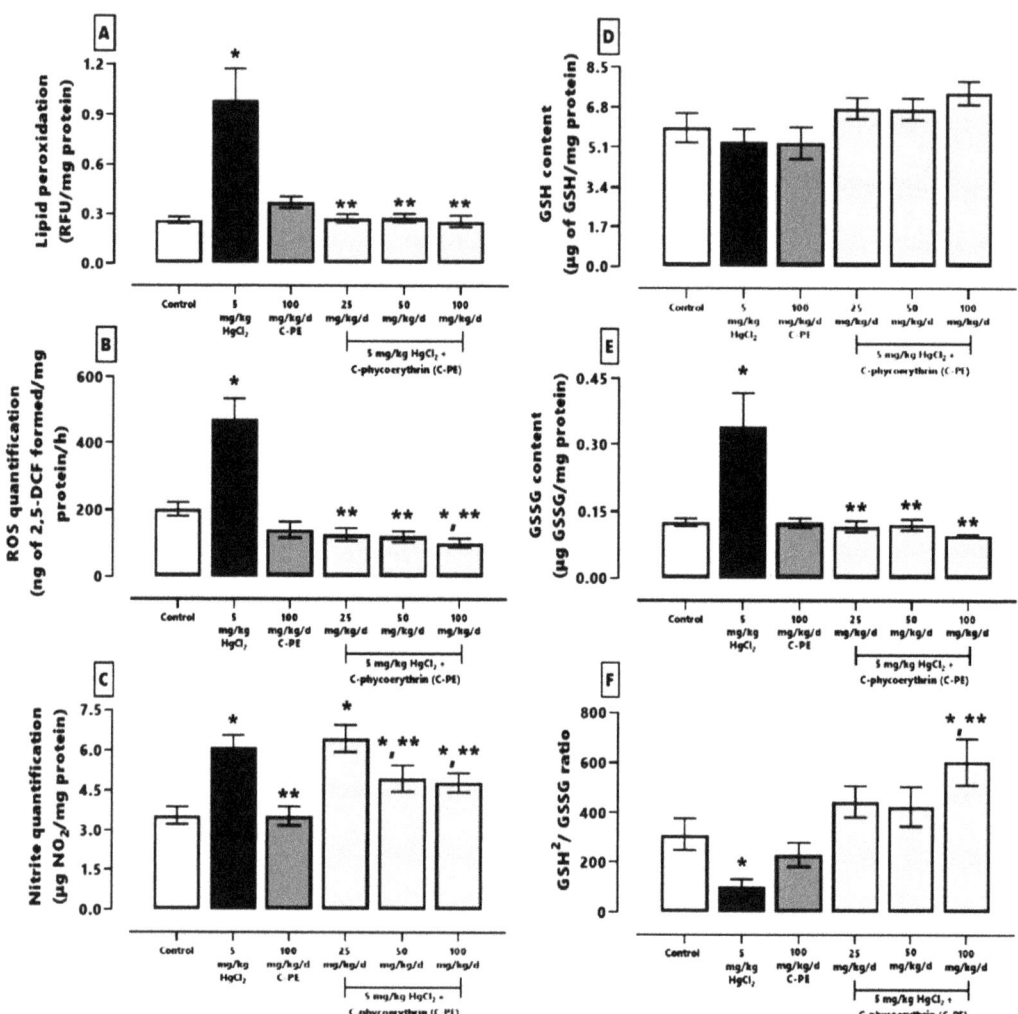

Figure 4. Effect of C-phycoerythrin (C-PE) on HgCl$_2$-induced oxidative stress and alterations in the redox environment of the kidney. Oxidative stress markers (**A–C**). Redox environment markers (**D–F**). Data are expressed as the mean ± SEM (n = 6 mice/group). One-way ANOVA and the Student-Newman-Keuls post hoc test. RFU, relative fluorescence units. * $p < 0.05$ vs. the control group. ** $p < 0.05$ vs. the HgCl$_2$ group.

Regarding the proteins associated with glomerular damage (Figure 5), mercury decreased the expression of nephrin (A) and podocin (B) by ~65% and ~71%, respectively. Treatment with C-PE partially reduced, by ~36% and ~48%, the downregulation of nephrin and podocin, respectively. These changes can be appreciated by the corresponding Western blots (Figure 5C).

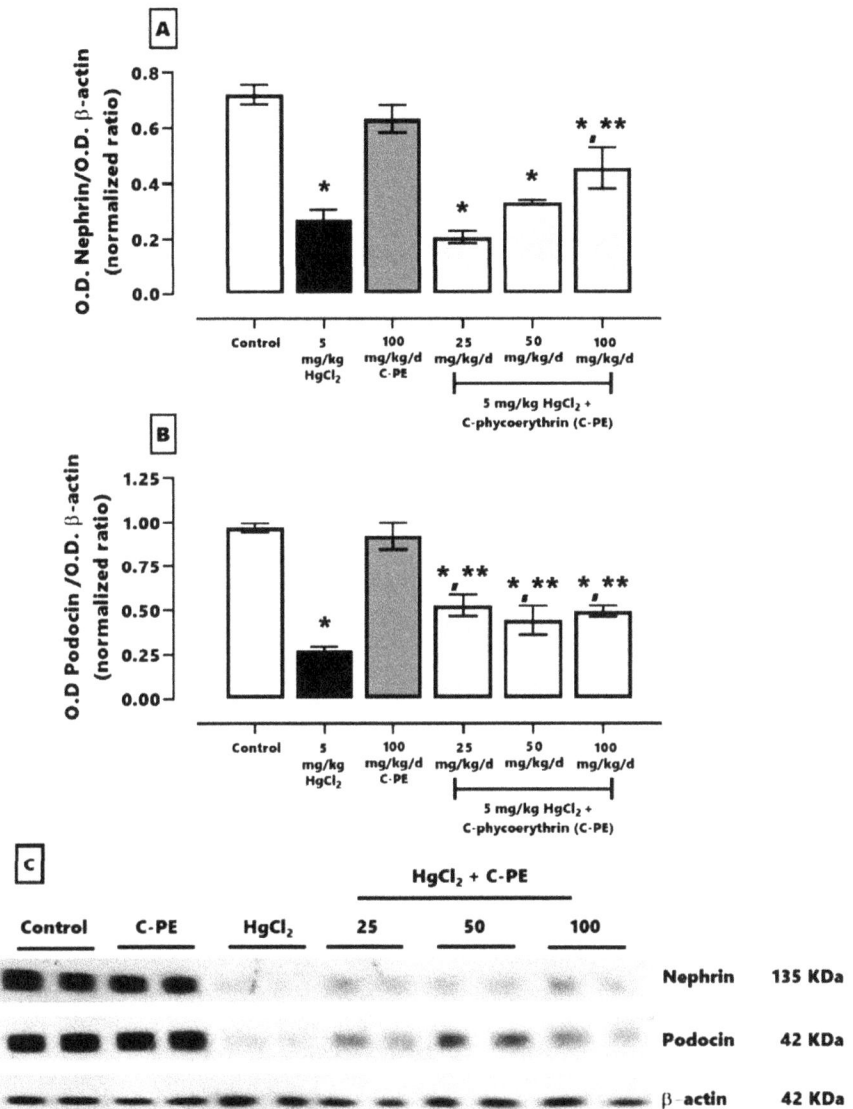

Figure 5. Effect of C-phycoerythrin (C-PE) on the decreased expression of nephrin (**A**) and podocin (**B**) in the kidneys that results from the exposure of mice to $HgCl_2$. (**C**) Representative Western blots of each experimental group. Data are expressed as the mean ± SEM (n = 6 mice/group). OD, optical density. One-way ANOVA and the Student-Newman-Keuls post hoc test. * $p < 0.05$ vs. the control group. ** $p < 0.05$ vs. the $HgCl_2$ group.

According to typical photomicrographs of the renal cortex stained with hematoxylin-eosin (H&E) (Figure 6), the control (vehicle only) and C-PE only groups had normal cytoarchitecture, which is characterized by glomeruli and the surrounding tubules with cuboidal epithelium. The photomicrographs of the group treated with mercury only display edema, cellular atrophy of distal and proximal tubules, distortion of cellular continuity, loss of the cell nucleus, hyperchromatic nuclei, and glomerulosclerosis. The AKI mice treated with C-PE exhibited a dose-dependent nutraceutical effect capable of preventing cellular damage.

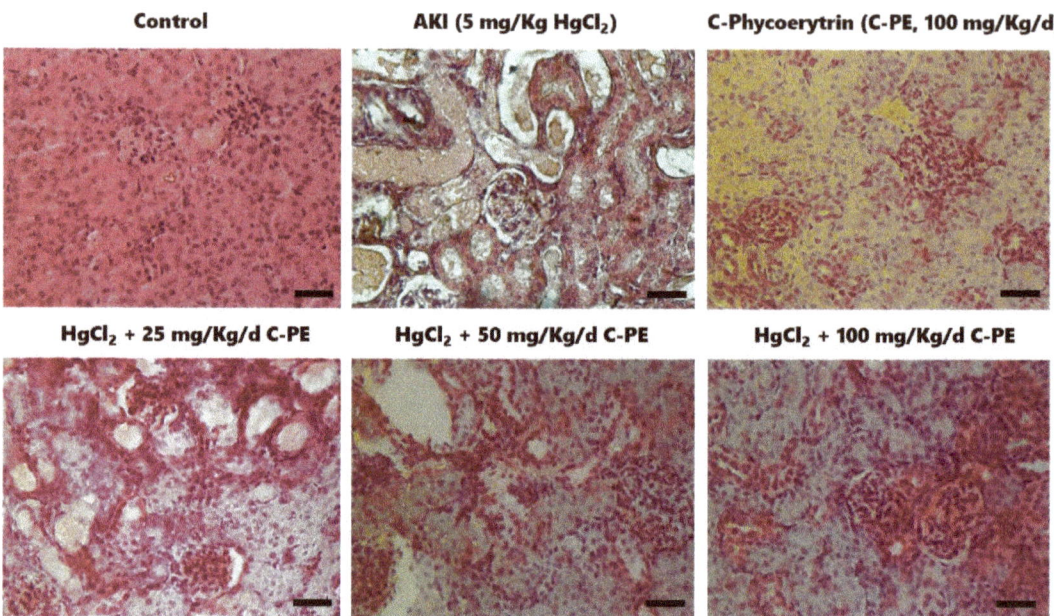

Figure 6. Representative photomicrographs of the renal cortex of animals intoxicated with $HgCl_2$ and treated with C-phycoerythrin (C-PE). $HgCl_2$ causes cell atrophy, hyperchromatic nuclei, and edema. Histological alterations were ameliorated in groups treated with C-PE. The tissue was stained with hematoxylin-eosin. The lower right bar represents 250 µm.

The effect of C-PE on the activity of caspases 3 and 9 is shown in Figure 7 (panels A and B, respectively). $HgCl_2$ generated an increase of ~511% and ~347% in the level of caspases 3 and 9, respectively. These results indicate grade 4 histological damage (panel C), affecting over 75% of the tubules and glomerulus. C-PE diminished damage in a dose-dependent manner (panel C). The highest C-PE dose (100 mg/kg/day) led to grade 1–2 kidney damage, affecting 25–50% of the tubules and glomerulus.

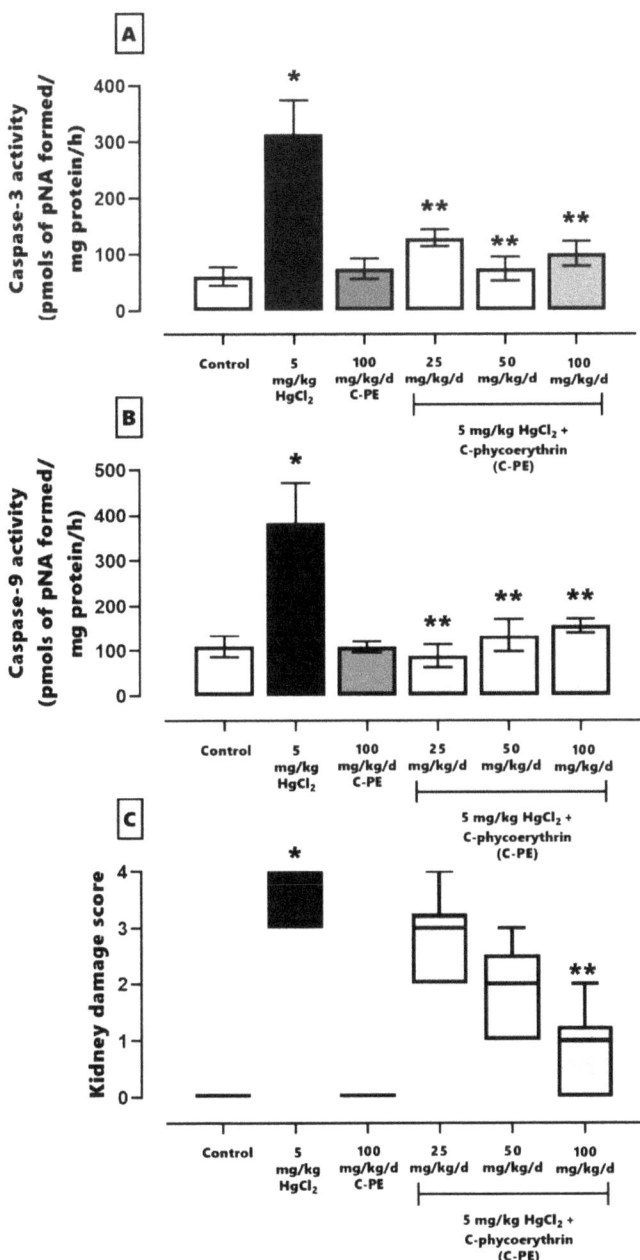

Figure 7. The effect of C-phycoerythrin (C-PE) on the activity of caspases 3 (**A**) and 9 (**B**) and the kidney damage score (**C**) in mice with $HgCl_2$-induced AKI. In (**A**) and (**B**), data are expressed as the mean ± SEM (n = 6 mice/group). Data were analyzed with one-way ANOVA and the Student-Newman-Keuls post hoc test. * $p < 0.05$ vs. the control group. ** $p < 0.05$ vs. the $HgCl_2$ group. In (**C**), each box represents the median ± interquartile space. Data were examined with the Kruskal–Wallis test and Dunn post hoc test. * $p < 0.05$ vs. the control group. ** $p < 0.05$ vs. the $HgCl_2$ group.

2.3. Evaluation of ER Stress

The effects of C-PE on the PERK/p-eIF2α (Ser52)/ATF4 and PERK/p-eIF2α (Ser52)/ATF6α signaling pathways is portrayed in Figure 8. $HgCl_2$-induced AKI was manifested as an overexpression of PERK (A), p-eIF2α (Ser 52) (B), ATF4 (C), GADD153 (D), GADD34 (E), and ATF6α (F). The C-PE treatment did not prevent the alteration in the expression of these proteins in both pathways. A representative Western blot of the marker for the PERK/eIF2α/ATF4 and PERK/eIF2α/ATF6α signaling pathways is shown in Figure 9.

Figure 10 shows the effect of C-PE on the IRE1α pathway and the proteins associated with cellular damage. $HgCl_2$ exposure generated an overexpression of IRE1α (panel A), XBP1 (panel B), caspase 12 (panel C), Bax (panel D), p-p53 (Thr 155) (panel G), and p53 (panel H). It also increased the Bax/Bcl2 and p-p53 (Thr 155)/p53 ratios (panels F and I, respectively) and reduced the expression of Bcl2 (panel E). With C-PE treatment, there was no alteration in the level of any of the proteins evaluated, which is observed in the corresponding Western blot depicted in Figure 11.

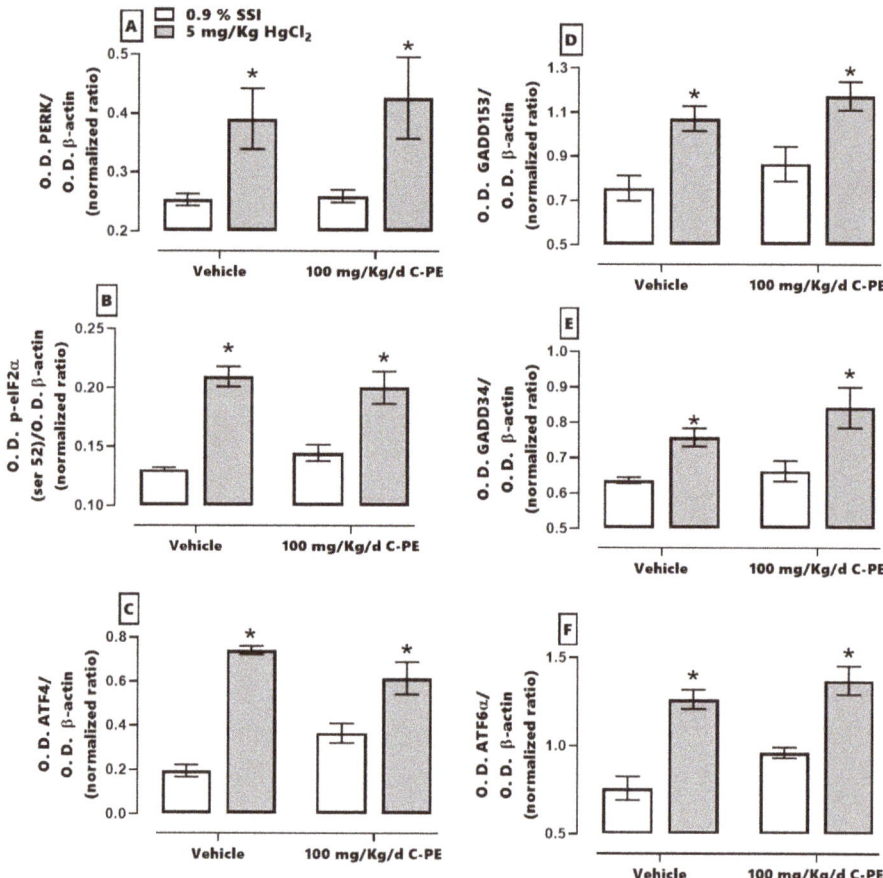

Figure 8. Effect of C-phycoerythrin (C-PE) on $HgCl_2$-induced endoplasmic reticulum stress through the PERK/p-eIF2α (Ser 52)/ATF4-GADD153 and PERK/p-eIF2α (Ser 52)/ATF6α/GADD153 pathways in the kidney. An evaluation was made of the expression of PERK (**A**), p-eIF2α (Ser 52) (**B**), ATF4 (**C**), GADD153 (**D**), GADD34 (**E**), and ATF6α (**F**). Data are expressed as the mean ± SEM (n = 3 mice/group). OD, optical density. * $p < 0.05$ vs. the control group.

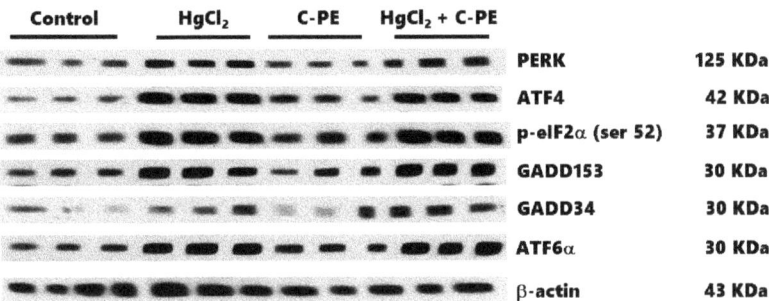

Figure 9. Representative Western blot of the effect of C-phycoerythrin (C-PE) on HgCl$_2$-induced endoplasmic reticulum stress through the PERK/p-eIF2α (Ser 52)/ATF4/GADD153 and PERK/p-eIF2α (Ser 52)/ATF6α/GADD153 pathways.

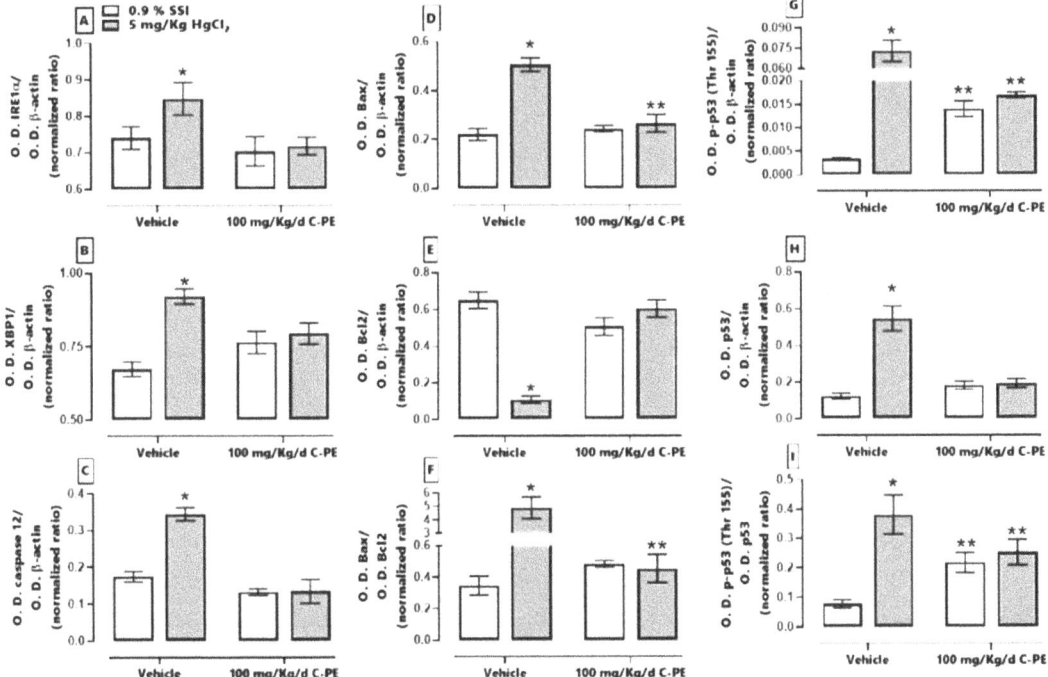

Figure 10. Effect of C-phycoerythrin (C-PE) on HgCl$_2$-induced endoplasmic reticulum stress and cell death. Protein expression was evaluated for IRE1α (**A**), XBP1 (**B**), caspase 12 (**C**), Bax (**D**), Bcl2 (**E**), the Bax/Bcl2 ratio (**F**), p53 (**G**), p-p53 (Thr 155) (**H**), and the p53/p-p53 (Thr 155) ratio (**I**). Data are expressed as the mean ± SEM (n = 3 mice/group). OD, optical density. * $p < 0.05$ vs. the control group. ** $p < 0.05$ vs. the HgCl$_2$ group.

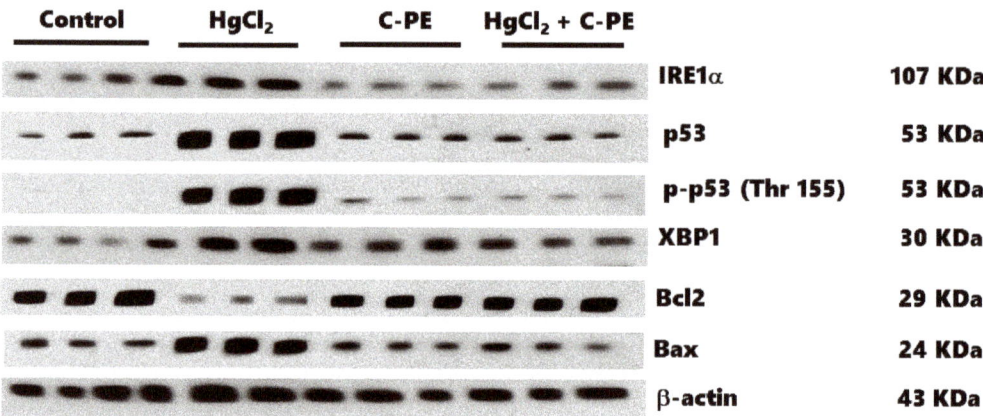

Figure 11. Representative Western blot of the effect of C-phycoerythrin (C-PE) on HgCl$_2$-induced endoplasmic reticulum stress through the IRE1α pathway and the attenuation of cell death.

3. Discussion

C-PE is reported to have nutraceutical activity against the damage resulting from cell insult [12,13]. Our group has demonstrated that treatment with a protein extract rich in C-PE prevented oxidative stress and cellular damage in an animal model of HgCl$_2$-induced AKI [16]. This model was chosen because mercury produces ER stress, which leads to renal damage. However, the aforementioned study only associated the nutraceutical properties of C-PE with scavenging and antioxidant activity. Thus, the aim of the current contribution was to explore the molecular mechanism of action of C-PE (purified from *P. persicinum*) by examining its nephroprotective activity against HgCl$_2$-induced ER stress, oxidative stress, and alterations in the redox environment in the same animal model.

HgCl$_2$ produces oxidative stress and alterations in the redox environment by three mechanisms: Fenton and Haber-Weiss reactions that generate free radicals and ROS [17], the activation of ER stress [3], and the binding of Hg^{2+} with intracellular sulfhydryl-containing proteins and low-molecular-weight compounds (e.g., GSH) capable of affecting the redox environment and protein function [18]. As a consequence of these reactions, nephrin and podocin are downregulated, and the slit diaphragm is injured, which is observed as HgCl$_2$-induced AKI. The resulting inflammatory process participates in the progression of AKI [19].

In recent years, the use of nutraceuticals from cyanobacteria and their metabolites has proven effective against renal damage (e.g., AKI) stemming from toxicants or chronic kidney disease [16,20–22]. Purified C-PE presently demonstrated nephroprotective activity when tested against HgCl$_2$-induced AKI, as evidenced by the reduction found in oxidative stress and ER stress.

C-PE, a protein with a molecular weight of ~240 KDa, has nutraceutical properties in vitro as an ROS scavenger [23]. Moreover, it prevents oxidative stress and cellular damage in vivo [12,13]. All reports on C-PE suggest that it is a potent antioxidant. By scavenging ROS, it avoids alterations in the redox environment and therefore impedes cellular damage [12,13,24]. However, animal studies have not yet completely defined the nutraceutical protection mechanism.

C-PE may act as a prodrug that leads to the release of the phycoerythrobilin moiety into the gastrointestinal tract, as previously demonstrated by our group for C-PC and phycocyanobilin [22]. C-PC is known to break down into chromo-peptides that contain phycocyanobilin, followed by the apparent absorption of linear tetrapyrrole compounds facilitated by the action of intestinal peptidases [24,25]. Once in serum, phycoerythrobilin could bind to albumin due to its low water solubility, which would extend its therapeutic activity into the entire organism [26].

The protective effect of C-PE against HgCl$_2$-induced AKI is associated with antioxidant, anti-inflammatory, and chelation mechanisms. C-PE acts as an antioxidant because it contains PEB. In addition, the chemical structure of phycoerythrobilin acts as a nucleophilic compound, neutralizing free radicals and ROS [24]. According to an in vitro model, the chelation of Hg^{2+} by PEB suppresses the degranulation of RBL-2H3 mast cells and decreases the intracellular concentration of Ca^{2+} [27], giving rise to anti-inflammatory and nephroprotective effects. Hg^{2+} binds to PEB thioether bridges in C-PE, which assume a cyclic helical form capable of chelation [28]. The antioxidant and chelating activity of C-PE can avoid Fenton and Haber-Weiss reactions and consequently ameliorate the production of free radicals, the generation of oxidative stress, and the alteration of the redox environment in kidney cells. All the aforementioned mechanisms of C-PE are related to the maintenance of the redox environment and therefore prevent the dysfunction of organelles such as the ER.

In the current evaluation of proteostasis, HgCl$_2$-induced ER stress was found to activate the IRE1α pathway and promote cell death. At the same time, mercury activated the PERK pathway, which restored proteostasis through PERK/eIF2α/ATF-4/GADD153. When the cell was incapable of compensating for imbalances in proteostasis, the activation of ATF4 and GADD153 in the same pathway led to the expression of proapoptotic proteins and the triggering of cell death. As can be appreciated, PERK and IRE1α have a synergic effect in prompting kidney cell death by increasing the Bax/Bcl-2 ratio and the level of caspases 3, 8, 9, and 12 [3,10]. Hence, HgCl$_2$ was capable of generating AKI in the present study by fomenting oxidative stress, an alteration in the redox environment, and ER stress. The resulting histological damage was considerable (grade 4), affecting over 75% of tubular and glomerular cells.

C-PE treatment enhanced the canonical ER response through the PERK/p-eIF2α (ser 52)/ATF-4/GADD153 pathway, involving ER-associated degradation (ERAD), known to process misfolded and unfolded proteins. The phosphorylation of eIF2α (ser 52) is able to suppress the overall translation of mRNA, thus reducing protein stress in the ER. Furthermore, the moderate increment in ATF6α upregulates several genes that participate in the adaptative phase of the unfolded protein response [29]. C-PE treatment is herein proposed to have activated the PERK and ATF6 signaling pathways, maintaining proteostasis by avoiding oxidative stress and alterations in the redox environment and by activating the unfolded protein response [30,31].

The response elicited by C-PE is distinct from that of other phycobiliproteins. For instance, C-PC averts the overexpression of GADD34 by activating GADD153, which is related to the inhibition of apoptosis [11,32]. On the other hand, both C-PC and C-PE maintain proteostasis. The differences between these two responses should be explored in depth in future research.

C-PE and C-PC have a similar effect on the IREα pathway, decreasing cell death mediated by caspases 3, 9, and 12 as well as reducing the disruption in p53 activation and the alteration of the Bax/Bcl2 ratio [10,11]. This idea is supported by neurotoxicological models, where C-PE prevents ER stress linked to calcium deregulation and mitochondrial dysfunction [33].

In the control group, interestingly, C-PE per se increased the phosphorylation of p53 (Thr 155), which is a genome gatekeeper because it is a master transcriptional factor that induces cellular senescence and suppresses cell growth and tumor formation. Exposure to various cellular stressors, however, causes p53 to be overexpressed and phosphorylated in several regions, leading to cell cycle arrest or apoptosis. Accordingly, p53 is phosphorylated by the C-Jun activation domain-binding protein-1 (Jab1) in Thr 155, promoting its translocation into the cytoplasm to favor interaction with the COP9 signalosome complex. These nuclear export mechanisms of p53 provide a practical future approach to a possible C-PE-induced activation of anti-cancer therapy by p53 [34], as evidenced by the lack of histological irregularities in the C-PE control group as well as the capacity of C-PE treatment of AKI mice to prevent oxidative stress, ER stress, and alterations in the redox environment and cell death markers.

4. Materials and Methods

4.1. Animals

Forty-eight male albino NIH Swiss mice (25–30 g) were kept in a cool room (21 ± 2 °C) with 40–60% relative humidity under a 12/12 h light/dark cycle (lights on at 8 AM). Food and water were provided ad libitum. The experimental procedures were in accordance with the Official Mexican Norm (NOM-062-ZOO-1999, technical specifications for the production, care, and use of laboratory animals) [35]. The protocol was approved by the institutional Internal Bioethics Committee (ZOO-013-2021).

The animals were divided into two lots to carry out distinct protocols, one to assess oxidative stress and kidney damage and another to analyze ER stress. For the evaluation of oxidative stress and kidney damage, 36 mice were randomly allocated to 6 groups (n = 6). Three were control groups: (1) the vehicle (negative control), with 100 mM of phosphate buffer (PB, at pH 7.4) administered by oral gavage (og) + 0.9% of saline solution (SS) applied intraperitoneally (ip), (2) AKI induced by a single application of 5 mg/kg $HgCl_2$ ip + the vehicle (PB) og, and (3) C-PE treatment, consisting of 100 mg/kg/day C-PE og + 0.9% SS ip. The other three groups received a single application of $HgCl_2$ ip as well as 25, 50, or 100 mg/kg/day C-PE og. For the analysis of ER stress, twelve mice were randomly allocated to four groups with the following treatments (n = 3): (1) the control (vehicle), (2) mercury-induced AKI, (3) the C-PE treatment, and (4) the AKI + C-PE treatment (a single application of $HgCl_2$ ip and 100 mg/kg/day C-PE og).

C-PE or the vehicle was administered 30 min before the injection of $HgCl_2$ or 0.9% of SS. C-PE was administered once daily for five days (the first protocol) or for three days (the second protocol) at the same time (12:00 AM) each day. Whereas the mice assigned to the evaluation of oxidative stress and renal damage were euthanized 5 days after mercury intoxication, those employed for assessing ER stress were euthanized 3 days after the same event. The right kidneys were frozen at −70 °C to await examination of the markers of oxidative stress and the redox environment by Western blot, while the left kidneys were put into paraformaldehyde in PBS (4% v/v) to appraise cell damage.

4.2. Cultivation, Purification, and Characterization of C-PE from Phormidium persicinum

P. persicinum was obtained from the culture collection of the Centro de Investigaciones Biológicas del Noroeste, S. C. (CIB 84). It was grown in a synthetic medium (denominated NM), created and optimized by our group (composition: 29 g/L of commercial sea salt, 0.8 g/L $NaHCO_3$, 0.05 g/L K_2HPO_4, 2.16 g/L $NaNO_3$, 5 mg/L $MgSO_4$, 1 mg/L $FeSO_4$, and 1 mL of a micronutrient solution containing 0.2 mM EDTA, 46.2 mM H_3BO_3, 9.3 mM $MnCl_2$, 0.95 mM $ZnSO_4$, 2.03 mM Na_2MoO_4, 0.49 mM $Ca(NO_3)_2$, and 0.77 mM $CuSO_4$). Incubation was carried out at 21 ± 2 °C with constant aeration provided by an air pump, under green LED illumination (24 W, 3000 Lx) and a 12/12 h light/dark cycle (lights on at 8:00 AM).

Regarding the purification of C-PE, the cyanobacterial biomass was centrifuged at 10,000× g for 1 min and 5–10 g of the resulting cell pellet was re-suspended in 20 mL of distilled water. Subsequently, three freeze–thaw cycles were performed, freezing at −20 °C and thawing at 4 °C during 24 h. The resulting slurry was centrifuged in 4 cycles at 21,400× g for 10 min at 4 °C to remove the cell debris. An aliquot of 20 mL of the phycobiliprotein-rich extract was injected into a column (33 cm long × 4.7 cm in diameter) containing Sephadex G-250 gel previously equilibrated with 10 mM of PB (pH 7.4). The pink fractions were obtained and precipitated with a saturated solution of $(NH_4)_2SO_4$ at 4 °C for 24 h in the dark. This mixture was centrifuged at 21,400× g for 2 min at 4 °C, and the resulting pellet was resuspended in 100 mM of PB at pH 7.4. The membrane was then dialyzed with PB for 24 h, after which time an aliquot of C-PE was immediately lyophilized to construct a calibration curve, obtain an absorption spectrum, and characterize the extract fluorometrically with an EEM. The C-PE extract was solubilized in PB and 5 mM of sucrose and frozen at −20 °C to await administration to the animals [36].

The EEM was recorded by scanning excitation and emission simultaneously in a Luminescent Spectrometer (Perkin Elmer LS 55) equipped with a Xenon discharge lamp and an excitation/emission slit 5/5. The scans were processed by 3D View Perkin Elmer software to produce 3D fingerprint contour maps by using fluorescence lines (with emission plotted on the X-axis and excitation on the Y-axis), as previously reported [37].

The calibration curve of 0.6–6 mg/mL of C-PE solubilized in PB was calculated as follows:

$$CPE\left(\frac{mg}{dL}\right) = \frac{[Absorbance_{562\ nm} - 0.1374]}{0.3540}; r^2 = 0.9899; r = 0.9949;$$
$$\in Absorbance_{562\ nm}\ [0.330 - 2.245]$$

The purity index was calculated as the ratio of the maximum absorbance peak to the absorbance peak of the proteins (A_{562}/A_{280}) [38].

4.3. Evaluation of Oxidative Stress, the Redox Environment, and the Activity of Effector Caspases 3 and 9

Kidneys were homogenized in 3.5 mL of 10 mM PB for all assays. The quantification of oxidative stress, the redox environment, and the activity of effector caspases 3 and 9 was performed with a previously described method [3,22].

The lipid peroxidation technique employed an aliquot of 500 µL of homogenate, which was added to 4 mL of chloroform-methanol (2:1, *v/v*). The mixture was agitated and kept at 4 °C for 30 min (protected from light) to allow for the separation of the polar and nonpolar phases. Afterwards, the aqueous phase was aspirated and discarded. With an aliquot of 2 mL of the organic phase (chloroform), fluorescence was determined at 370 nm (excitation) and 430 nm (emission). The results were expressed as relative fluorescence units (RFU) per mg of protein.

The level of ROS was quantified by the formation of 2,7-dichlorofluorescein (DCF), and 10 µL of the homogenate was added to 1945 µL of TRIS-HEPES (18:1 *v/v*) and incubated in the presence of 50 µL of 2,7-dichlorofluorescin diacetate (DCFH-DA) at 37 °C for 1 h. The reaction was stopped by freezing, and the fluorescence was measured at 488 nm (excitation) and 525 nm (emission).

Nitrites were assessed as indirect markers of nitrergic stress. An aliquot of 500 µL of homogenate was added to 500 µL of concentrated chlorhydric acid and 500 µL of 20% zinc suspension. The mixture was stirred and incubated at 37 °C for 1 h, followed by centrifugation at 4000× *g* for 2 min. The supernatant (50 µL) was added to a 96-well polystyrene plate containing 50 µL of 0.6% sulfanilamide and 0.12% *N*-(naftyl)-ethylenediamine, and then incubated for 15 min at room temperature. The absorbance was measured at 530 nm in a Multiscan Go® plate spectrophotometer.

A determination was made of two redox environment markers, GSH and GSSG, in a sample of 300 µL, treated with 500 µL of 30% phosphoric acid and centrifuged at 10,000× *g* for 30 min at 4 °C. To analyze GSH, an aliquot of 30 µL of the supernatant was diluted in 1.9 mL of FEDTA (1:10, 100 mM phosphate and 5 mM EDTA), and the mixture was reacted with 100 µL of o-phthaldialdehyde. To assess GSSG, 130 µL of the supernatant was added to 60 µL of N-ethylmaleimide and left for 30 min. Subsequently, an aliquot of 60 µL of the mixture was combined with 1.84 mL of FEDTA and 100 µL of o-phthaldialdehyde. The two chemical species were measured at 350 nm (excitation) and 420 nm (emission).

The activity of caspases 3 and 9 was evaluated using a commercial colorimetric assay kit as specified in the manufacturer's instructions (Millipore, APT165 and APT173, respectively). Accordingly, *p*-nitroaniline (*p*NA) was cleaved from the substrate *N*-Acetyl-Asp-Glu-Val-Asp *p*-nitroaniline (DEVD-*p*NA, caspase 3) or *N*-Acetyl-Leu-Glu-His-Asp *p*-nitroaniline (LEHD-*p*NA, caspase 9), and then the samples were measured spectrophotometrically at 405 nm.

4.4. Examination of Kidney Damage

Histopathological analysis was performed to appraise kidney damage. The kidneys were fixed for 48 h in 4% paraformaldehyde in PBS. Afterwards, they were embedded in paraffin to obtain 5 μm slices on a standard microtome. Each section was stained with H&E, dehydrated, and mounted in resin. The presence or absence of kidney cell damage was evaluated with a histopathological graded scale [6,20,22] as follows: 0, undamaged (indistinguishable from the controls); 1, minimal (affecting ≤25% of the tubules and glomerulus); 2, mild (affecting >25% and ≤50% of the tubules and glomerulus); 3, moderate (affecting >50% and ≤75% of the tubules and glomerulus); 4, severe (affecting >75% of the tubules and glomerulus).

4.5. Western Blot Analysis for Nephrin, Podocin, and ER Stress Markers

The expression of proteins was determined with Western blot assays. Briefly, the samples were prepared with 100 μL of the homogenate mixed with 50 μL of a complete protease inhibitor cocktail® (MilliporeSigma, Burlington, MA, USA) in lysis buffer, and then 150 μL of the 2× Laemmli sample buffer (Biorad, Hercules, CA, USA, 161-0737) was added. The samples were homogenized by vortex, placed in a boiling water bath for 3 min, and then kept at -20 °C to await processing. Fifty μg of protein samples were loaded in 15% polyacrylamide gel with sodium dodecyl sulfate (SDS-PAGE) and separated by electrophoresis (90 V for 60 min). Subsequently, the proteins were electrotransferred from the gels to PVDF membranes in a Trans-Blot Turbo system (Biorad) at 25 V and 2.05 A for 7 min. Upon completing this time, the membranes were blocked for 1 h under constant stirring in PBST (PBS with 0.05% Tween 20 and 5% low-fat milkSvelty®), followed by incubation overnight at 4 °C in a blocking buffer containing the primary antibodies. The primary antibodies (Santa Cruz Biotechnology, Dallas, TX, USA), diluted 1:1000, were PERK (sc-377400), p-eIF2α (Ser 52, sc-12412), ATF-4 (sc-200), GADD153 (sc-56107), ATF-6α (sc-166659), IRE-1α (sc-390960), p-p53 (Thr 155, sc-377567), XBP1 (sc-7160), Bax (sc-20067), and Bcl2 (sc-7382). Podocin (orb337389), nephrin (orb11107), GADD34 (orb13417), and p53 (orb14498) were acquired from Byorbit (Cambridgeshire, Cambridge, UK) and diluted 1:500. After incubation, membranes were washed three times with fresh PBST (20 min/wash) and then incubated in a secondary antibody diluted 1:1500 (HPR-conjugated goat anti-rabbit; Life Technologies, Rockford, IL, USA, 65-6120) at room temperature for 1 h under constant stirring. Membranes were washed three times with fresh PBST. Finally, the protein bands were revealed on photographic plates (JUAMA, Mexico City, Mexico) by chemiluminescence, using Luminata TM Forte® (MilliporeSigma, Burlington, MA, USA). β-Actin protein expression served as the loading control and constitutive protein (Santa Cruz Biotechnology; sc-1615, dilution 1:4000). The optical density (OD) of all bands was quantified by the Image J program (NIH, Bethesda, MD, USA) and described as the protein/β-actin ratio.

4.6. Statistical Analysis

All data are expressed as the mean ± standard error, except for the kidney damage score. The latter is described as the median ± interquartile spaces, with the values analyzed with the Kruskal–Wallis method. The variables in the first protocol (to evaluate oxidative stress and the redox environment) were examined by one-way analysis of variance (ANOVA). Two-way ANOVA was utilized to assess ER stress, considering the treatment and absence/presence of AKI as factors. ANOVA was followed by the Student-Newman-Keuls post hoc test. Statistical significance was considered at $p < 0.05$.

5. Conclusions

The nutraceutical effect of C-PE on $HgCl_2$-induced AKI stems from its antioxidant activity, which reduces the level of oxidative stress markers and maintains the redox environment. Additionally, C-PE modulates intracellular signaling pathways involved in proteostasis, avoiding the disruption of podocytes and damage to glomerular and tubular cells. Hence, the nephroprotective activity of C-PE is related to the prevention of oxidative stress and ER stress in the kidney of animals intoxicated with mercury. The nutraceutical effect may also be related to anti-inflammatory activity, possibly triggering autophagy as a survival pathway linked to the unfolded protein response. This mechanism is worthy of greater attention in future research.

Author Contributions: V.B.-V. and P.R.-F.: Methodology, data curation, writing of the original draft and funding acquisition; J.I.S.-C.: Writing of the original draft, reviewing and editing; A.A.S.: Methodology, data curation, reviewing and editing the manuscript; C.G.-H.: Methodology; M.F.-C. and E.C.-E.: Conceptualization, supervision, project administration, funding acquisition, writing of the original draft, review and editing. All authors have read and agreed to the published version of the manuscript.

Funding: This study was supported by SIP-IPN (grant numbers 20210052, 20210080, 20210787, and 20210743). The APC was funded by Imperial College London.

Institutional Review Board Statement: The experimental procedures were in accordance with the Official Mexican Norm (NOM-062-ZOO-1999, technical specifications for the production, care, and use of laboratory animals) [35]. The protocol was approved by the institutional Internal Bioethics Committee (ZOO-013-2021).

Data Availability Statement: Publicly available datasets were analyzed in this study. This data can be found here: [https://drive.google.com/file/d/15HqGDpXfEdC6_lv9RdAO3cq8glJocEbF/view?usp=sharing, accessed on 2 October 2021].

Acknowledgments: We thank the Instituto Politécnico Nacional, Secretaría de Investigación y Posgrado-IPN, for financial support. The Mexican researchers are fellows of EDI, COFAA, and SNI. JISC is supported by the NIHR Imperial Biomedical Research Centre (BRC).

Conflicts of Interest: The authors declare no conflict of interest.

References

1. Ronco, C.; Bellomo, R.; Kellum, J.A. Acute kidney injury. *Lancet* **2019**, *394*, 1949–1964. [CrossRef]
2. Peyrou, M.; Hanna, P.E.; Cribb, A.E. Cisplatin, gentamicin, and p-aminophenol induce markers of endoplasmic reticulum stress in the rat kidneys. *Toxicol. Sci.* **2007**, *99*, 346–353. [CrossRef]
3. Rojas-Franco, P.; Franco-Colín, M.; Torres-Manzo, A.P.; Blas-Valdivia, V.; Thompson-Bonilla, M.R.; Kandir, S.; Cano-Europa, E. Endoplasmic reticulum stress participates in the pathophysiology of mercury-caused acute kidney injury. *Ren. Fail.* **2019**, *41*, 1001–1010. [CrossRef]
4. Bridges, C.C.; Zalups, R.K. Transport of inorganic mercury and methylmercury in target tissues and organs. *J. Toxicol. Environ. Health-Part B Crit. Rev.* **2010**, *13*, 385–410. [CrossRef]
5. Zalups, R.K. Molecular interactions with mercury in the kidney. *Pharmacol. Rev.* **2000**, *52*, 113–144.
6. Rodriguez-Sánchez, R.; Ortiz-Butrón, R.; Blas-Valdivia, V.; Hernández-García, A.; Cano-Europa, E.; Rodríguez-Sánchez, R.; Ortiz-Butrón, R.; Blas-Valdivia, V.; Hernández-García, A.; Cano-Europa, E.; et al. Phycobiliproteins or C-phycocyanin of *Arthrospira (Spirulina) maxima* protect against $HgCl_2$-caused oxidative stress and renal damage. *Food Chem.* **2012**, *135*, 2359–2365. [CrossRef]
7. Smedley, G.D.; Walker, K.E.; Yuan, S.H. The role of PERK in understanding development of neurodegenerative diseases. *Int. J. Mol. Sci.* **2021**, *22*, 8146. [CrossRef]
8. Almanza, A.; Carlesso, A.; Chintha, C.; Creedican, S.; Doultsinos, D.; Leuzzi, B.; Luís, A.; McCarthy, N.; Montibeller, L.; More, S.; et al. Endoplasmic reticulum stress signalling from basic mechanisms to clinical applications. *FEBS J.* **2019**, *286*, 241–278. [CrossRef] [PubMed]
9. Hetz, C.; Zhang, K.; Kaufman, R.J. Mechanisms, regulation and functions of the unfolded protein response. *Nat. Rev. Mol. Cell Biol.* **2020**, *21*, 421–438. [CrossRef] [PubMed]

10. Rojas-Franco, P.; Franco-Colín, M.; Camargo, M.E.; Estévez Carmona, M.M.; Ortíz-Butrón, M.R.; Blas-Valdivia, V.; Cano-Europa, E. Phycobiliproteins and phycocyanin of *Arthrospira maxima (Spirulina)* reduce apoptosis promoters and glomerular dysfunction in mercury-related acute kidney injury. *Toxicol. Res. Appl.* **2018**, *2*, 2397847318805070. [CrossRef]
11. Rojas-Franco, P.; Franco-Colín, M.; Blas-Valdivia, V.; Melendez-Camargo, M.E.; Cano-Europa, E. *Arthrospira maxima (Spirulina)* prevents endoplasmic reticulum stress in the kidney through its C-phycocyanin. *J. Zhejiang Univ. Sci. B* **2021**, *22*, 603–608. [CrossRef]
12. Soni, B.; Visavadiya, N.P.; Madamwar, D. Attenuation of diabetic complications by C-phycoerythrin in rats: Antioxidant activity of C-phycoerythrin including copper-induced lipoprotein and serum oxidation. *Br. J. Nutr.* **2009**, *102*, 102–109. [CrossRef] [PubMed]
13. Soni, B.; Visavadiya, N.P.; Madamwar, D. Ameliorative action of cyanobacterial phycoerythrin on CCl_4-induced toxicity in rats. *Toxicology* **2008**, *248*, 59–65. [CrossRef] [PubMed]
14. Sonani, R.R.; Sharma, M.; Gupta, G.D.; Kumar, V.; Madamwar, D. *Phormidium* phycoerythrin forms hexamers in crystals: A crystallographic study. *Acta Crystallogr. Sect. F Struct. Biol. Commun.* **2015**, *71*, 998–1004. [CrossRef] [PubMed]
15. Sonani, R.R.; Singh, N.K.; Kumar, J.; Thakar, D.; Madamwar, D. Concurrent purification and antioxidant activity of phycobiliproteins from *Lyngbya* sp. A09DM: An antioxidant and anti-aging potential of phycoerythrin in *Caenorhabditis elegans*. *Process Biochem.* **2014**, *49*, 1757–1766. [CrossRef]
16. Cano-Europa, E.; Ortiz-Butrón, R.; Gallardo-Casas, C.A.; Blas-Valdivia, V.; Pineda-Reynoso, M.; Olvera-Ramírez, R.; Franco-Colin, M. Phycobiliproteins from *Pseudanabaena tenuis* rich in c-phycoerythrin protect against $HgCl_2$-caused oxidative stress and cellular damage in the kidney. *J. Appl. Phycol.* **2010**, *22*, 495–501. [CrossRef]
17. Valko, M.; Morris, H.; Cronin, M. Metals, toxicity and oxidative stress. *Curr. Med. Chem.* **2005**, *12*, 1161–1208. [CrossRef]
18. Patrick, L. Mercury toxicity and antioxidants: Part I: Role of glutathione and alpha-lipoic acid in the treatment of mercury toxicity. *Altern. Med. Rev.* **2002**, *7*, 456–471.
19. Nechemia-arbely, Y.; Barkan, D.; Pizov, G.; Shriki, A.; Rose-john, S.; Galun, E.; Axelrod, J.H. IL-6/IL-6R axis plays a critical role in acute kidney injury. *J. Am. Soc. Nephrol.* **2008**, *19*, 1106–1115. [CrossRef]
20. Sharma, M.K.; Sharma, A.; Kumar, A.; Kumar, M. Evaluation of protective efficacy of Spirulina fusiformis against mercury induced nephrotoxicity in Swiss albino mice. *Food Chem. Toxicol.* **2007**, *45*, 879–887. [CrossRef]
21. Memije-Lazaro, I.N.I.N.; Blas-Valdivia, V.; Franco-Colín, M.; Cano-Europa, E. *Arthrospira maxima (Spirulina)* and C-phycocyanin prevent the progression of chronic kidney disease and its cardiovascular complications. *J. Funct. Foods* **2018**, *43*, 37–43. [CrossRef]
22. Garcia-Pliego, E.; Franco-Colin, M.; Rojas-Franco, P.; Blas-Valdivia, V.; Serrano-Contreras, J.I.; Pentón-Rol, G.; Cano-Europa, E. Phycocyanobilin is the molecule responsible for the nephroprotective action of phycocyanin in acute kidney injury caused by mercury. *Food Funct.* **2021**, *12*, 2985–2994. [CrossRef] [PubMed]
23. Patel, S.N.; Sonani, R.R.; Jakharia, K.; Bhastana, B.; Patel, H.M.; Chaubey, M.G.; Singh, N.K.; Madamwar, D. Antioxidant activity and associated structural attributes of *Halomicronema* phycoerythrin. *Int. J. Biol. Macromol.* **2018**, *111*, 359–369. [CrossRef] [PubMed]
24. Yabuta, Y.; Fujimura, H.; Kwak, C.S.; Enomoto, T.; Watanabe, F. Antioxidant activity of the phycoerythrobilin compound formed from a dried Korean purple laver (*Porphyra* sp.) during *in vitro* digestion. *Food Sci. Technol. Res.* **2010**, *16*, 347–352. [CrossRef]
25. Minic, S.L.; Stanic-Vucinic, D.; Mihailovic, J.; Krstic, M.; Nikolic, M.R.; Cirkovic Velickovic, T. Digestion by pepsin releases biologically active chromopeptides from C-phycocyanin, a blue-colored biliprotein of microalga *Spirulina*. *J. Proteom.* **2016**, *147*, 132–139. [CrossRef]
26. Radibratovic, M.; Minic, S.; Stanic-Vucinic, D.; Nikolic, M.; Milcic, M.; Cirkovic Velickovic, T. Stabilization of human serum albumin by the binding of phycocyanobilin, a bioactive chromophore of blue-green alga *Spirulina*: Molecular dynamics and experimental study. *PLoS ONE* **2016**, *11*, e0167973. [CrossRef]
27. Sakai, S.; Komura, Y.; Nishimura, Y.; Sugawara, T.; Hirata, T. Inhibition of mast cell degranulation by phycoerythrin and its pigment moiety phycoerythrobilin, prepared from *Porphyra yezoensis*. *Food Sci. Technol. Res.* **2011**, *17*, 171–177. [CrossRef]
28. Ghosh, T.; Chatterjee, S.; Bhayani, K.; Mishra, S. A natural cyanobacterial protein C-phycoerythrin as an Hg^{2+} selective fluorescent probe in aqueous systems. *New J. Chem.* **2020**, *44*, 6601–6609. [CrossRef]
29. Carreras-Sureda, A.; Pihán, P.; Hetz, C. Calcium signaling at the endoplasmic reticulum: Fine-tuning stress responses. *Cell Calcium* **2018**, *70*, 24–31. [CrossRef]
30. Sprenkle, N.T.; Sims, S.G.; Sánchez, C.L.; Meares, G.P. Endoplasmic reticulum stress and inflammation in the central nervous system. *Mol. Neurodegener.* **2017**, *12*, 42. [CrossRef]
31. Bhardwaj, M.; Leli, N.M.; Koumenis, C.; Amaravadi, R.K. Regulation of autophagy by canonical and non-canonical ER stress responses. *Semin. Cancer Biol.* **2020**, *66*, 116–128. [CrossRef]
32. Marciniak, S.J.; Yun, C.Y.; Oyadomari, S.; Novoa, I.; Zhang, Y.; Jungreis, R.; Nagata, K.; Harding, H.P.; Ron, D. CHOP induces death by promoting protein synthesis and oxidation in the stressed endoplasmic reticulum. *Genes Dev.* **2004**, *18*, 3066. [CrossRef]
33. Oh, J.H.; Kim, E.-Y.; Nam, T.-J. Phycoerythrin peptide from *Pyropia yezoensis* Alleviates endoplasmic reticulum stress caused by perfluorooctane sulfonate-induced calcium dysregulation. *Mar. Drugs* **2018**, *16*, 44. [CrossRef]
34. Lee, E.-W.; Oh, W.; Song, H.P.; Kim, W.K. Phosphorylation of p53 at threonine 155 is required for Jab1-mediated nuclear export of p53. *BMB Rep.* **2017**, *50*, 373–378. [CrossRef]
35. Norma Oficial Mexicana NOM-062-ZOO-1999: Especificaciones Técnicas para la Producción, Cuidado y Uso de los Animales de Laboratorio. 1999. Available online: https://www.fmvz.unam.mx/fmvz/principal/archivos/062ZOO.PDF (accessed on 12 October 2021).

36. Kannaujiya, V.K.; Sinha, R.P. Thermokinetic stability of phycocyanin and phycoerythrin in food-grade preservatives. *J. Appl. Phycol.* **2016**, *28*, 1063–1070. [CrossRef]
37. Sfriso, A.A.; Gallo, M.; Baldi, F. Phycoerythrin productivity and diversity from five red macroalgae. *J. Appl. Phycol.* **2018**, *30*, 2523–2531. [CrossRef]
38. Madamwar, D.; Patel, D.K.; Desai, S.N.; Upadhyay, K.K.; Devkar, R. V Apoptotic potential of C-phycoerythrin from *Phormidium* sp. A27DM and *Halomicronema* sp. A32DM on human lung carcinoma cells. *EXCLI J.* **2015**, *14*, 527–539. [PubMed]

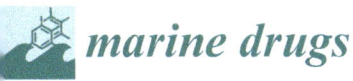

Article

Astaxanthin Protects Dendritic Cells from Lipopolysaccharide-Induced Immune Dysfunction

Yinyan Yin [1,2,*,†], Nuo Xu [1,†], Yi Shi [1], Bangyue Zhou [1], Dongrui Sun [1,3], Bixia Ma [4], Zhengzhong Xu [5], Jin Yang [3,*] and Chunmei Li [4,*]

1. College of Medicine, Yangzhou University, Yangzhou 225009, China; kf56xunuo58@126.com (N.X.); sy15365888238@163.com (Y.S.); zby18252737828@163.com (B.Z.); sun1316561047@163.com (D.S.)
2. Jiangsu Key Laboratory of Experimental and Translational Non-Coding RNA Research, Yangzhou University, Yangzhou 225009, China
3. Clinical Medical College, Yangzhou University, Yangzhou 225001, China
4. College of Food Science and Engineering, Yangzhou University, Yangzhou 225009, China; mabixia@vazyme.com
5. Jiangsu Key Laboratory of Zoonosis, Yangzhou University, Yangzhou 225009, China; zzxu@yzu.edu.cn
* Correspondence: yyyin@yzu.edu.cn (Y.Y.); yzyangjin@hotmail.com (J.Y.); licm@yzu.edu.cn (C.L.)
† These authors contributed equally.

Citation: Yin, Y.; Xu, N.; Shi, Y.; Zhou, B.; Sun, D.; Ma, B.; Xu, Z.; Yang, J.; Li, C. Astaxanthin Protects Dendritic Cells from Lipopolysaccharide-Induced Immune Dysfunction. *Mar. Drugs* **2021**, *19*, 346. https://doi.org/10.3390/md19060346

Academic Editors: Donatella Degl'Innocenti and Marzia Vasarri

Received: 21 May 2021
Accepted: 15 June 2021
Published: 17 June 2021

Publisher's Note: MDPI stays neutral with regard to jurisdictional claims in published maps and institutional affiliations.

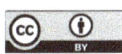

Copyright: © 2021 by the authors. Licensee MDPI, Basel, Switzerland. This article is an open access article distributed under the terms and conditions of the Creative Commons Attribution (CC BY) license (https://creativecommons.org/licenses/by/4.0/).

Abstract: Astaxanthin, originating from seafood, is a naturally occurring red carotenoid pigment. Previous studies have focused on its antioxidant properties; however, whether astaxanthin possesses a desired anti-inflammatory characteristic to regulate the dendritic cells (DCs) for sepsis therapy remains unknown. Here, we explored the effects of astaxanthin on the immune functions of murine DCs. Our results showed that astaxanthin reduced the expressions of LPS-induced inflammatory cytokines (TNF-α, IL-6, and IL-10) and phenotypic markers (MHCII, CD40, CD80, and CD86) by DCs. Moreover, astaxanthin promoted the endocytosis levels in LPS-treated DCs, and hindered the LPS-induced migration of DCs via downregulating CCR7 expression, and then abrogated allogeneic T cell proliferation. Furthermore, we found that astaxanthin inhibited the immune dysfunction of DCs induced by LPS via the activation of the HO-1/Nrf2 axis. Finally, astaxanthin with oral administration remarkably enhanced the survival rate of LPS-challenged mice. These data showed a new approach of astaxanthin for potential sepsis treatment through avoiding the immune dysfunction of DCs.

Keywords: astaxanthin; dendritic cells; sepsis; immune dysfunction; lipopolysaccharide

1. Introduction

The immune system, as a tight and dynamic regulatory network, maintains an immune homeostasis, which keeps a balance between the response to heterogenic antigens and tolerance to self-antigens [1]. However, in some diseases, such as sepsis, rheumatoid arthritis (RA), multiple sclerosis (MS), systemic lupus erythematosus (SLE), and inflammatory bowel disease (IBD), this immune homeostasis is broken [2]. Sepsis is a highly heterogeneous clinical syndrome that mainly results from the dysregulated inflammatory response to infection, which continues to cause considerable morbidity and accounts for 5.3 million deaths per year in high income countries [3]. Recently, the incidence of sepsis is progressively increased and sepsis-related mortality cases remain at a high level in China [4]. The host immune response induced by sepsis is a complex and dynamic process. After infection, the conserved motifs of pathogens, termed the pathogen-associated molecular patterns (PAMPs), such as lipopolysaccharide (LPS, cell wall component of gram-negative bacteria) or lipoteichoic acid (cell wall component of gram-positive bacteria), are recognized by the pattern recognition receptors (PRRs) expressed by immune cells, and an overwhelming innate immune response is triggered in septic patients [5,6]. Under physiological conditions, the immune activation contributes to eliminating pathogens and clearing infected cells. However, when driven by sepsis, the immune homeostasis appears imbalanced and initiates a life-threatening "cytokine storm". Currently, no drugs have been approved specifically for the treatment of sepsis, and clinical trials of potential therapies have failed to reduce mortality; therefore, new approaches are needed. Immunemodulatory intervention is the main potential therapeutic strategy against sepsis [7]. For instance, single cytokine, or a combination of multiple cytokines, including G-CSF, GM-CSF, IFN-γ, IL-3, IL-7, and IL-15, were introduced into sepsis therapy, according to a diseasespecific progression and patient immune responses [8]. Some immunosuppressive agents, such as bursopentin [9], curcumin [10], and oleuropein [11], provided protection against inflammatory injury in the LPS-induced sepsis models.

Dendritic cells (DCs), as the most important potent antigen-presenting cells, link the innate and adaptive immune response. The maturation/activation of DCs is followed by the transformations of phenotype and function, improving their migration ability to draining the lymph node, resulting in the activation of downstream T lymphocyte cells [12]. In fact, DCs reside in all the tissues of the host mainly in an antigen-capturing state and maintain immune tolerance by migrating to the lymph nodes for presenting self-antigens to lymphocytes in a tolerogenic manner [13]. Therefore, DCs also balance the immune homeostasis in the host, and guide the skewing of the downstream immune response [14]. Notably, the abnormalities of DC homeostasis are implicated in sepsis. The differentiation level of monocytes into DCs is improved during sepsis [15]. The expression levels of surface molecules related to the DC function are changed [16]. Considering the critical role of DCs in the immune regulation in sepsis, the modification of the DC system is becoming an increasingly important target for sepsis therapy [15]. Modificatory DCs by adenovirus/IL-10 transduction maintained an immature state with low expressions of IL-12, CD86, and MHCII, and the survival rate of septic mice remarkably increased [17,18]. Bursopentin inhibited the LPS-induced phenotypic and the functional maturation of DCs [9,19]. These studies indicated that compartmental modification of DC function can alter the sepsisinduced immune response.

Astaxanthin, 3,3′-dihydroxy-β,β′-carotene-4,4′-dione, is a naturally occurring red carotenoid pigment classified as a xanthophyll, found in microalgae and seafood such as salmon, trout, and shrimp [20,21]. The lipid-soluble carotenoid, with a polar–nonpolar–polar structure, is able to help astaxanthin easily pass through and fix into the double layers of the cell membrane. Moreover, free radicals inside and outside of the cell membrane can be scavenged by the polar structure of astaxanthin, and radicals located in the cell membrane can be captured by its polyene chain [22]. Therefore, astaxanthin has a strong antioxidant property, and is regarded as a potential candidate agent against many diseases [23–26]. Recent studies have shown that astaxanthin had a variety of pharmacological effects against inflammatory injury [27–29]. Astaxanthin provided a neuroprotection against diabetes-induced sickness behavior through inhibiting inflammation [30]. Astaxanthin also can attenuate monosodium urate crystal-induced arthritis by suppressing the level of pro-inflammatory cytokines [31]. Moreover, astaxanthin was shown to suppress LPS-induced inflammatory factors increase, MAPK phosphorylation, and NF-kB activation in vivo [32]. These studies demonstrated to us that astaxanthin have a great potential as a therapeutic agent of sepsis by an anti-inflammatory strategy.

In this study, we attempted to characterize the effects of astaxanthin on the immune activation and functional properties of the LPS-induced DCs for potential sepsis therapy. Our data suggested that astaxanthin protected DCs from LPS-induced immune dysfunction, which might be a simple, inexpensive, and highly effective anti-inflammatory strategy via regulating DC activity in sepsis.

2. Results

2.1. Astaxanthin Inhibited LPS-Induced Cytokine Production by DCs

Firstly, the biosafety of astaxanthin was evaluated in the murine DCs. The cells were treated with astaxanthin and the cell viability was analyzed by the CCK-8 assay. The results revealed that the cellular viability was not changed until 24 h after treatment with astaxanthin up to 50 µM (Figure 1A). Next, we examined the expression of CD69, which is a critical activation marker of DCs. After exposure to LPS (100 ng/mL) for 24 h, the expression of CD69 was upregulated, whereas they were significantly inhibited with treatment of astaxanthin (Figure 2A,B). In addition, we tested whether astaxanthin affected the production of cytokines in LPS-induced DCs. Significantly, pro-inflammatory cytokines (TNF-α and IL-6) were downregulated by astaxanthin in a dose-dependent manner (Figure 2C,D). Surprisingly, the secretion of IL-10 was not increased (Figure 2E), implying that the suppressive effect of astaxanthin probably was not mediated through anti-inflammatory cytokine. These results indicated that astaxanthin attenuated the cytokines secreted by LPS-induced DCs.

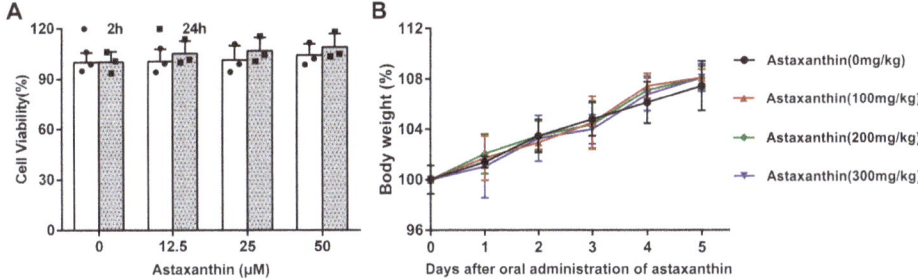

Figure 1. Biosafety evaluation of astaxanthin in vitro and in vivo. (**A**) The cytotoxicity of astaxanthin with different doses was performed in the DCs by using the CCK-8 assay. (**B**) Astaxanthin with different concentrations was given orally for five days every 24 h; the data represent the change of body weight in each group ($n = 10$/group). The data shown are the means ± s.d. of three replicates and are representative of three independent experiments. Statistical significance is assessed by unpaired Student's two-sided *t*-test to compare astaxanthin (0 µM).

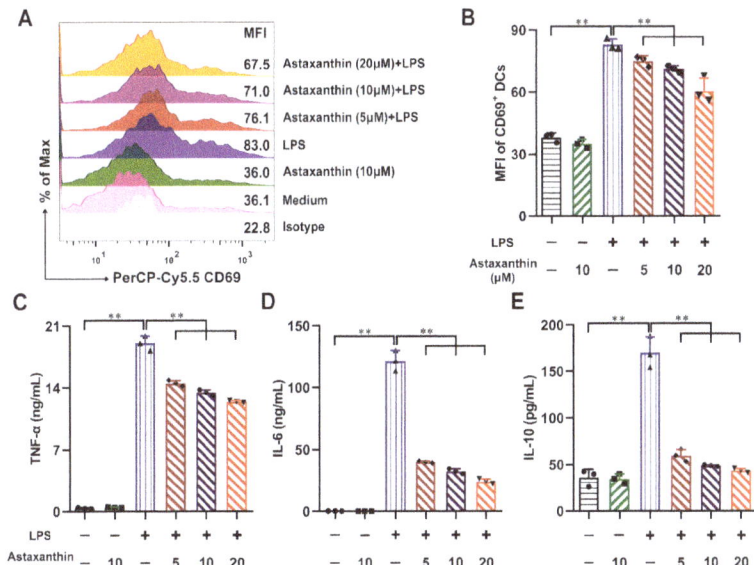

Figure 2. Astaxanthin suppressed the secretion of cytokines from LPS-stimulated DCs. DCs were incubated with the astaxanthin or plus 100 ng/mL LPS for 24 h. (**A,B**) The expression of activation marker CD69 on DCs was analyzed by FCM. (**C–E**) Supernatants were collected and TNF-α, IL-6, and IL-10 were detected by ELISA. The data shown are the means ± s.d. of three replicates and are representative of three independent experiments. Statistical significance is assessed by one-way ANOVA analysis to compare the results between different groups. ** $p < 0.01$.

2.2. Astaxanthin Reversed the Morphological Changes in LPS-Activated DCs

Mature DCs were easily aggregated to form larger clusters and longer extensions [33]. Upon LPS stimulation alone, the size of clusters and the extension morphologies of DCs were increased, compared with the untreated and the astaxanthin-alone group. However, these processes were impaired by astaxanthin (Figure 3A,C). Meanwhile, the size of clusters and the cell shape index (major axis/minor axis) of each group were measured. As shown in Figure 3B,D, these two indexes were markedly increased after LPS stimulation. Treatment of astaxanthin significantly suppressed the increase of two indexes in LPS-induced DCs. These results indicated that astaxanthin attenuated the morphological changes of LPS-activated DCs.

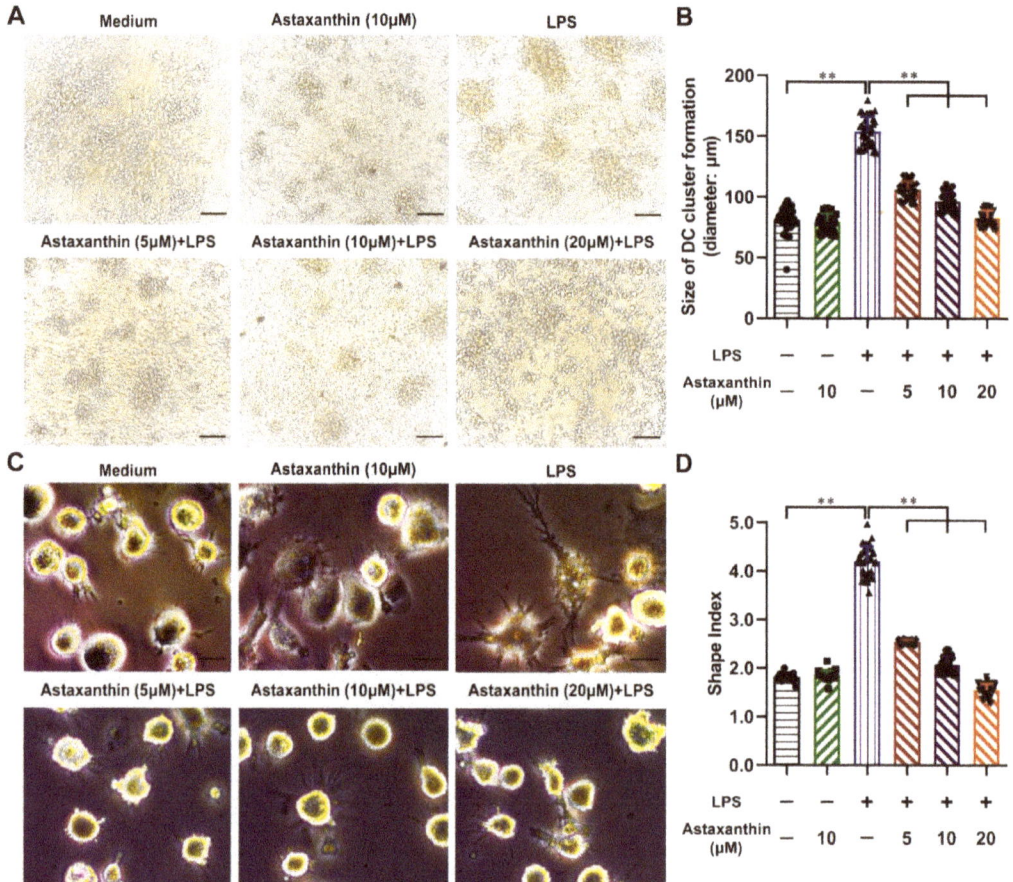

Figure 3. Astaxanthin decreased the morphological changes of LPS-stimulated DCs. After stimulation for 24 h with astaxanthin or plus 100 ng/mL LPS, DC aggregation (**A**) and dendrites (**C**) were observed by microscopy. (**B,D**) Statistical results on the size of DC cluster formation and the cellular shape indices in each group. Data shown are the means ± s.d. of 40 clusters or DCs randomly selected from 3 separate experiments. Statistical significance is assessed by one-way ANOVA analysis to compare the results between different groups. ** $p < 0.01$. Bars: (**A**) 100 µm; (**C**) 20 µm.

2.3. Astaxanthin Impaired the Phenotypic Maturation of LPS-Induced DCs

Maturation is the key step in the DC-mediated regulation of immune responses. To investigate whether astaxanthin modulated the DC maturation, the expression levels of MHCII and costimulatory molecules in DCs were analyzed by FCM. With LPS treatment alone, the expressions of MHCII, CD40, CD80, and CD86 were markedly upregulated, whereas they were down-regulated remarkably with the treatment of astaxanthin (Figure 4). These data suggested that astaxanthin diminished LPS-activated DC phenotypic maturation and compromised the immunostimulation of the activated DCs.

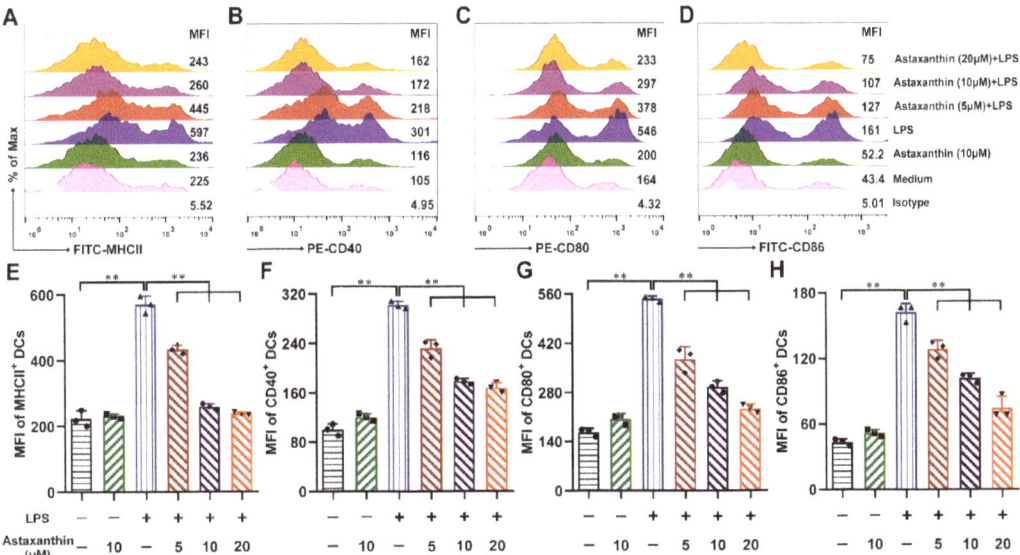

Figure 4. Astaxanthin suppressed the expression of phenotypic markers by LPS-stimulated DCs in vitro. After stimulation for 24 h with astaxanthin or plus 100 ng/mL LPS, the expressions of phenotypic markers on DCs, including MHCII (**A**,**E**), CD40 (**B**,**F**), CD80 (**C**,**G**), and CD86 (**D**,**H**), were analyzed by FCM. Data shown are the means ± s.d. of three replicates and are representative of three independent experiments. Statistical significance is assessed by one-way ANOVA analysis to compare the results between different groups. ** $p < 0.01$.

2.4. Astaxanthin Increased the Endocytosis Capability of LPS-Induced DCs

In response to inflammatory stimuli, DCs trigger the process of maturation; down-regulation of endocytosis is a hallmark of maturation [34]. To investigate whether astaxanthin modulated the endocytosis of DCs, the fluorescent marker dextran was used. As shown in Figure 5A,B, LPS alone significantly decreased the endocytosis capability of DCs compared to the untreated control, while astaxanthin enhanced the uptake of dextran in LPS-induced DCs. Moreover, confocal laser scanning microscopy (CLSM) images displayed the amount of Alexa Fluor 647-dextran existing in the body of LPS-induced DCs and was enhanced after the treatment of astaxanthin (Figure 5C). These results suggested that astaxanthin significantly increased the endocytosis capability of LPS-induced DCs.

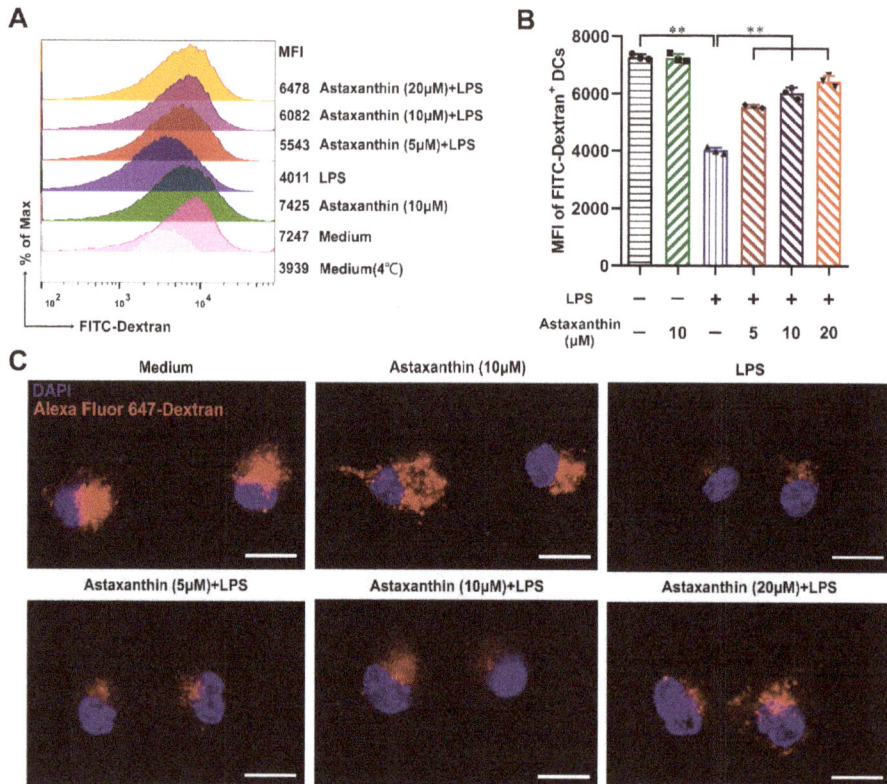

Figure 5. Astaxanthin enhanced the endocytosis ability of DCs after LPS treatment in vitro. After stimulation for 24 h with astaxanthin or plus 100 ng/mL LPS, the treated DCs were incubated with 1 mg/mL FITC-Dextran (**A**,**B**) or Alexa Fluor 647-Dextran (**C**) at 37 °C for 30 min. After incubation, the cells were washed three times with cold PBS and analyzed by FCM (**A**) or were observed by using confocal laser scanning microscopy (CLSM). Parallel experiments were performed at 4 °C to determine the nonspecific binding. The data shown are the means ± s.d. of three replicates and are representative of three independent experiments. (**C**) Dextran (Alexa Fluor 647; red) and Nuclei (4′,6-diamidino-2-phenylindole (DAPI); blue). The results are from one representative experiment of three performed. Bars: 10 μm. Statistical significance is assessed by one-way ANOVA analysis to compare the results between different groups. ** $p < 0.01$.

2.5. Astaxanthin Inhibited the Migration Capability of LPS-Induced DCs

DCs that are stimulated with inflammatory mediators can mature and migrate from nonlymphoid regions to lymphoid organs for initiating T cell-mediated immune responses. This migratory step is closely related to the CCR7 expression of DCs [35]. To investigate whether astaxanthin modulated the DC migration, the expression levels of CCR7 in DCs were analyzed by FCM. With LPS treatment alone, CCR7 expression was significantly increased, whereas they remarkably declined after the treatment of astaxanthin (Figure 6A,B). Moreover, chemotaxis assay in transwell chambers was used to examine the DC migration on the basis of attraction of mature DCs for CCL19 or CCL21. The migration of LPS-induced DCs was remarkably inhibited after the treatment of astaxanthin in response to CCL19 (Figure 6C,D). These results suggested that astaxanthin significantly inhibited the migration capability of LPS-induced DCs.

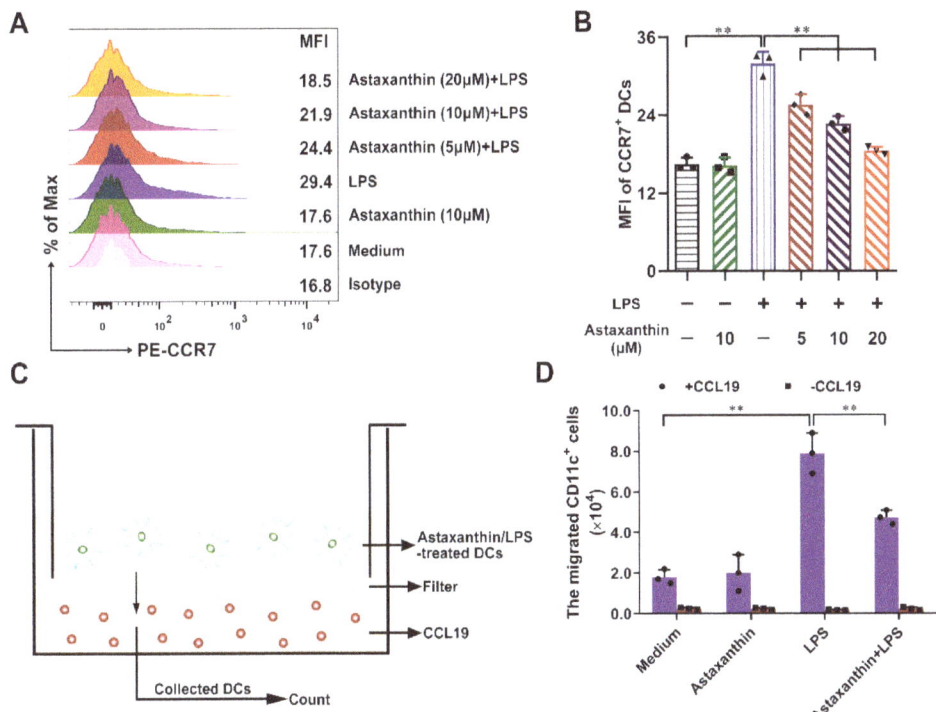

Figure 6. Astaxanthin decreased the LPS-induced CCR7 expression and DC's migration ability in vitro. DCs were incubated by astaxanthin or plus 100 ng/mL LPS for 24 h. (**A,B**) FCM analysis of CCR7 expression. Data shown are the means ± s.d. of three replicates and are representative of three independent experiments. (**C,D**) DCs from astaxanthin (10 μM) alone, LPS (100 ng/mL) alone, astaxanthin (10 μM) plus LPS (100 ng/mL) groups were seeded into the upper wells of a 24-well transwell chamber, and CCL19 (200 ng/mL) was included in lower chamber. After 4 h, the number of DCs that were transferred from the upper to the lower wells was counted by FCM. The spontaneous migration of cells (absence of CCL19) was also shown. Data shown are the means ± s.d. of three replicates and are representative of three independent experiments. Statistical significance is assessed by one-way ANOVA analysis to compare the results between different groups. ** $p < 0.01$.

2.6. Astaxanthin Impaired the Allostimulatory Capacity of LPS-Induced DCs

Mature DCs are potent stimulators of allogeneic T cell proliferation in the mixed lymphocyte reaction (MLR) [36]. To determine the effects of astaxanthin on the ability of LPS-induced DCs to stimulate the MLR, DCs were collected and incubated with allogeneic CD4[+] T cells. As shown in Figure 7, LPS-induced DCs stimulated proliferative responses more effectively than untreated DCs, while astaxanthin-treated DCs impaired proliferative responses derived from the LPS stimulation at all ratios of DC: T cell tests. These results suggested that astaxanthin strongly impaired the allostimulatory capacity of LPS-induced DCs.

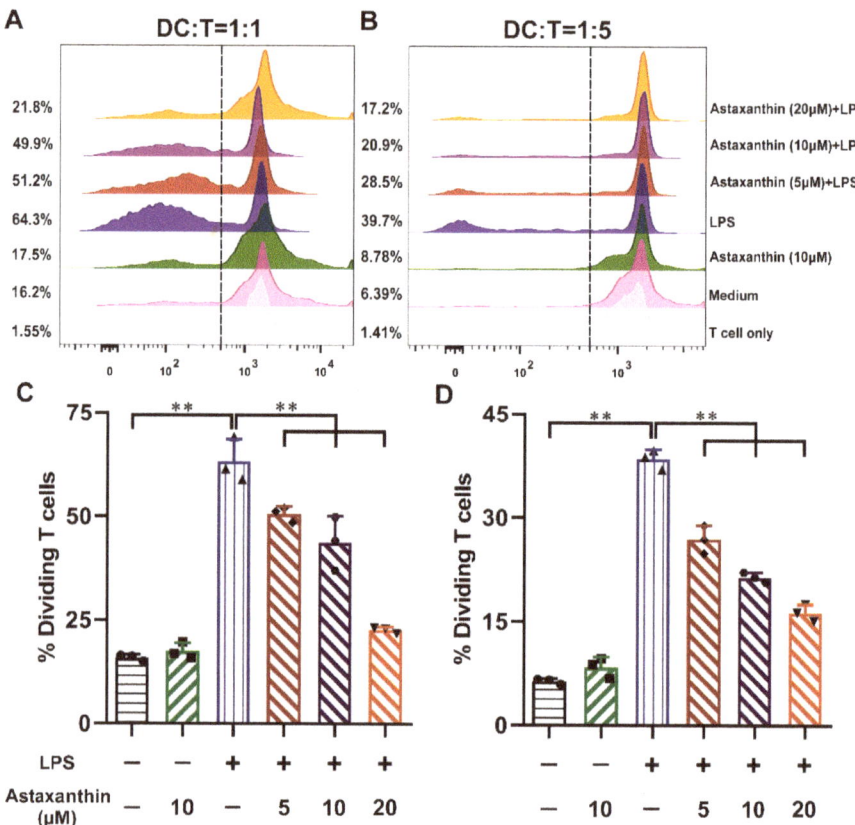

Figure 7. Astaxanthin decreased LPS-induced DCs to increase the proliferation of allogeneic T cells. After incubation with astaxanthin or plus 100 ng/mL LPS for 24 h, the collected DCs were used in two graded cell numbers (DC/T-cell ratios: 1:1 (**A,C**) and 1:5 (**B,D**)) to stimulate CFSE-labeled naive CD4$^+$ allogeneic T cells (5×10^5 responder cells per well). After 5 days, proliferation was detected by FCM. Data shown are the means ± s.d. of three replicates and are representative of three independent experiments. Statistical significance is assessed by one-way ANOVA analysis to compare the results between different groups. ** $p < 0.01$.

2.7. Astaxanthin Protected the LPS-Induced Immune Dysfunction of DCs via Activation of HO-1/Nrf2 Axis

To investigate whether astaxanthin modulated the DC maturation by the HO-1/Nrf2 pathway, the expression levels of HO-1 and Nrf2 on DCs were analyzed by FCM. As shown in Figure 8A–D, treatment of LPS-induced DCs with astaxanthin, HO-1, and Nrf2 were significantly upregulated, compared with the LPS-only group. Next, to study whether HO-1 played an important role in the suppression of DC maturation, the cytokine release (TNF-α and IL-10) (Figure 8I,J) and phenotypic markers (CD80 and CD86) (Figure 8E–H) were detected. The results showed that the effects of astaxanthin in the LPS-induced DCs were diminished when DCs were pretreated with SnPP (a HO-1 inhibitor) (Figure 8E–J). However, CoPP (a HO-1 inducer) aggravated the inhibitory effect of astaxanthin in the LPS-induced DCs (Figure 8E–J). Therefore, the Nrf2/HO-1 pathway played an important role in the inhibition of LPS-induced DCs maturation by astaxanthin.

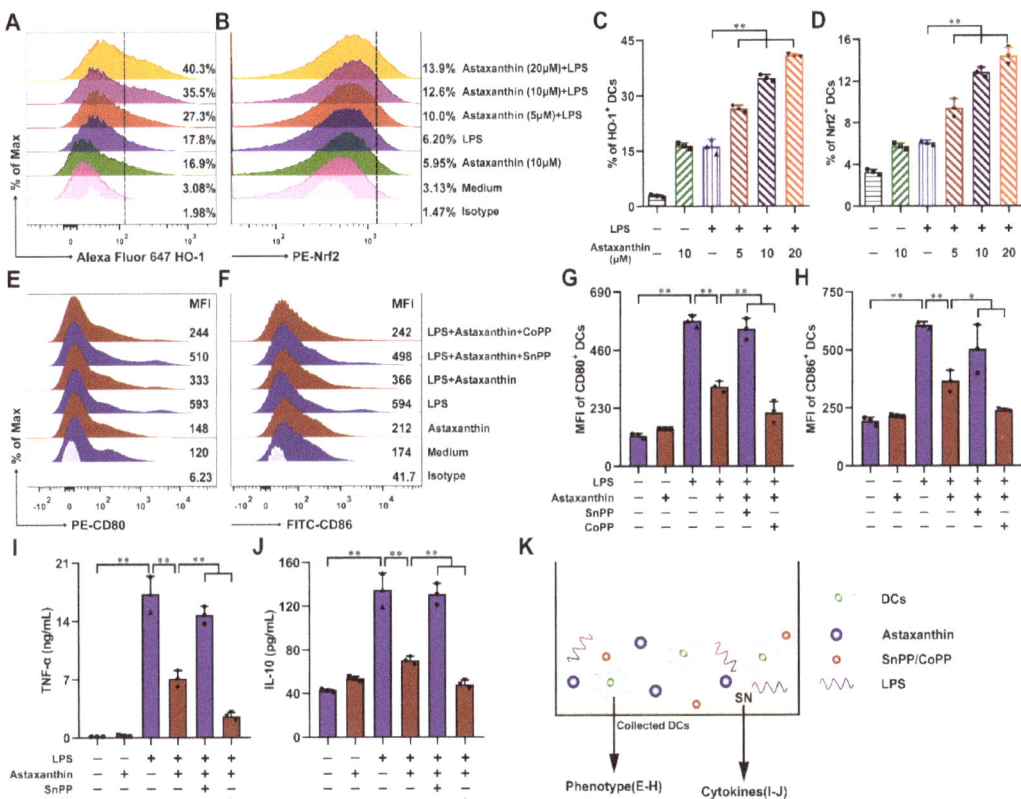

Figure 8. Astaxanthin enhanced the expression of HO-1 and Nrf2 protein in the LPS-induced DCs. (**A–D**) DCs were incubated by astaxanthin or plus 100 ng/mL LPS for 24 h. FCM analysis of HO-1 and Nrf2 expression. Data shown are the means ± s.d. of three replicates and are representative of three independent experiments. (**K**) Experimental setting to study DC maturation, DCs were treated with 10 µM astaxanthin or plus 100 ng/mL LPS in the presence or absence of SnPP (25 µM) or CoPP (50 µM) for 24 h. (**E–H**) The expressions of CD80 (**E,G**) and CD86 (**F,H**) were detected by FCM. (**I,J**) TNF-α and IL-10 released from supernatants were detected by ELISA. The data shown are the means ± s.d. of three replicates and are representative of three independent experiments. Statistical significance is assessed by one-way ANOVA analysis to compare the results between different groups. * $p < 0.05$; ** $p < 0.01$. SN: supernatant.

2.8. Astaxanthin Protected LPS-Induced Sepsis in Mice

The overwhelming production of pro-inflammatory cytokines and mediators results in tissue damage or lethality. To determine the effects of astaxanthin on the LPS-induced septic lethal rate and production of cytokines in LPS-challenged mice, firstly, the biosafety of astaxanthin was evaluated in mice. As shown in Figure 1B, the body weight of mice was not changed in the astaxanthin group compared with the control group, even if the dose used was up to 300 mg/kg. Next, the changes in body weight and survival rates were monitored after LPS injection for 3 days or 40 h, respectively. As shown in Figure 9A, LPS administration markedly increased the loss of body weight in mice. However, the astaxanthin recovered the change of body weight in the LPS-challenged mice. Moreover, the astaxanthin decreased the mortality of the LPS-treated mice (Figure 9B). Next, the levels of cytokines in mice serum were detected by ELISA. The results showed that administration of astaxanthin significantly decreased the production of TNF-α, IL-6, and IL-10 (Figure 9C–E). Taken together, these data demonstrated that astaxanthin effectively protected LPS-induced sepsis in mice.

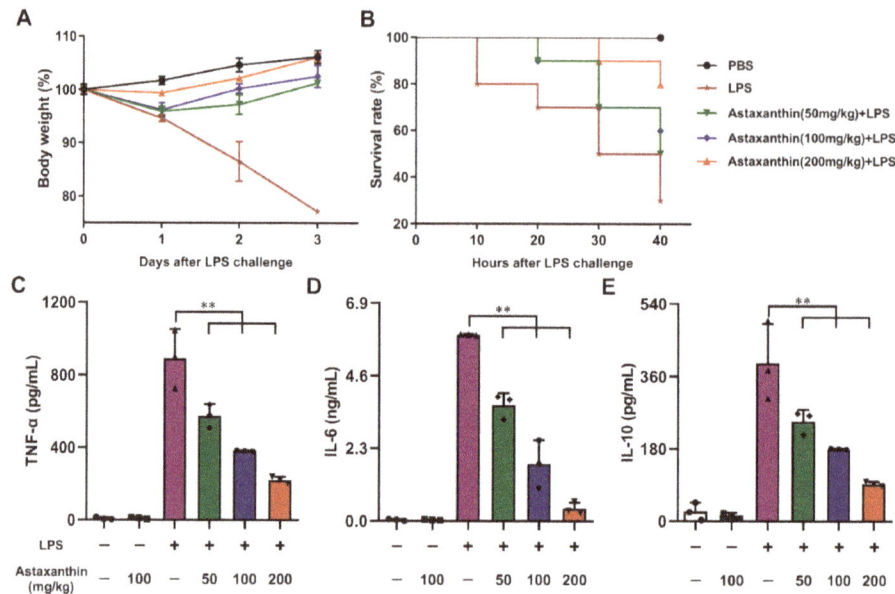

Figure 9. Astaxanthin recovered the changes in body weight and decreased the cytokines secretion in LPS-challenged mice. (**A,B**) The data represent the body weight changes and survival rates of each group ($n = 10$/group). (**C–E**) The level of cytokines in plasma was measured by ELISA. Data shown are the means ± s.d. of three replicates and are representative of three independent experiments. Statistical significance is assessed by one-way ANOVA analysis to compare the results between different groups. ** $p < 0.01$.

3. Discussion

Here, we explored the immunosuppressive properties of astaxanthin on the activation and maturation of DCs for the first time. Our data indicated that astaxanthin reduced the expression of activation markers (CD69), LPS-induced pro-inflammatory (TNF-α and IL-6), and anti-inflammatory (IL-10) cytokines by DCs; reversed the morphological changes of LPS-activated DCs; decreased the LPS-induced expression of phenotypic markers by DCs, including MHCII, CD40, CD80, and CD86; promoted the endocytosis levels in LPS-treated DCs; and hindered the LPS-induced migration of DCs via downregulating CCR7 expression. Furthermore, astaxanthin abrogated allogeneic T cell proliferation by LPS-induced DCs. Finally, astaxanthin enhanced the survival rate of LPS-challenged mice and inhibited the production of inflammatory cytokines in serum, suggesting that astaxanthin can strongly protect LPS-induced sepsis (Figure 10).These results powerfully implied that astaxanthin may have a potential application in the treatment of sepsis.

Toll-like receptor (TLR) 4 signaling, leading to secretion of inflammatory productions, has been considered as a critical pathway in sepsis pathophysiology. LPS from gram-negative bacteria interacted with TLR4 to cause phagocytic cells to robustly generate a variety of proinflammatory cytokines [37]. CD69, as a type II C-type lectin, is known as a very early activation marker, which is first upregulated upon primary activation [38,39]. In our study, we found that astaxanthin reduced the activation level of LPS-treated DCs by downregulating CD69 expression, suggesting that the immunosuppressive ability of astaxanthin was involved in the early inflammatory response. After DC activation, a mass of inflammatory cytokines was released. TNF-α, as a rapid proinflammatory cytokine, can strongly accelerate DC maturation [40]. Furthermore, TNF-α also can regulate other inflammatory cytokines, especially for IL-6 [41], implying that astaxanthin might suppress the secretion of TNF-α, and then result in the down-expression of IL-6 in DCs. At the late stage of sepsis, the anti-inflammatory state may appear, showing a high expression of

IL-10, which may result in a further impaired immune response with an increased risk of nosocomial infections [42]. Therefore, we evaluated the effects of astaxanthin treatment in LPS-induced IL-10 expression, and found that IL-10 was also decreased, and thereby, astaxanthin plays a remarkable inhibition role on both pro- and anti-inflammatory stages.

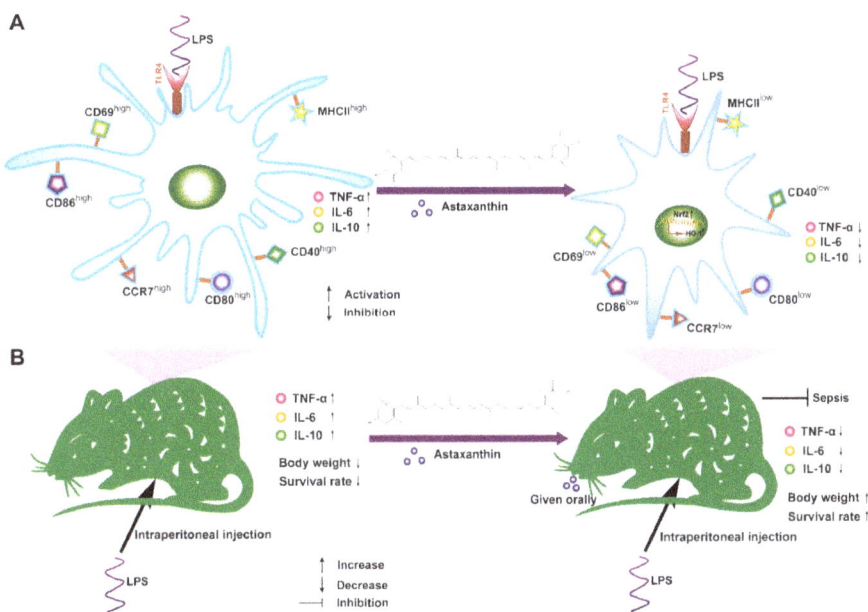

Figure 10. Schematic of the proposed mechanism for astaxanthin, rescuing the LPS-induced immune dysfunction of DCs and protecting LPS-induced sepsis in mice. (A) Astaxanthin firstly activated the Nrf2 signaling pathway, and then significantly upregulated HO-1 expression, which suppressed the immune functions of LPS-induced DCs, including activation markers (CD69), the cytokines release (TNF-α, IL-6, and IL-10), phenotypic marker (MHCII, CD40, CD80, and CD86) and migration marker (CCR7). (B) Astaxanthin decreased the production of TNF-α, IL-6, and IL-10 in serum, recovered the change in body weight and decreased the mortality of the LPS-treated mice.

DCs possess two major states, including immature DCs (iDCs) and mature DCs (mDCs). The iDCs have a strong antigen capture ability with lower expression of phenotypic markers. After antigen uptake, iDCs were transformed into mDCs, which have a strong ability to stimulate the proliferation and differentiation of T cells by upregulating the surface levels of MHCII and costimulatory molecules. Moreover, DCs can easily mature into inflammatory DCs, thereby sustaining a continuous activation of the adaptive immune response at inflammation sites [43]. However, iDCs were able to induce immune tolerance, and have therefore been introduced as a therapy for systemic lupus erythematosus (SLE) [44,45]. In our data, astaxanthin can effectively inhibit LPS-induced phenotypic markers of DCs, including MHCII, CD40, CD80, and CD86, suggesting that astaxanthin was able to prevent the transformation from iDCs into mDCs. In addition, LPS-induced DCs with astaxanthin treatment possessed a strong antigen capture ability, indicating that the DCs remain in an immature state. Furthermore, once DCs mature, the chemokine receptor CCR7 displays a high-upregulation, which will guide the DCs to migrate toward a draining lymph node, a T cell-rich area with a high expression of CCL19 and CCL21 (CCR7 ligands), for an expanded immune response [46]. Our data suggested that astaxanthin could probably block the connection between DCs and draining lymph nodes via down-regulating CCR7 expression, and lead to limit extensive immune responses. Even if contact happened, LPS-induced DCs with astaxanthin treatment were hardly promoted to a proliferation of allogeneic T cells in our allogeneic mixed lymphocyte reaction assay, which might be associated with the down-regulation of MHCII, costimulatory molecules, and cytokines.

Inflammation is the most common feature of many chronic diseases and complications. Previous studies have revealed that the transcription nuclear factor erythroid 2-related factor 2 (Nrf2) contributes to the anti-inflammatory process by orchestrating the recruitment of inflammatory cells and regulating gene expression through the antioxidant response element (ARE) [47]. Heme oxygenase-1 (HO-1) is the inducible isoform and rate-limiting enzyme that catalyzes the degradation of heme into carbon monoxide (CO) and free iron, and biliverdin to bilirubin [48]. Several studies have demonstrated that HO-1 and its metabolites have significant anti-inflammatory effects mediated by Nrf2 [49]. It has been reported that activation of Nrf2 prevents LPS-induced transcriptional upregulation of pro-inflammatory cytokines, including IL-6 and IL-1β [50]. Here, we have demonstrated that astaxanthin inhibited the maturation of LPS-induced DCs via the activation of the HO-1/Nrf2 axis. Interestingly, astaxanthin is a potential antioxidant, and the HO-1/Nrf2 axis is also a key known antioxidative pathway; whether astaxanthin utilizes its antioxidant property to activate the HO-1/Nrf2 pathway and then to initiate an anti-inflammatory response needs to be further investigated.

LPS and other PAMPs are related in the pathogenesis of sepsis and the activation of immune responses, resulting in tissue pathological injury and multiple organ failure [51]. Management of excessive inflammatory response is a key strategy for sepsis treatment [52]. In the present study, we performed a series of experiments to determine the anti-inflammatory activities of astaxanthin using LPS-challenged mice. Our results showed that administration of astaxanthin promoted the survival rate of LPS-challenged mice. Additionally, administration of astaxanthin reduced the levels of inflammatory cytokines in serum, including TNF-α, IL-6, and IL-10, which was in line with the result of DCs in vitro. These results implied that DC-targeted anti-inflammatory strategies have great potential in the treatment of sepsis.

4. Materials and Methods

4.1. Ethics Statement

The Jiangsu Administrative Committee for Laboratory Animals approved all of the animal studies according to the guidelines of Jiangsu Laboratory Animal Welfare and Ethical of Jiangsu Administrative Committee of Laboratory Animals (Permission number: SYXKSU-2007-0005).

4.2. Reagents

Astaxanthin (mol wt 596.84), LPS derived from *Escherichia coli* 026: B6, FITC-Dextran (mol wt 40,000) and Cobalt protoporphyrin (CoPP, a HO-1 inducer) were from Sigma-Aldrich. Alexa Fluor 647-Dextran (mol wt 10,000) was from Thermo Fisher. Carboxyfluorescein succinimidylester (CFSE) and RPMI 1640 medium were from Invitrogen. Fetal bovine serum (FBS) was from Hyclone. Recombinant CCL19, GM-CSF, and IL-4 were from Peprotech. CCK-8 kit was from Beyotime. $CD4^+$ T cell isolation kit was from Miltenyi Biotech. Fluorescent-labeled anti-mouse mAbs, PerCP-Cy5.5 CD69, FITC-MHCII, PE-CD40, PE-CD80, FITC-CD86, PE-CCR7 or respective isotype controls, were from BD PharMingen. Alexa Fluor 647 HO-1 or respective isotype was from Abcam. PE-Nrf2 or respective isotype was from Cell Signaling Technology. Tin protoporphyrin IX (SnPP, a HO-1 inhibitor) was from MedChemExpress.

4.3. Generation of DCs

Male C57BL/6 mice, 4–6 weeks old, were from the Animal Research Center of Yangzhou University (Jiangsu, China). The mice were housed under specific pathogen-free conditions for at least 1 week before use. DCs were isolated and cultured as our improved method [53]. Briefly, bone marrow cells were extracted from the tibias and femurs of mice, and then cultured in complete medium (RPMI 1640 supplemented with 10% FBS, 1%

streptomycin and penicillin, 10 ng/mL GM-CSF and 10 ng/mL IL-4). After 60 h of culture, medium was gently discarded and fresh medium was added. On day 6, non-adherent and loosely adherent DC aggregates were harvested and sub-cultured overnight. On day 7, only cultures with >90% cells expressing CD11c by flow cytometry (FCM) were used.

4.4. Cell Viability Assay

The cytotoxicity assay of astaxanthin with different doses was performed in DCs using the CCK-8 kit in accordance with the manufacturer's instructions. Briefly, 5×10^3 cells were cultured in 96-well plate. After treatment, 10 µL CCK-8 was added to each well, and the cells were incubated for an additional 1 h. The absorbance was measured at 450 nm, and the results were compared as a percentage of the control group.

4.5. Cytokine Assay

In vitro, the DCs were incubated with astaxanthin and/or LPS for 24 h. Next, the levels of TNF-α, IL-6, and IL-10 in the culture supernatants were measured by using ELISA kits (eBioscience) and were performed according to the manufacturer's instruction.

4.6. Phenotype Assay

DCs were harvested and washed twice with PBS, and incubated with FITC-MHCII, PE-CD40, PE-CD80, FITC-CD86, or their respective isotypes, at 4 °C for 30 min as per the manufacturer's guidelines. After being washed three times with PBS, DCs were analyzed by FCM.

4.7. Endocytosis Assay

The harvested DCs were incubated with 1 mg/mL FITC-Dextran at 37 °C for 30 min as previously described [54]. After incubation, DCs were washed twice with PBS and analyzed by FCM. In addition, 4 °C control was also performed to exclude adhesion.

4.8. Migration Assay

The chemotaxis of DCs was performed in a 24-well transwell chamber (pore size, 5 µm; Corning) as described previously [55]. DCs (1×10^5 cells) were then seeded onto the upper chambers and CCL19 (200 ng/mL) was added in the lower chamber. After incubation for 4 h, the migrated cells were collected from the lower chamber, and the number of cells was counted by FCM.

4.9. Allogeneic Mixed Lymphocyte Reaction Assay

Male BALB/c mice, 6 weeks old, were from the Animal Research Center of Yangzhou University (Jiangsu, China). Responder T cells were purified from mice splenic lymphocytes using a $CD4^+$ T cell isolation kit and labeled with CFSE according to the manufacturer's instructions. Next, these cells were cocultured in duplicate with DCs (DC/T cell ratios of 1:1 or 1:5) in 5% CO_2 incubator at 37 °C for 5 days and detected by FCM.

4.10. HO-1 and Nrf2 Protein Expression Assay

The treated DCs were incubated with Alexa Fluor 647 HO-1, PE-Nrf2, or the respective isotypes for 30 min at 4 °C. The cells were analyzed using FCM.

4.11. Body Weight Change Assay

Six-week-old C57BL/6 mice were divided into five groups (n = 10/group). In the treatment group, the mice were given astaxanthin orally for 4 days every 24 h, and the doses of astaxanthin were 50, 100, and 200 mg/kg, respectively; 48 h after the firstly oral administration, the mice received LPS (10 mg/kg body weight) by intraperitoneal injection, body weight changes were monitored for 3 days.

4.12. Survival Rate and Cytokine Assay

48 h after 1st oral administration, the mice received LPS (20 mg/kg body weight) by intraperitoneal injection, survival rates were monitored for 40 h as described previously [56]. The mice were euthanized and blood was collected at 4 h after LPS injection, the levels of cytokines (TNF-α, IL-6, and IL-10) in plasma were measured by an ELISA kit according to the manufacturer's protocol.

4.13. Statistical Analysis

Results were expressed as the means ± SD. Statistical significance between the 2 groups was determined by unpaired Student's two-sided *t*-test. To compare multiple groups, one-way ANOVA with Tukey's post hoc test was performed by using SPSS 17.0. * $p < 0.05$, ** $p < 0.01$.

5. Conclusions

In summary, our findings showed that astaxanthin inhibited the immune dysfunction of DCs induced by LPS via the activation of HO-1/Nrf2 axis in vitro, and enhanced the survival rate of LPS-challenged mice in vivo, which might be used as a potential candidate strategy for clinical sepsis.

Author Contributions: Conceptualization, Y.Y., C.L. and J.Y.; methodology, Y.Y., N.X., Y.S. and B.M.; software, Y.Y., B.Z. and D.S.; validation, Y.Y., C.L. and J.Y.; formal analysis, Y.Y., N.X., C.L. and J.Y.; investigation, Y.Y., N.X. and Z.X.; resources, Y.Y., C.L. and J.Y.; data curation, Y.Y., N.X.; writing—original draft preparation, Y.Y., C.L. and J.Y.; writing—review and editing, Y.Y., C.L. and J.Y.; visualization, Y.Y., N.X.; supervision, Y.Y., C.L. and J.Y.; project administration, Y.Y., C.L. and J.Y.; funding acquisition, Y.Y., C.L. All authors have read and agreed to the published version of the manuscript.

Funding: This research was funded by the National Natural Science Foundation of China (31600113, 31800284), the Agricultural Science and Technology Independent Innovation Fund of Jiangsu Province (CX(20)3092), a project funded by the Priority Academic Program Development of Jiangsu Higher Education (PAPD), and the Open Project Program of Jiangsu Key Laboratory of Zoonosis (R1909).

Institutional Review Board Statement: The study was conducted according to the guidelines of Jiangsu Laboratory Animal Welfare and Ethical, and approved by the Jiangsu Administrative Committee of Laboratory Animals (Permission number: SYXKSU-2007-0005).

Conflicts of Interest: The authors declare no conflict of interest.

References

1. Crimeen-Irwin, B.; Scalzo, K.; Gloster, S.; Mottram, P.L.; Plebanski, M. Failure of immune homeostasis—The consequences of under and over reactivity. *Curr. Drug Targets Immune Endocr. Metab. Disord.* **2005**, *5*, 413–422. [CrossRef]
2. Horwitz, D.A.; Fahmy, T.M.; Piccirillo, C.A.; La Cava, A. Rebalancing Immune Homeostasis to Treat Autoimmune Diseases. *Trends Immunol.* **2019**, *40*, 888–908. [CrossRef]
3. Fleischmann, C.; Scherag, A.; Adhikari, N.K.; Hartog, C.S.; Tsaganos, T.; Schlattmann, P.; Angus, D.C.; Reinhart, K.; International Forum of Acute Care Trialists. Assessment of Global Incidence and Mortality of Hospital-treated Sepsis. Current Estimates and Limitations. *Am. J. Respir. Crit. Care Med.* **2016**, *193*, 259–272. [CrossRef]
4. Liao, X.; Du, B.; Lu, M.; Wu, M.; Kang, Y. Current epidemiology of sepsis in mainland China. *Ann. Transl. Med.* **2016**, *4*, 324. [CrossRef]
5. van der Poll, T.; van de Veerdonk, F.L.; Scicluna, B.P.; Netea, M.G. The immunopathology of sepsis and potential therapeutic targets. *Nat. Rev. Immunol.* **2017**, *17*, 407–420. [CrossRef]
6. Baccala, R.; Gonzalez-Quintial, R.; Lawson, B.R.; Stern, M.E.; Kono, D.H.; Beutler, B.; Theofilopoulos, A.N. Sensors of the innate immune system: Their mode of action. *Nat. Rev. Rheumatol.* **2009**, *5*, 448–456. [CrossRef]
7. Steinhagen, F.; Schmidt, S.V.; Schewe, J.C.; Peukert, K.; Klinman, D.M.; Bode, C. Immunotherapy in sepsis—Brake or accelerate? *Pharm. Ther.* **2020**, *208*, 107476. [CrossRef] [PubMed]
8. Delano, M.J.; Ward, P.A. Sepsis-induced immune dysfunction: Can immune therapies reduce mortality? *J. Clin. Investig.* **2016**, *126*, 23–31. [CrossRef]
9. Yin, Y.; Qin, T.; Yu, Q.; Yang, Q. Bursopentin (BP5) from chicken bursa of fabricius attenuates the immune function of dendritic cells. *Amino Acids* **2014**, *46*, 1763–1774. [CrossRef]

10. Zhong, W.; Qian, K.; Xiong, J.; Ma, K.; Wang, A.; Zou, Y. Curcumin alleviates lipopolysaccharide induced sepsis and liver failure by suppression of oxidative stress-related inflammation via PI3K/AKT and NF-kappaB related signaling. *Biomed. Pharm.* **2016**, *83*, 302–313. [CrossRef]
11. Alsharif, K.F.; Almalki, A.A.; Al-Amer, O.; Mufti, A.H.; Theyab, A.; Lokman, M.S.; Ramadan, S.S.; Almeer, R.S.; Hafez, M.M.; Kassab, R.B.; et al. Oleuropein protects against lipopolysaccharide-induced sepsis and alleviates inflammatory responses in mice. *IUBMB Life* **2020**, *72*, 2121–2132. [CrossRef]
12. Banchereau, J.; Briere, F.; Caux, C.; Davoust, J.; Lebecque, S.; Liu, Y.J.; Pulendran, B.; Palucka, K. Immunobiology of dendritic cells. *Annu. Rev. Immunol.* **2000**, *18*, 767–811. [CrossRef]
13. Gallo, P.M.; Gallucci, S. The dendritic cell response to classic, emerging, and homeostatic danger signals. Implications for autoimmunity. *Front. Immunol.* **2013**, *4*, 138. [CrossRef]
14. Tisch, R. Immunogenic versus tolerogenic dendritic cells: A matter of maturation. *Int. Rev. Immunol.* **2010**, *29*, 111–118. [CrossRef]
15. Wu, D.D.; Li, T.; Ji, X.Y. Dendritic Cells in Sepsis: Pathological Alterations and Therapeutic Implications. *J. Immunol. Res.* **2017**, *2017*, 3591248. [CrossRef] [PubMed]
16. Fan, X.; Liu, Z.; Jin, H.; Yan, J.; Liang, H.P. Alterations of dendritic cells in sepsis: Featured role in immunoparalysis. *Biomed. Res. Int.* **2015**, *2015*, 903720. [CrossRef] [PubMed]
17. Oberholzer, A.; Oberholzer, C.; Efron, P.A.; Scumpia, P.O.; Uchida, T.; Bahjat, K.; Ungaro, R.; Tannahill, C.L.; Murday, M.; Bahjat, F.R.; et al. Functional modification of dendritic cells with recombinant adenovirus encoding interleukin 10 for the treatment of sepsis. *Shock* **2005**, *23*, 507–515. [PubMed]
18. Oberholzer, A.; Oberholzer, C.; Bahjat, K.S.; Ungaro, R.; Tannahill, C.L.; Murday, M.; Bahjat, F.R.; Abouhamze, Z.; Tsai, V.; LaFace, D.; et al. Increased survival in sepsis by in vivo adenovirus-induced expression of IL-10 in dendritic cells. *J. Immunol.* **2002**, *168*, 3412–3418. [CrossRef]
19. Qin, T.; Yin, Y.; Yu, Q.; Yang, Q. Bursopentin (BP5) protects dendritic cells from lipopolysaccharide-induced oxidative stress for immunosuppression. *PLoS ONE* **2015**, *10*, e0117477. [CrossRef] [PubMed]
20. Kishimoto, Y.; Yoshida, H.; Kondo, K. Potential Anti-Atherosclerotic Properties of Astaxanthin. *Mar. Drugs* **2016**, *14*, 35. [CrossRef]
21. Li, C.; Ma, B.; Chen, J.; Jeong, Y.; Xu, X. Astaxanthin Inhibits p70 S6 Kinase 1 Activity to Sensitize Insulin Signaling. *Mar. Drugs* **2020**, *18*, 495. [CrossRef]
22. Augusti, P.R.; Quatrin, A.; Somacal, S.; Conterato, G.M.; Sobieski, R.; Ruviaro, A.R.; Maurer, L.H.; Duarte, M.M.; Roehrs, M.; Emanuelli, T. Astaxanthin prevents changes in the activities of thioredoxin reductase and paraoxonase in hypercholesterolemic rabbits. *J. Clin. Biochem. Nutr.* **2012**, *51*, 42–49. [CrossRef] [PubMed]
23. Yang, Y.; Bae, M.; Kim, B.; Park, Y.K.; Koo, S.I.; Lee, J.Y. Astaxanthin prevents and reverses the activation of mouse primary hepatic stellate cells. *J. Nutr. Biochem.* **2016**, *29*, 21–26. [CrossRef] [PubMed]
24. Otsuka, T.; Shimazawa, M.; Inoue, Y.; Nakano, Y.; Ojino, K.; Izawa, H.; Tsuruma, K.; Ishibashi, T.; Hara, H. Astaxanthin Protects Against Retinal Damage: Evidence from In Vivo and In Vitro Retinal Ischemia and Reperfusion Models. *Curr. Eye Res.* **2016**, *41*, 1465–1472. [CrossRef] [PubMed]
25. Kim, B.; Farruggia, C.; Ku, C.S.; Pham, T.X.; Yang, Y.; Bae, M.; Wegner, C.J.; Farrell, N.J.; Harness, E.; Park, Y.K.; et al. Astaxanthin inhibits inflammation and fibrosis in the liver and adipose tissue of mouse models of diet-induced obesity and nonalcoholic steatohepatitis. *J. Nutr. Biochem.* **2017**, *43*, 27–35. [CrossRef]
26. Jia, Y.; Wu, C.; Kim, J.; Kim, B.; Lee, S.J. Astaxanthin reduces hepatic lipid accumulations in high-fat-fed C57BL/6J mice via activation of peroxisome proliferator-activated receptor (PPAR) alpha and inhibition of PPAR gamma and Akt. *J. Nutr. Biochem.* **2016**, *28*, 9–18. [CrossRef]
27. Zhang, L.; Wang, H. Multiple Mechanisms of Anti-Cancer Effects Exerted by Astaxanthin. *Mar. Drugs* **2015**, *13*, 4310–4330. [CrossRef]
28. Brown, D.R.; Gough, L.A.; Deb, S.K.; Sparks, S.A.; McNaughton, L.R. Astaxanthin in Exercise Metabolism, Performance and Recovery: A Review. *Front. Nutr.* **2017**, *4*, 76. [CrossRef]
29. Fang, Q.; Guo, S.; Zhou, H.; Han, R.; Wu, P.; Han, C. Astaxanthin protects against early burn-wound progression in rats by attenuating oxidative stress-induced inflammation and mitochondria-related apoptosis. *Sci. Rep.* **2017**, *7*, 41440. [CrossRef]
30. Ying, C.J.; Zhang, F.; Zhou, X.Y.; Hu, X.T.; Chen, J.; Wen, X.R.; Sun, Y.; Zheng, K.Y.; Tang, R.X.; Song, Y.J. Anti-inflammatory Effect of Astaxanthin on the Sickness Behavior Induced by Diabetes Mellitus. *Cell. Mol. Neurobiol.* **2015**, *35*, 1027–1037. [CrossRef] [PubMed]
31. Peng, Y.J.; Lu, J.W.; Liu, F.C.; Lee, C.H.; Lee, H.S.; Ho, Y.J.; Hsieh, T.H.; Wu, C.C.; Wang, C.C. Astaxanthin attenuates joint inflammation induced by monosodium urate crystals. *FASEB J.* **2020**, *34*, 11215–11226. [CrossRef] [PubMed]
32. Cai, X.; Chen, Y.; Xie, X.; Yao, D.; Ding, C.; Chen, M. Astaxanthin prevents against lipopolysaccharide-induced acute lung injury and sepsis via inhibiting activation of MAPK/NF-κB. *Am. J. Transl. Res.* **2019**, *11*, 1884–1894.
33. Zeng, X.; Wang, T.; Zhu, C.; Xing, X.; Ye, Y.; Lai, X.; Song, B.; Zeng, Y. Topographical and biological evidence revealed FTY720-mediated anergy-polarization of mouse bone marrow-derived dendritic cells in vitro. *PLoS ONE* **2012**, *7*, e34830. [CrossRef]
34. Platt, C.D.; Ma, J.K.; Chalouni, C.; Ebersold, M.; Bou-Reslan, H.; Carano, R.A.; Mellman, I.; Delamarre, L. Mature dendritic cells use endocytic receptors to capture and present antigens. *Proc. Natl. Acad. Sci. USA* **2010**, *107*, 4287–4292. [CrossRef] [PubMed]
35. Yanagihara, S.; Komura, E.; Nagafune, J.; Watarai, H.; Yamaguchi, Y. EBI1/CCR7 is a new member of dendritic cell chemokine receptor that is up-regulated upon maturation. *J. Immunol.* **1998**, *161*, 3096–3102. [PubMed]

36. Freudenthal, P.S.; Steinman, R.M. The distinct surface of human blood dendritic cells, as observed after an improved isolation method. *Proc. Natl. Acad. Sci. USA* **1990**, *87*, 7698–7702. [CrossRef]
37. Bosmann, M.; Ward, P.A. The inflammatory response in sepsis. *Trends Immunol.* **2013**, *34*, 129–136. [CrossRef]
38. Kimura, M.Y.; Koyama-Nasu, R.; Yagi, R.; Nakayama, T. A new therapeutic target: The CD69-Myl9 system in immune responses. *Semin. Immunopathol.* **2019**, *41*, 349–358. [CrossRef]
39. Alari-Pahissa, E.; Notario, L.; Lorente, E.; Vega-Ramos, J.; Justel, A.; Lopez, D.; Villadangos, J.A.; Lauzurica, P. CD69 does not affect the extent of T cell priming. *PLoS ONE* **2012**, *7*, e48593. [CrossRef] [PubMed]
40. Ding, X.; Yang, W.; Shi, X.; Du, P.; Su, L.; Qin, Z.; Chen, J.; Deng, H. TNF receptor 1 mediates dendritic cell maturation and CD8 T cell response through two distinct mechanisms. *J. Immunol.* **2011**, *187*, 1184–1191. [CrossRef]
41. Trevejo, J.M.; Marino, M.W.; Philpott, N.; Josien, R.; Richards, E.C.; Elkon, K.B.; Falck-Pedersen, E. TNF-alpha -dependent maturation of local dendritic cells is critical for activating the adaptive immune response to virus infection. *Proc. Natl. Acad. Sci. USA* **2001**, *98*, 12162–12167. [CrossRef]
42. Hibbert, J.E.; Currie, A.; Strunk, T. Sepsis-Induced Immunosuppression in Neonates. *Front. Pediatr.* **2018**, *6*, 357. [CrossRef] [PubMed]
43. Jensen, S.S.; Gad, M. Differential induction of inflammatory cytokines by dendritic cells treated with novel TLR-agonist and cytokine based cocktails: Targeting dendritic cells in autoimmunity. *J. Inflamm.* **2010**, *7*, 37. [CrossRef]
44. Huang, C.; Zhang, L.; Ling, F.; Wen, S.; Luo, Y.; Liu, H.; Liu, J.; Zheng, W.; Liang, M.; Sun, J.; et al. Effect of immune tolerance induced by immature dendritic cells and CTLA4-Ig on systemic lupus erythematosus: An in vivo study. *Exp. Ther. Med.* **2018**, *15*, 2499–2506. [CrossRef] [PubMed]
45. Mok, M.Y. Tolerogenic dendritic cells: Role and therapeutic implications in systemic lupus erythematosus. *Int. J. Rheum. Dis.* **2015**, *18*, 250–259. [CrossRef]
46. Alvarez, D.; Vollmann, E.H.; von Andrian, U.H. Mechanisms and consequences of dendritic cell migration. *Immunity* **2008**, *29*, 325–342. [CrossRef]
47. Kim, J.H.; Yu, S.; Chen, J.D.; Kong, A.N. The nuclear cofactor RAC3/AIB1/SRC-3 enhances Nrf2 signaling by interacting with transactivation domains. *Oncogene* **2013**, *32*, 514–527. [CrossRef]
48. Otterbein, L.E.; Soares, M.P.; Yamashita, K.; Bach, F.H. Heme oxygenase-1: Unleashing the protective properties of heme. *Trends Immunol.* **2003**, *24*, 449–455. [CrossRef]
49. Ahmed, S.M.; Luo, L.; Namani, A.; Wang, X.J.; Tang, X. Nrf2 signaling pathway: Pivotal roles in inflammation. *Biochim. Biophys. Acta Mol. Basis Dis.* **2017**, *1863*, 585–597. [CrossRef] [PubMed]
50. Kobayashi, E.H.; Suzuki, T.; Funayama, R.; Nagashima, T.; Hayashi, M.; Sekine, H.; Tanaka, N.; Moriguchi, T.; Motohashi, H.; Nakayama, K.; et al. Nrf2 suppresses macrophage inflammatory response by blocking proinflammatory cytokine transcription. *Nat. Commun.* **2016**, *7*, 11624. [CrossRef]
51. Cohen, J. The immunopathogenesis of sepsis. *Nature* **2002**, *420*, 885–891. [CrossRef] [PubMed]
52. Toner, P.; McAuley, D.F.; Shyamsundar, M. Aspirin as a potential treatment in sepsis or acute respiratory distress syndrome. *Crit. Care* **2015**, *19*, 374. [CrossRef]
53. Yin, Y.; Qin, T.; Wang, X.; Lin, J.; Yu, Q.; Yang, Q. CpG DNA assists the whole inactivated H9N2 influenza virus in crossing the intestinal epithelial barriers via transepithelial uptake of dendritic cell dendrites. *Mucosal Immunol.* **2015**, *8*, 799–814. [CrossRef]
54. Lutz, M.B.; Assmann, C.U.; Girolomoni, G.; Ricciardi-Castagnoli, P. Different cytokines regulate antigen uptake and presentation of a precursor dendritic cell line. *Eur. J. Immunol.* **1996**, *26*, 586–594. [CrossRef]
55. Qin, T.; Ma, S.; Miao, X.; Tang, Y.; Huangfu, D.; Wang, J.; Jiang, J.; Xu, N.; Yin, Y.; Chen, Y.; et al. Mucosal Vaccination for Influenza Protection Enhanced by Catalytic Immune-Adjuvant. *Adv. Sci.* **2020**, *7*, 2000771. [CrossRef]
56. Marton, A.; Kolozsi, C.; Kusz, E.; Olah, Z.; Letoha, T.; Vizler, C.; Pecze, L. Propylene-glycol aggravates LPS-induced sepsis through production of TNF-alpha and IL-6. *Iran. J. Immunol.* **2014**, *11*, 113–122.

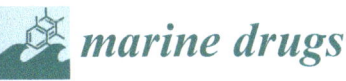

Article

Astaxanthin Provides Antioxidant Protection in LPS-Induced Dendritic Cells for Inflammatory Control

Yinyan Yin [1,2,*,†], Nuo Xu [1,†], Tao Qin [3], Bangyue Zhou [1], Yi Shi [1], Xinyi Zhao [3], Bixia Ma [4], Zhengzhong Xu [5] and Chunmei Li [4,*]

1. College of Medicine, Yangzhou University, Yangzhou 225009, China; kf56xunuo58@126.com (N.X.); zby18252737828@163.com (B.Z.); sy15365888238@163.com (Y.S.)
2. Jiangsu Key Laboratory of Experimental and Translational Non-Coding RNA Research, Yangzhou University, Yangzhou 225009, China
3. College of Veterinary Medicine, Yangzhou University, Yangzhou 225009, China; qintao@yzu.edu.cn (T.Q.); yangzhoudaxuezxy@163.com (X.Z.)
4. College of Food Science and Engineering, Yangzhou University, Yangzhou 225009, China; mabixia@vazyme.com
5. Jiangsu Key Laboratory of Zoonosis, Yangzhou University, Yangzhou 225009, China; zzxu@yzu.edu.cn
* Correspondence: yyyin@yzu.edu.cn (Y.Y.); licm@yzu.edu.cn (C.L.)
† These authors contributed equally.

Abstract: Astaxanthin, originating from marine organisms, is a natural bioactive compound with powerful antioxidant activity. Here, we evaluated the antioxidant ability of astaxanthin on dendritic cells (DCs), a key target of immune regulation, for inflammatory control in a sepsis model. Our results showed that astaxanthin suppressed nitric oxide (NO) production, reactive oxygen species (ROS) production, and lipid peroxidation activities in LPS-induced DCs and LPS-challenged mice. Moreover, the reduced glutathione (GSH) levels and the GSH/GSSG ratio were increased, suggesting that astaxanthin elevated the level of cellular reductive status. Meanwhile, the activities of antioxidant enzymes, including glutathione peroxidase (GPx), catalase (CAT), and superoxide dismutase (SOD), were significantly upregulated. Astaxanthin also inhibited the LPS-induced secretions of IL-1β, IL-17, and TGF-β cytokines. Finally, we found that the expressions of heme oxygenase 1 (HO-1) and nuclear factor erythroid 2-related factor 2 (Nrf2) were significantly upregulated by astaxanthin in LPS-induced DCs, suggesting that the HO-1/Nrf2 pathway plays a significant role in the suppression of oxidative stress. These results suggested that astaxanthin possesses strong antioxidant characteristics in DC-related inflammatory responses, which is expected to have potential as a method of sepsis treatment.

Keywords: astaxanthin; oxidative stress; sepsis; dendritic cells; inflammation

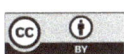

1. Introduction

Sepsis is an organic dysfunction caused by a disordered host response to infection by viruses, fungi, and bacteria [1–4], which remains a major cause of morbidity and mortality worldwide, with increased burden in low- and middle-resource settings [5]. In the United States, the treatment of sepsis accounted for more than USD 20 billion (5.2%) in total hospital expenses in 2011 [6]. An extrapolation from high-income country data suggests that on a yearly basis, there are an estimated 31.5 million sepsis and 19.4 million severe sepsis cases, with a potential 5.3 million deaths globally [7]. Although more than 100 clinical therapeutic trials have been conducted, no treatment options for sepsis are currently approved by the US Food and Drug Administration (FDA) [8].

After infection, the components of the pathogen, such as lipopolysaccharide (LPS), a key component of the bacterial cell wall, are recognized by macrophages, dendritic cells (DCs), and other immune cells, and then the overloaded inflammatory immune response is activated in early septic patients [9]. Historically, direct anti-hyperinflammatory strategies that attempt to block cytokines, such as interleukin-1 (IL-1) and tumor necrosis factor (TNF), have been the main therapeutic pathway against sepsis. However, the outcome of life-threatening infection is determined by the endogenous complicated inflammatory response. Therefore, using a conventional anti-inflammatory strategy in sepsis cases has to date failed to improve outcomes [8]. Notably, exposure to LPS can induce the rapid and robust production of reactive oxygen species (ROS), which is also a critical pathological feature in septic patients [10]. Oxidative stress is induced by an imbalanced redox state, involving either the excessive generation of ROS or dysfunction of the antioxidant system [11], resulting in the induction of cellular damage, impairment of the DNA repair system, and mitochondrial dysfunction [12]. A growing number of studies agree that interdependence and interconnection are not to be neglected between oxidative stress and inflammation, which co-exist in the inflamed microenvironment. Abundant ROS are released by inflammatory cells at the inflammatory site, which results in exaggerated oxidative injury. Meanwhile, a large amount of ROS and oxidative stress products strengthen proinflammatory responses [13]. Therefore, versatile antioxidants need to be developed to help control overwhelming oxidative stress and hyperinflammatory responses.

DCs are key regulators of innate and adaptive immunity [14]. The maturation of DCs is directed by signal transduction events downstream of Toll-like receptors (TLRs) and other pattern recognition receptors, following an increase in the production of cytokines, chemokines, and costimulatory molecules [15]. Just as importantly, DCs that possess strong antioxidant systems not only regulate the balance of oxidative stress but also influence the levels of inflammatory responses through the polarization of T cells. Therefore, DCs are an ideal target to manage both oxidative stress and inflammatory responses by some multifunctional antioxidants. Astaxanthin originates from seafood, such as microalgae, trout, yeasts, salmon, and krill [16,17]. Of note, a freshwater unicellular alga, named *Haematococcus pluvialis* (*H. pluvialis*), contains abundant natural astaxanthin [17,18]. Its structure is a xanthophyll carotenoid with hydroxyl and keto moieties on both ends (Figure 1) [19], which effectively scavenges free radicals, thereby protecting fatty acid and biological membranes from oxidative damage [20]. Astaxanthin also can attenuate inflammatory injury caused by diabetes-induced sickness and urate crystal-induced arthritis [21,22].

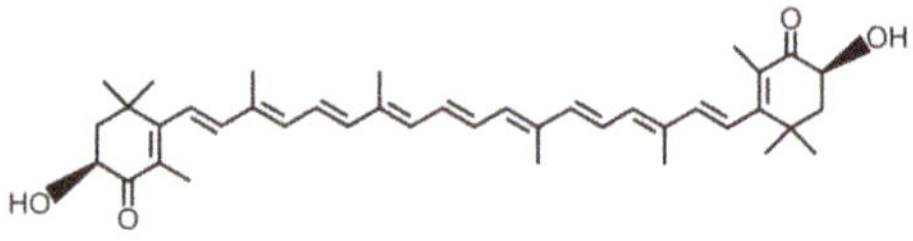

Figure 1. Chemical structure of astaxanthin.

Here, the antioxidant ability of astaxanthin was systematically evaluated on DCs for inflammatory control, which provides evidence that a DC-targeting strategy could be effectively applied in sepsis treatment.

2. Results

2.1. Astaxanthin Suppressed NO Production in LPS-Induced DCs and LPS-Challenged Mice

Nitric oxide (NO) plays a significant role in killing pathogens; however, excessive NO production has been identified as a key pathogenic factor in most immune-mediated diseases [23]. As shown in Figure 2A, LPS was shown to strongly stimulate NO production in DCs compared with an untreated group. Of note, astaxanthin was shown to remarkably suppress NO production in LPS-induced DCs. Many studies have documented an increase in NO production in response to severe sepsis or LPS administration [24]. Therefore, we further examined whether astaxanthin could affect NO levels in LPS-challenged mice. Mice were pre-treated with astaxanthin for 2 days and then injected with LPS. After LPS injection for 4 h, serum samples were collected for NO detection. We found that the administration of astaxanthin significantly decreased NO production in serum after LPS challenge (Figure 2B).

Collectively, these findings suggested that astaxanthin strongly inhibited NO production in LPS-induced DCs and LPS-challenged mice.

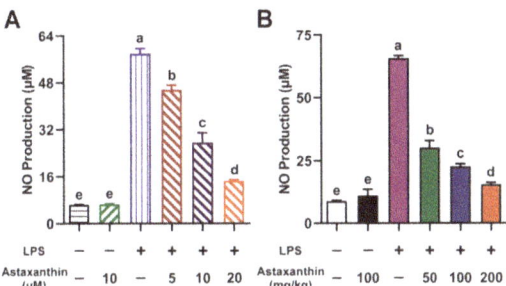

Figure 2. Astaxanthin suppressed the NO production in LPS-induced DCs and LPS-challenged mice. (**A**) DCs were incubated with the indicated concentrations of astaxanthin and LPS (100 ng/mL) for 24 h. (**B**) C57BL/6 mice were orally given astaxanthin before LPS injection. NO production in DC supernatants and serum was detected using the Griess reagent. Results are from one representative experiment of three performed. All of the data are presented as means ± SD. The comparisons were performed with analysis of variance (ANOVA) (multiple groups). Different lowercase letters indicate significant differences between groups ($p < 0.05$).

2.2. Astaxanthin Decreased ROS Levels in LPS-Induced DCs

Oxidative stress refers to elevated intracellular levels of ROS, which result in damage to cellular lipids, proteins, and DNA. Next, intracellular ROS was measured as described previously, with some modifications [25]. As shown in Figure 3, ROS levels were remarkably increased after exposure to LPS for 24 h, whereas astaxanthin strongly attenuated the LPS-induced ROS production in a dose-dependent manner.

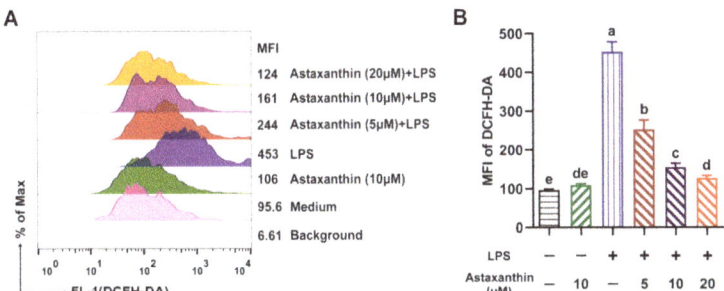

Figure 3. Astaxanthin suppressed the ROS production in LPS-induced DCs. (**A**) After stimulation for 24 h with astaxanthin and LPS (100 ng/mL), DCs were stained with 2′,7′ dichlorofluorescein diacetate (DCFH-DA) and analyzed by flow cytometry (FCM) for ROS detection. (**B**) Results are from one representative experiment of three performed. All of the data are presented as means ± SD. The comparisons were performed with analysis of variance (ANOVA) (multiple groups). Different lowercase letters indicate significant differences between groups ($p < 0.05$).

2.3. Astaxanthin Exhibited Anti-Lipid Peroxidation Activities in LPS-Induced DCs and LPS-Challenged Mice

Maleic dialdehyde (MDA) is commonly known as a marker of oxidative stress and antioxidant status in cells [26]. To investigate whether astaxanthin modulated lipid peroxidation activities in LPS-induced DCs, the intracellular level of MDA was measured. Compared with the control group, the MDA level was significantly elevated in the LPS-only group, while it was remarkably inhibited by the treatment of astaxanthin in a dose-dependent manner (Figure 4A). The serum MDA is a marker of lipid peroxidation in sepsis [27]. Our murine serum results showed a significant decrease in MDA levels after the administration of astaxanthin in LPS-challenged mice (Figure 4B).

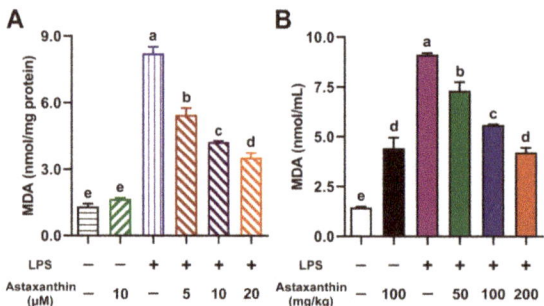

Figure 4. Astaxanthin suppressed lipid peroxidation in LPS-induced DCs and LPS-challenged mice. (**A**) DCs were incubated with the indicated concentrations of astaxanthin and LPS (100 ng/mL) for 24 h. (**B**) C57BL/6 mice were orally given astaxanthin before LPS injection. Blood was sampled at 4 h after LPS injection. The MDA contents in DC lysate supernatants and murine serum were measured as described in the Materials and Methods section. Results are from one representative experiment of three performed. The comparisons were performed with analysis of variance (ANOVA) (multiple groups). Different lowercase letters indicate significant differences between groups ($p < 0.05$).

2.4. Astaxanthin Exhibited Modulating Effects on Intracellular GSH, GSSG, and the GSH/GSSG Ratio in LPS-Induced DCs

We further investigated the effects of astaxanthin on the cellular levels of reduced glutathione (GSH), oxidized glutathione (GSSG), and their ratio (GSH/GSSG) in LPS-induced DCs. As shown in Figure 5, LPS significantly decreased the GSH level, increased the GSSG level, and reduced the GSH/GSSG ratio compared with the control. However, astaxanthin remarkably reversed this process in a dose-dependent manner.

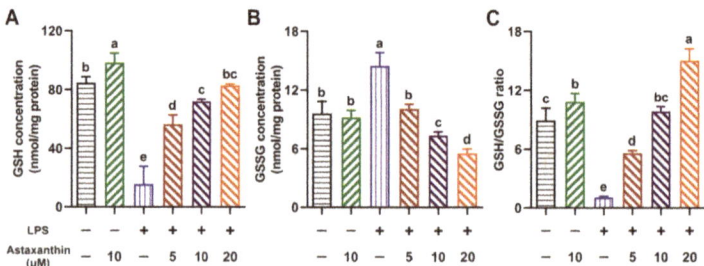

Figure 5. Astaxanthin modulated the intracellular GSH, GSSG, and GSH/GSSG ratio in LPS-induced DCs. After stimulation for 24 h with astaxanthin and LPS (100 ng/mL), the levels of GSH (**A**) and GSSG (**B**), and the ratio of GSH/GSSG (**C**), in DCs were measured as described in the Materials and Methods section. Results are from one representative experiment of three performed. The comparisons were performed with analysis of variance (ANOVA) (multiple groups). Different lowercase letters indicate significant differences between groups ($p < 0.05$).

2.5. Astaxanthin Exhibited Enhancing Effects on Antioxidant Enzyme Activities in LPS-Induced DCs and LPS-Challenged Mice

The cells are equipped with a variety of antioxidants, such as glutathione peroxidase (GPx), catalase (CAT), and superoxide dismutase (SOD), which served to counterbalance the effect of oxidants [28]. Therefore, we evaluated the effects of astaxanthin on the activities of antioxidative enzymes (GPx, CAT, and SOD) in LPS-induced DCs. As shown in

Figure 6A–C, LPS destroyed the antioxidant system of DCs through decreases in GPx, CAT, and SOD activity. Surprisingly, astaxanthin possessed the ability to increase the activities of these antioxidative enzymes in a dose-dependent manner. Meanwhile, the activities of serum GPx, CAT, and SOD were also detected in LPS-challenged mice. As expected, the administration of astaxanthin remarkably upregulated the serum GPx, CAT, and SOD activities in LPS-challenged mice (Figure 6D–F). Collectively, these results indicated that astaxanthin strongly elevated the activities of the antioxidant enzymes in LPS-induced DCs and LPS-challenged mice.

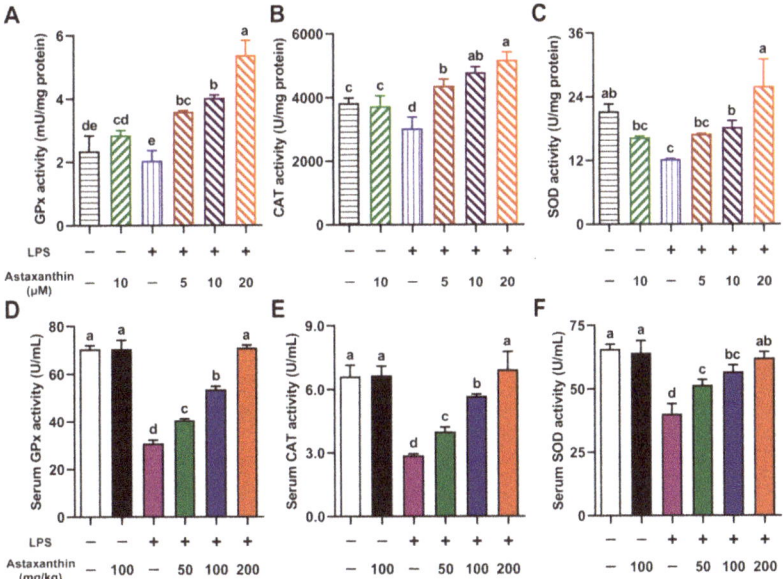

Figure 6. Astaxanthin enhanced the activities of antioxidant enzymes in LPS-induced DCs and LPS-challenged mice. (**A**–**C**) DCs were incubated with the indicated concentrations of astaxanthin and LPS (100 ng/mL) for 24 h. (**D**–**F**) C57BL/6 mice were orally given astaxanthin before LPS injection. Serum was sampled at 4 h after LPS injection. The levels of GPx, CAT, and SOD in the lysate of DCs or serum were measured as described in the Materials and Methods section. Results are from one representative experiment of three performed. Data are presented as means ± SD. The comparisons were performed with analysis of variance (ANOVA) (multiple groups). Different lowercase letters indicate significant differences between groups ($p < 0.05$).

2.6. Astaxanthin Exhibited Inhibitive Effects on Cytokine Production in LPS-Induced DCs and LPS-Challenged Mice

To investigate whether astaxanthin modulated the production of cytokines in LPS-induced DCs, the levels of interleukin-1β (IL-1β), interleukin-17 (IL-17), and transforming growth factor-beta (TGF-β) in supernatants of DCs were measured by an enzyme-linked immunosorbent assay (ELISA). After being exposed to LPS (100 ng/mL) for 24 h, the secretion of IL-1β, IL-17, and TGF-β cytokines was upregulated, whereas it was significantly inhibited by the treatment of astaxanthin in a dose-dependent manner (Figure 7A–C). LPS-induced sepsis is associated with overloaded cytokines [29]; therefore, serum samples were collected from mice. As shown in Figure 7D–F, LPS administration markedly increased the levels of IL-1β, IL-17, and TGF-β in mice. As expected, astaxanthin treatment significantly decreased the expression of these cytokines in a dose-dependent manner. These results suggested that astaxanthin strongly inhibited cytokine production in LPS-induced DCs and LPS-challenged mice.

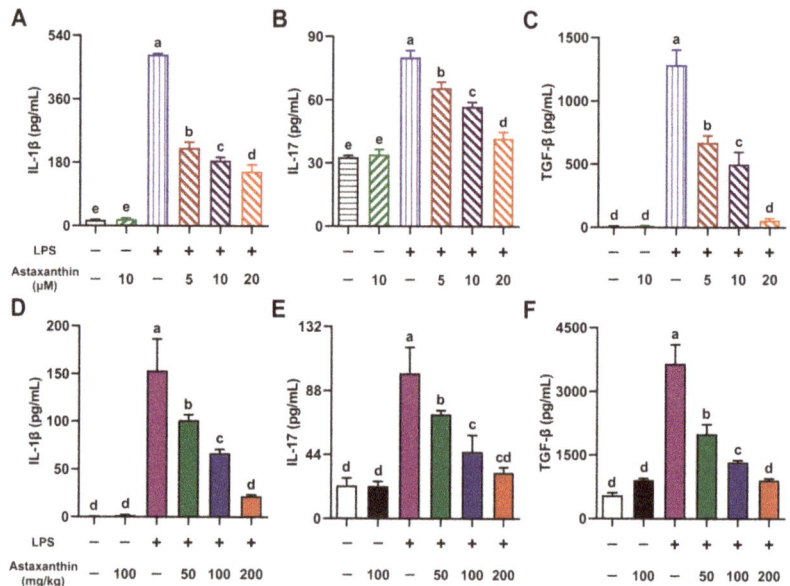

Figure 7. Astaxanthin efficiently impaired the secretion of cytokines in LPS-induced DCs and LPS-challenged mice. (**A–C**) DCs were incubated with the indicated concentrations of astaxanthin and LPS (100 ng/mL) for 24 h. (**D–F**) C57BL/6 mice were orally given astaxanthin before LPS injection, and then serum was sampled at 4 h after LPS injection. Levels of IL-1β, IL-17, and TGF-β in DC supernatants or serum were measured by ELISA. Results are from one representative experiment of three performed. Data are presented as means ± SD. The comparisons were performed with analysis of variance (ANOVA) (multiple groups). Different lowercase letters indicate significant differences between groups ($p < 0.05$).

2.7. HO-1/Nrf2 Axis Played a Key Role in Suppression of Oxidative Stress in LPS-Induced DCs

Heme oxygenase 1 (HO-1) and its products can also provide beneficial protection against oxidative injury. Nuclear factor erythroid 2-related factor 2 (Nrf2) is a cytoprotective factor that regulates gene expression for antioxidant and anti-inflammatory properties [30]. Therefore, we detected the expression levels of HO-1 and Nrf2 in DCs by Western blot. Our results demonstrated that astaxanthin treatment significantly upregulated the expression of HO-1 and Nrf2 in LPS-induced DCs (Figure 8A–C). We further investigated whether HO-1 played a significant role in the antioxidant effects of astaxanthin in LPS-induced DCs. We detected the NO production (Figure 8D), intracellular GSH (Figure 8E), GSSG (Figure 8F), the GSH/GSSG ratio (Figure 8G), and the SOD activity (Figure 8H). Significantly, tin protoporphyrin IX (SnPP, an inhibitor of HO-1) reversed the antioxidant effects of astaxanthin in LPS-induced DCs (Figure 8D–H), whereas the suppressive effect of astaxanthin was further aggravated by cobalt protoporphyrin (CoPP, an inducer of HO-1) (Figure 8D–H). Taken together, this showed that the HO-1/Nrf2 axis played a key role in the suppression of oxidative stress in LPS-induced DCs.

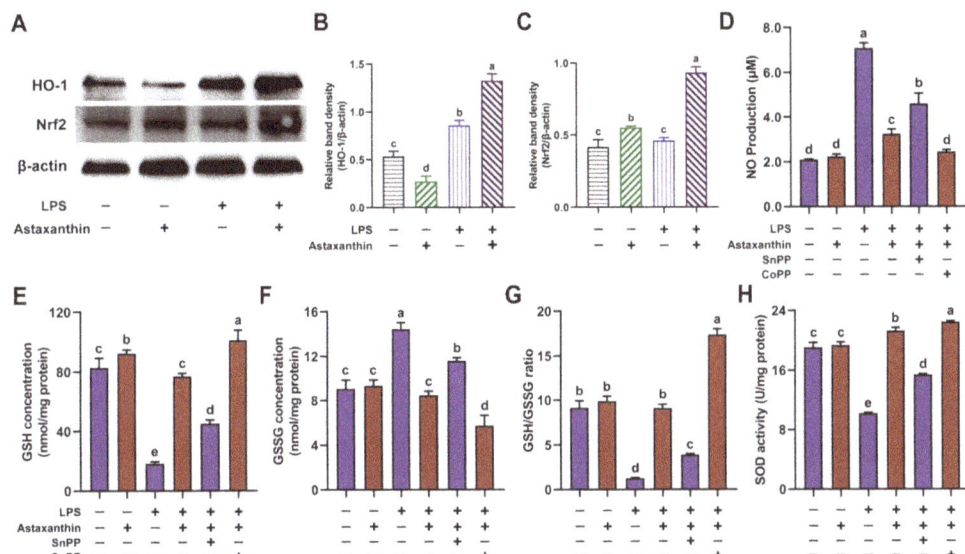

Figure 8. Astaxanthin suppressed oxidative stress via HO-1/Nrf2 axis in LPS-induced DCs. (**A–C**) After stimulation for 24 h with astaxanthin and LPS (100 ng/mL), HO-1 and Nrf2 levels were assessed by Western blot. (**D–H**) DCs were incubated with astaxanthin (10 µM) and LPS (100 ng/mL) in the presence or absence of SnPP (25 µM) or CoPP (50 µM) for 24 h. (**D**) NO production in DC supernatants was measured using the Griess reagent. (**E–H**) The levels of GSH (**E**), GSSG (**F**), and SOD (**H**), and the ratio of GSH/GSSG (**G**), in DCs were measured as described in the Materials and Methods section. Results are from one representative experiment of three performed. Data are presented as means ± SD. The comparisons were performed with analysis of variance (ANOVA) (multiple groups). Different lowercase letters indicate significant differences between groups ($p < 0.05$).

3. Discussion

Previously, we found that astaxanthin strongly inhibited the immune dysfunction of DCs induced by LPS [31]. Here, our work further shows the antioxidative effects of astaxanthin in DCs and mice, which is a potential key aspect of inflammatory control in the sepsis model (Figure 9). These investigational results demonstrated that astaxanthin reduced NO production, ROS production, and lipid peroxidation activities in LPS-induced DCs and LPS-challenged mice. Meanwhile, the GSH level, the GSH/GSSG ratio, and antioxidant enzyme (GPx, CAT, and SOD) activities were upregulated during the above processes. Based on these antioxidant properties, astaxanthin strongly inhibited the cytokine production (IL-1β, IL-17, and TGF-β) in LPS-induced DCs and LPS-challenged mice. Furthermore, we found that the antioxidation mechanism of astaxanthin depended on the HO-1/Nrf2 axis.

NO, an intracellular messenger, regulates cellular functions, such as inflammation and pathogen elimination [32]. However, excess NO can combine with O_2^- to form $ONOO^-$, which results in oxidative stress and cellular injury [33]. ROS, generated through a variety of extracellular and intracellular actions, have gained attention as novel signal mediators which are involved in growth, differentiation, progression, and cell death [34]. However, the overproduction of ROS induces significant oxidative stress, resulting in the damage of cell structures, including lipids, membranes, proteins, and DNA [35]. Lipid peroxidation can directly affect the biophysical properties and alter other biophysical characteristics of cell membranes. In addition, cell membrane fluidity is decreased by lipid peroxidation [36]. Meanwhile, ROS can react with polyunsaturated fatty acids of lipid membranes and induce lipid peroxidation [37]. In this study, our results suggested that astaxanthin exerts powerful suppressive effects on NO production, ROS levels, and lipid peroxidation in vitro and in vivo, which play a key role in reversing overloaded LPS-induced oxidative stress.

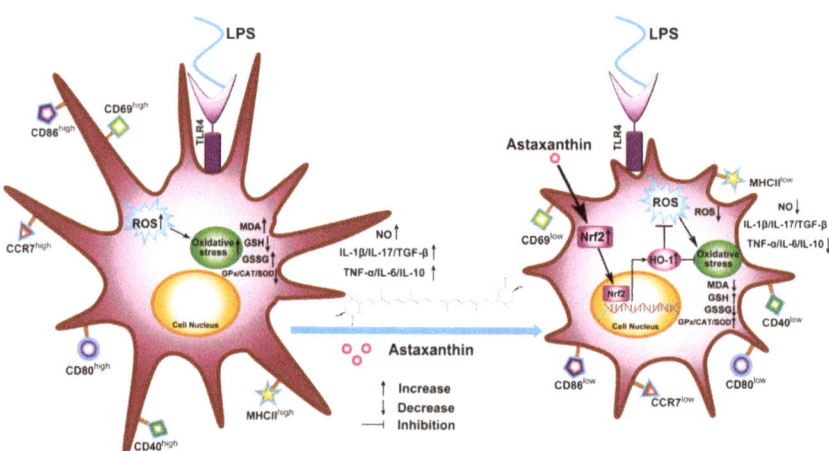

Figure 9. Schematic of proposed mechanism of antioxidant protection of astaxanthin for inflammatory control in LPS-induced DCs. The HO-1/Nrf2 axis was activated by astaxanthin, which inhibited the oxidative stress of LPS-induced DCs, including NO production, ROS production, the lipid peroxidation activities, the GSH level, the GSH/GSSG ratio, and antioxidant enzyme (GPx, CAT, and SOD) activities. These antioxidant properties are conducive to inflammatory controls in DCs, including decreases in levels of activation marker (CD69), the release of cytokines (IL-1β, IL-17, TGF-β, TNF-α, IL-6, and IL-10), phenotypic markers (MHCII, CD40, CD80, and CD86), and a migration marker (CCR7) by astaxanthin.

Previous studies have found that high concentrations of glutathione within cells provide protection against different ROS [32]. GSH, a ubiquitous tripeptide thiol, is known as a vital intracellular and extracellular protective antioxidant, which plays a series of key roles in the control of signaling processes, detoxifying certain xenobiotics and heavy metals [38]. Furthermore, GSH is considered to be one of the most important scavengers of ROS, and its ratio with GSSG may be used as a marker of oxidative stress [38]. The GSH/GSSG redox couple can readily interact with most of the physiologically relevant redox couples, undergoing reversible oxidation or reduction reactions, thereby maintaining the appropriate redox balance in the cells [39]. Under oxidative stress conditions, the GSH can convert itself to GSSG, and the reduction of H_2O_2 is catalyzed by the GPx enzyme [40]. Importantly, the addition of astaxanthin to DCs was shown to dramatically attenuate intracellular oxidative stress, indicative of an increase in GSH levels, the GSH/GSSG ratio, and GPx enzyme activity.

Apart from the GPx, other antioxidant enzymes, including CAT and SOD, also play a very important role in the defense of cells against oxygen-derived free radicals. CAT is a ubiquitous enzyme found in all known organisms, and can transform two H_2O_2 into two H_2O and O_2 [41]. SOD activity was discovered by McCord and Fridovich in 1969, which can dismutate two superoxide anions (O_2^-) into H_2O_2 and O_2 [42]. Our results indicated that astaxanthin significantly upregulates the activities of CAT and SOD, suggesting that the increase in antioxidative enzyme activity might be beneficial to the suppression of oxidative stress.

LPS, derived from Gram-negative bacteria, interacts with Toll-like receptor 4 (TLR4) to cause phagocytic cells to robustly generate a variety of proinflammatory cytokines [43]. Interleukin-1β (IL-1β) is a key proinflammatory cytokine involved in host responses to pathogens and tissue injury [44]. Monocytes, macrophages, and DCs are major IL-1β sources and release this cytokine in response to stimuli such as pathogen-associated or danger-associated molecular patterns (PAMPs or DAMPs) mediated by signaling via several TLR pathways [45]. IL-17 is not only a proinflammatory cytokine, but also a potent mediator of inflammatory responses in various tissues [46]. IL-17 induces multiple genes associated with inflammation, including interleukin-6 (IL-6), and granulocyte-macrophage colony-stimulating factor (GM-CSF) [47–49]. In addition, IL-17 enhances the proinflammatory responses induced by IL-1β [50,51], implying that astaxanthin might downregulate the production of IL-1β and IL-17 to protect LPS-induced sepsis. TGF-β is required for IL-17 to produce T helper cell (Th-17 cell) differentiation [52]. In our data, astaxanthin reduced the production of IL-1β, IL-17, and TGF-β in LPS-induced DCs and in LPS-challenged mice, which is in line with our previous findings that showed a decrease in TNF-α, IL-6, and IL-10 caused by astaxanthin in an LPS-induced DC model [31]. These data suggest that astaxanthin, as an antioxidant, can effectively mitigate overloaded cytokine production in vitro and in vivo. The TLR family of receptors can activate the innate immune system by DAMPs that are released during conditions of oxidative stress [53]. ROS from NADPH oxidase can signal the commencement of inflammatory pathways through TLRs. Therefore, we speculated that astaxanthin utilizes its antioxidant property to control inflammation, which might be a promising strategy for treating sepsis. However, the mechanism needs to be further investigated.

Previously, astaxanthin was shown to suppress an LPS-induced increase in inflammatory factors via mitogen-activated protein kinase (MAPK) phosphorylation and nuclear factor-κB (NF-κB) activation in vivo [54]. Here, we demonstrated that astaxanthin inhibited the oxidative stress in LPS-induced DCs and LPS-challenged mice via the activation of the HO-1/Nrf2 pathway. Nrf2 is a transcription factor responsible for the regulation of cellular redox balance and protective antioxidant and phase II detoxification responses [55,56]. Several studies have demonstrated that HO-1 genes are regulated through Nrf2 and play a crucial role in the development of oxidative stress [57]. HO-1, a stress-inducible enzyme, cooperates with NADPH cytochrome P450 to degrade heme in order to produce three bioactive products: iron ions, carbon monoxide (CO), and biliverdin, with the latter being rapidly converted to bilirubin. Biliverdin and bilirubin are potent antioxidants; meanwhile, the other products of HO-1 activity regulate inflammation, apoptosis, and angiogenesis [30]. In addition, CO, an end product of HO-1, can also inhibit NO production and inducible nitric oxide synthase (iNOS) expression via the inactivation of NF-κB [58]. It has been reported that the activation of Nrf2 may prevent an increase in ROS generation through NADPH oxidase [59]. Additionally, the overexpression of HO-1 was also able to inhibit NO production and iNOS expression [58]. Therefore, the activation of the Nrf2/HO-1 axis plays a significant role in protecting host cells against oxidative stress [60].

4. Materials and Methods

4.1. Ethics Statement

Animal studies were approved by the Jiangsu Administrative Committee for Laboratory Animals (permission number: SYXK(SU)2017-0044) and complied with the guidelines for laboratory animal welfare and ethics of the Jiangsu Administrative Committee for Laboratory Animals.

4.2. Materials

Astaxanthin, cobalt protoporphyrin (CoPP, an inducer of HO-1), and LPS (from *Escherichia coli* 026: B6) were obtained from Sigma-Aldrich (St. Louis, MO, USA). Tin protoporphyrin IX (SnPP, an inhibitor of HO-1) was obtained from MedChemExpress (Monmouth Junction, NJ, USA). Rabbit anti-mouse β-actin, rabbit anti-mouse HO-1, and goat anti-rabbit IgG-horseradish peroxidase (HRP) were sourced from Bioworld (St. Louis Park, MN, USA). Recombinant mouse GM-CSF and interleukin-4 (IL-4) were obtained from Peprotech (Rocky Hill, NJ, USA). RPMI 1640 medium and fetal bovine serum (FBS) were sourced from Thermo Fisher Scientific (Waltham, MA, USA). Streptomycin and penicillin were obtained from Invitrogen (Grand Island, NY, USA).

4.3. Generation of Bone Marrow-Derived DCs (BMDCs)

BMDCs were isolated and cultured using our improved method [61]. In brief, bone marrow cells were obtained from the tibias and femurs of C57BL/6 mice and cultured in complete medium (RPMI 1640 with 10% FBS, 1% streptomycin and penicillin (Invitrogen, Grand Island, NY, USA), 10 ng/mL GM-CSF and IL-4). The nonadherent cells were discarded and fresh medium was added after 60 h of culture. On day 6, nonadherent and loosely adherent cells were harvested and then cultured overnight. Only cultures with >90% cells expressing CD11c by FCM were used for the experiments.

4.4. LPS-Induced Sepsis

C57BL/6 mice, aged 6 weeks old, were randomly divided into five groups ($n = 10$/group), as described previously [31]. Astaxanthin (50, 100, and 200 mg/kg body weight) was orally administered for 2 days every 24 h; 48 h after the 1st oral administration, the mice were injected intraperitoneally with LPS (20 mg/kg body weight). Serum specimens were harvested 4 h after LPS treatment and were stored at $-20\ °C$ until use.

4.5. Cytokine Assays by ELISA

In vitro, the DCs were incubated with the indicated concentrations of astaxanthin and LPS (100 ng/mL) for 24 h. The culture supernatants were collected. IL-1β, IL-17, and TGF-β in supernatants or serum specimens were determined by using ELISA kits (eBioscience, San Diego, CA, USA) according to the manufacturer's instructions.

4.6. Determination of NO Production

Nitrite (NO_2^-) was measured as an indicator of NO synthesis and was estimated using the Griess reagent [62]. A NO detection kit (Beyotime, Shanghai, China) was used according to the manufacturer's instructions. In brief, 50 μL samples were mixed with an equal volume of Griess reagents I and II at room temperature. The absorbance was determined at 540 nm and calibrated with a nitrite standard curve to determine the nitrate concentration in samples.

4.7. Determination of ROS

In brief, after being treated with the indicated concentrations of astaxanthin or astaxanthin plus LPS (100 ng/mL) for 24 h, DCs were collected and incubated with 10 μM DCFH-DA (Beyotime, Shanghai, China) for 20 min at 37 °C. After being washed three times with PBS, ROS generation was analyzed by FCM.

4.8. Determination of the Lipid Peroxidation

MDA is the marker of lipid peroxidation [63]. In vitro, after stimulation for 24 h with astaxanthin or astaxanthin plus LPS, DCs were collected and lysed with RIPA buffer. The MDA content in the cell lysate supernatants or serum specimens was measured with thiobarbituric acid (TBA) according to the manufacturer's instructions (NJBC, Nanjing, China). Briefly, 100 μL samples were mixed with 1 ml of TBA working solution. After being heated for 40 min at 95 °C and cooled to room temperature, the absorbance of the organic layer was determined at 530 nm.

4.9. Determination of the GSH and GSSG

In vitro, after stimulation for 24 h with astaxanthin or astaxanthin plus LPS, DCs were lysed by sonication in ice-cold 5% metaphosphoric acid and centrifuged at $10,000 \times g$ for 20 min to remove debris. The total glutathione (T-GSH) content and GSSG content in the cell lysate supernatants were measured by T-GSH/GSSG kits (NJBC, Nanjing, China) according to the manufacturer's instructions. The GSH content was obtained by subtracting the $2 \times$ GSSG values from the T-GSH values.

4.10. Determination of the Antioxidant Enzyme Activity

In vitro, after stimulation for 24 h with astaxanthin or astaxanthin plus LPS, DCs were collected and lysed with RIPA buffer. The GPx activity in the cell lysate supernatants or serum specimens was measured by the GPx assay kit (NJBC, Nanjing, China). In brief, 10 µL samples were mixed with 10 µL of GPx assay working solution and 176 µL of GPx assay buffer at 25 °C for 5 min. Then, 4 µL of cumene hydroperoxide initiated the reaction and absorbance was measured at 340 nm for 3 min.

The SOD activity in the cell lysate supernatants or serum specimens was measured by the SOD assay kit (NJBC, Nanjing, China) according to the manufacturer's instructions. The absorbance was measured at 450 nm.

The CAT activity was detected in samples by the CAT assay kit (NJBC, Nanjing, China). Briefly, the samples were treated with excess H_2O_2 for an exact time, and a substrate coupled with the remaining H_2O_2. After treatment with peroxidase, the absorbance was measured at 520 nm.

4.11. Western Blot

Cells were washed once with ice-cold PBS and lysed with RIPA buffer. Protein concentrations were measured by the bicinchoninic acid (BCA) protein assay kit (Thermo Fisher Scientific, Waltham, MA, USA). Protein extracts were separated on an SDS-PAGE and then transferred to the poly (vinylidene fluoride) (PVDF) membrane. After blocking with 5% dry powdered milk for 2 h, the membrane was immunolabeled with rabbit anti-mouse HO-1 or rabbit anti-mouse β-actin overnight at 4 °C, followed by goat anti-rabbit IgG-HRP for 1 h at room temperature. The membranes were developed in order to visualize the protein by adding an enhanced chemiluminescence reagent (Pierce, Rockford, IL, USA). Autoradiograms were scanned and analyzed with Quantity One (Bio-Rad, Hercules, CA, USA) to quantify band densities.

4.12. Statistical Analysis

The results were expressed as the means ± SD and analyzed with GraphPad Prism 8 software (San Diego, CA, USA). One-way ANOVA analysis of variance was used to compare the variance between different groups. Differences were considered statistically significant when the value of p was <0.05.

5. Conclusions

In summary, astaxanthin protected LPS-induced DCs and LPS-challenged mice from oxidative stress via the HO-1/Nrf2 axis to achieve overloaded inflammatory control. These data indicate that astaxanthin is a potential candidate drug that could be applied to treat various inflammatory diseases.

Author Contributions: Conceptualization, Y.Y. and C.L.; methodology, Y.Y., N.X., T.Q., and B.M.; software, Y.Y., B.Z., and Y.S.; validation, Y.Y., X.Z., and Z.X.; formal analysis, Y.Y., N.X., and C.L.; investigation, Y.Y., N.X., and T.Q.; resources, Y.Y. and C.L.; data curation, Y.Y. and N.X.; writing—original draft preparation, Y.Y., C.L., and T.Q.; writing—review and editing, Y.Y., T.Q., and C.L.; visualization, Y.Y. and N.X.; supervision, Y.Y., T.Q., and C.L.; project administration, Y.Y. and C.L.; funding acquisition, Y.Y., C.L., and T.Q. All authors have read and agreed to the published version of the manuscript.

Funding: This research was funded by the National Natural Science Foundation of China (31600113, 31800284), the Agricultural Science & Technology Independent Innovation Fund of Jiangsu Province (CX(20)3092), the 2020 Interdisciplinary Project of Yangzhou University Veterinary Special Zone (yzuxk202004), the Jiangsu Provincial Natural Science Fund for Excellent Young Scholars (BK20200105), a project funded by the Priority Academic Program Development of Jiangsu Higher Education (PAPD), and the Open Project Program of Jiangsu Key Laboratory of Zoonosis (R1909).

Institutional Review Board Statement: The study was conducted according to the guidelines of Jiangsu Laboratory Animal Welfare and Ethical Committee, and approved by the Jiangsu Administrative Committee of Laboratory Animals (permission number: SYXK(SU)2017-0044).

Data Availability Statement: The data presented in this study are available upon request from the corresponding author.

Conflicts of Interest: The authors declare no conflict of interest.

References

1. Yuki, K.; Koutsogiannaki, S. Pattern recognition receptors as therapeutic targets for bacterial, viral and fungal sepsis. *Int. Immunopharmacol.* **2021**, *98*, 107909. [CrossRef]
2. Sands, K.; Carvalho, M.J.; Portal, E.; Thomson, K.; Dyer, C.; Akpulu, C.; Andrews, R.; Ferreira, A.; Gillespie, D.; Hender, T.; et al. Characterization of antimicrobial-resistant Gram-negative bacteria that cause neonatal sepsis in seven low- and middle-income countries. *Nat. Microbiol.* **2021**, *6*, 512–523. [CrossRef] [PubMed]
3. Singer, M.; Deutschman, C.S.; Seymour, C.W.; Shankar-Hari, M.; Annane, D.; Bauer, M.; Bellomo, R.; Bernard, G.R.; Chiche, J.D.; Coopersmith, C.M.; et al. The Third International Consensus Definitions for Sepsis and Septic Shock (Sepsis-3). *JAMA* **2016**, *315*, 801–810. [CrossRef] [PubMed]
4. Beltran-Garcia, J.; Osca-Verdegal, R.; Pallardo, F.V.; Ferreres, J.; Rodriguez, M.; Mulet, S.; Sanchis-Gomar, F.; Carbonell, N.; Garcia-Gimenez, J.L. Oxidative Stress and Inflammation in COVID-19-Associated Sepsis: The Potential Role of Anti-Oxidant Therapy in Avoiding Disease Progression. *Antioxidants* **2020**, *9*, 936. [CrossRef]
5. Salomao, R.; Ferreira, B.L.; Salomao, M.C.; Santos, S.S.; Azevedo, L.C.P.; Brunialti, M.K.C. Sepsis: Evolving concepts and challenges. *Braz. J. Med. Biol. Res.* **2019**, *52*, e8595. [CrossRef]
6. Torio, C.M.; Andrews, R.M. National Inpatient Hospital Costs: The Most Expensive Conditions by Payer, 2011: Statistical Brief #160. In *Healthcare Cost and Utilization Project (HCUP) Statistical Briefs*; Agency for Healthcare Research and Quality: Rockville, MD, USA, 2006.
7. Fleischmann, C.; Scherag, A.; Adhikari, N.K.; Hartog, C.S.; Tsaganos, T.; Schlattmann, P.; Angus, D.C.; Reinhart, K.; International Forum of Acute Care Trialists. Assessment of Global Incidence and Mortality of Hospital-treated Sepsis. Current Estimates and Limitations. *Am. J. Respir. Crit. Care Med.* **2016**, *193*, 259–272. [CrossRef]
8. Delano, M.J.; Ward, P.A. Sepsis-induced immune dysfunction: Can immune therapies reduce mortality? *J. Clin. Invest.* **2016**, *126*, 23–31. [CrossRef]
9. Van der Poll, T.; van de Veerdonk, F.L.; Scicluna, B.P.; Netea, M.G. The immunopathology of sepsis and potential therapeutic targets. *Nat. Rev. Immunol.* **2017**, *17*, 407–420. [CrossRef]
10. Xia, W.; Pan, Z.; Zhang, H.; Zhou, Q.; Liu, Y. Inhibition of ERRalpha Aggravates Sepsis-Induced Acute Lung Injury in Rats via Provoking Inflammation and Oxidative Stress. *Oxid. Med. Cell. Longev.* **2020**, *2020*, 2048632. [CrossRef] [PubMed]
11. Kim, G.H.; Kim, J.E.; Rhie, S.J.; Yoon, S. The Role of Oxidative Stress in Neurodegenerative Diseases. *Exp. Neurobiol.* **2015**, *24*, 325–340. [CrossRef]
12. Song, P.; Zou, M.H. Roles of Reactive Oxygen Species in Physiology and Pathology. In *Atherosclerosis: Risks, Mechanisms, and Therapies*; Wang, H., Patterson, C., Eds.; John Wiley & Sons Inc.: Hoboken, NJ, USA, 2015; p. 379392.
13. McGarry, T.; Biniecka, M.; Veale, D.J.; Fearon, U. Hypoxia, oxidative stress and inflammation. *Free Radic. Biol. Med.* **2018**, *125*, 15–24. [CrossRef]
14. Krawczyk, C.M.; Holowka, T.; Sun, J.; Blagih, J.; Amiel, E.; DeBerardinis, R.J.; Cross, J.R.; Jung, E.; Thompson, C.B.; Jones, R.G.; et al. Toll-like receptor-induced changes in glycolytic metabolism regulate dendritic cell activation. *Blood* **2010**, *115*, 4742–4749. [CrossRef]
15. Huang, Q.; Liu, D.; Majewski, P.; Schulte, L.C.; Korn, J.M.; Young, R.A.; Lander, E.S.; Hacohen, N. The plasticity of dendritic cell responses to pathogens and their components. *Science* **2001**, *294*, 870–875. [CrossRef]
16. Yuan, J.P.; Peng, J.; Yin, K.; Wang, J.H. Potential health-promoting effects of astaxanthin: A high-value carotenoid mostly from microalgae. *Mol. Nutr. Food Res.* **2011**, *55*, 150–165. [CrossRef] [PubMed]
17. Ambati, R.R.; Phang, S.M.; Ravi, S.; Aswathanarayana, R.G. Astaxanthin: Sources, extraction, stability, biological activities and its commercial applications—A review. *Mar. Drugs* **2014**, *12*, 128–152. [CrossRef]
18. Rammuni, M.N.; Ariyadasa, T.U.; Nimarshana, P.H.V.; Attalage, R.A. Comparative assessment on the extraction of carotenoids from microalgal sources: Astaxanthin from *H. pluvialis* and beta-carotene from *D. salina*. *Food Chem.* **2019**, *277*, 128–134. [CrossRef]
19. Kim, B.; Farruggia, C.; Ku, C.S.; Pham, T.X.; Yang, Y.; Bae, M.; Wegner, C.J.; Farrell, N.J.; Harness, E.; Park, Y.K.; et al. Astaxanthin inhibits inflammation and fibrosis in the liver and adipose tissue of mouse models of diet-induced obesity and nonalcoholic steatohepatitis. *J. Nutr. Biochem.* **2017**, *43*, 27–35. [CrossRef]
20. Augusti, P.R.; Quatrin, A.; Somacal, S.; Conterato, G.M.; Sobieski, R.; Ruviaro, A.R.; Maurer, L.H.; Duarte, M.M.; Roehrs, M.; Emanuelli, T. Astaxanthin prevents changes in the activities of thioredoxin reductase and paraoxonase in hypercholesterolemic rabbits. *J. Clin. Biochem. Nutr.* **2012**, *51*, 42–49. [CrossRef] [PubMed]

21. Ying, C.J.; Zhang, F.; Zhou, X.Y.; Hu, X.T.; Chen, J.; Wen, X.R.; Sun, Y.; Zheng, K.Y.; Tang, R.X.; Song, Y.J. Anti-inflammatory Effect of Astaxanthin on the Sickness Behavior Induced by Diabetes Mellitus. *Cell. Mol. Neurobiol.* **2015**, *35*, 1027–1037. [CrossRef] [PubMed]
22. Peng, Y.J.; Lu, J.W.; Liu, F.C.; Lee, C.H.; Lee, H.S.; Ho, Y.J.; Hsieh, T.H.; Wu, C.C.; Wang, C.C. Astaxanthin attenuates joint inflammation induced by monosodium urate crystals. *FASEB J.* **2020**, *34*, 11215–11226. [CrossRef] [PubMed]
23. Li, C.Y.; Suzuki, K.; Hung, Y.L.; Yang, M.S.; Yu, C.P.; Lin, S.P.; Hou, Y.C.; Fang, S.H. Aloe Metabolites Prevent LPS-Induced Sepsis and Inflammatory Response by Inhibiting Mitogen-Activated Protein Kinase Activation. *Am. J. Chin. Med.* **2017**, *45*, 847–861. [CrossRef] [PubMed]
24. Wizemann, T.M.; Gardner, C.R.; Laskin, J.D.; Quinones, S.; Durham, S.K.; Goller, N.L.; Ohnishi, S.T.; Laskin, D.L. Production of nitric oxide and peroxynitrite in the lung during acute endotoxemia. *J. Leukoc. Biol.* **1994**, *56*, 759–768. [CrossRef] [PubMed]
25. Qin, T.; Yin, Y.; Yu, Q.; Yang, Q. Bursopentin (BP5) protects dendritic cells from lipopolysaccharide-induced oxidative stress for immunosuppression. *PLoS ONE* **2015**, *10*, e0117477.
26. Del Rio, D.; Stewart, A.J.; Pellegrini, N. A review of recent studies on malondialdehyde as toxic molecule and biological marker of oxidative stress. *Nutr. Metab. Cardiovasc. Dis.* **2005**, *15*, 316–328. [CrossRef] [PubMed]
27. Lorente, L.; Martin, M.M.; Abreu-Gonzalez, P.; Dominguez-Rodriguez, A.; Labarta, L.; Diaz, C.; Sole-Violan, J.; Ferreres, J.; Borreguero-Leon, J.M.; Jimenez, A.; et al. Prognostic value of malondialdehyde serum levels in severe sepsis: A multicenter study. *PLoS ONE* **2013**, *8*, e53741.
28. Birben, E.; Sahiner, U.M.; Sackesen, C.; Erzurum, S.; Kalayci, O. Oxidative stress and antioxidant defense. *World Allergy Organ. J.* **2012**, *5*, 9–19. [CrossRef]
29. Wang, J.; Wang, H.; Zhu, R.; Liu, Q.; Fei, J.; Wang, S. Anti-inflammatory activity of curcumin-loaded solid lipid nanoparticles in IL-1beta transgenic mice subjected to the lipopolysaccharide-induced sepsis. *Biomaterials* **2015**, *53*, 475–483. [CrossRef]
30. Loboda, A.; Damulewicz, M.; Pyza, E.; Jozkowicz, A.; Dulak, J. Role of Nrf2/HO-1 system in development, oxidative stress response and diseases: An evolutionarily conserved mechanism. *Cell. Mol. Life Sci.* **2016**, *73*, 3221–3247. [CrossRef]
31. Yin, Y.; Xu, N.; Shi, Y.; Zhou, B.; Sun, D.; Ma, B.; Xu, Z.; Yang, J.; Li, C. Astaxanthin Protects Dendritic Cells from Lipopolysaccharide-Induced Immune Dysfunction. *Mar. Drugs* **2021**, *19*, 346. [CrossRef]
32. Li, D.Y.; Xue, M.Y.; Geng, Z.R.; Chen, P.Y. The suppressive effects of Bursopentine (BP5) on oxidative stress and NF-kB activation in lipopolysaccharide-activated murine peritoneal macrophages. *Cell. Physiol. Biochem.* **2012**, *29*, 9–20. [CrossRef]
33. Brown, G.C. Regulation of mitochondrial respiration by nitric oxide inhibition of cytochrome c oxidase. *Biochim. Biophys. Acta* **2001**, *1504*, 46–57. [CrossRef]
34. Zhang, H.; Gomez, A.M.; Wang, X.; Yan, Y.; Zheng, M.; Cheng, H. ROS regulation of microdomain Ca(2+) signalling at the dyads. *Cardiovasc. Res.* **2013**, *98*, 248–258. [CrossRef] [PubMed]
35. Valko, M.; Leibfritz, D.; Moncol, J.; Cronin, M.T.; Mazur, M.; Telser, J. Free radicals and antioxidants in normal physiological functions and human disease. *Int. J. Biochem. Cell. Biol.* **2007**, *39*, 44–84. [CrossRef] [PubMed]
36. Cheeseman, K.H. Mechanisms and effects of lipid peroxidation. *Mol. Aspects Med.* **1993**, *14*, 191–197. [CrossRef]
37. Barrera, G. Oxidative stress and lipid peroxidation products in cancer progression and therapy. *ISRN Oncol.* **2012**, *2012*, 137289. [CrossRef]
38. Zitka, O.; Skalickova, S.; Gumulec, J.; Masarik, M.; Adam, V.; Hubalek, J.; Trnkova, L.; Kruseova, J.; Eckschlager, T.; Kizek, R. Redox status expressed as GSH:GSSG ratio as a marker for oxidative stress in paediatric tumour patients. *Oncol. Lett.* **2012**, *4*, 1247–1253. [CrossRef]
39. Mari, M.; Colell, A.; Morales, A.; von Montfort, C.; Garcia-Ruiz, C.; Fernandez-Checa, J.C. Redox control of liver function in health and disease. *Antioxid. Redox Signal.* **2010**, *12*, 1295–1331. [CrossRef]
40. Mari, M.; Morales, A.; Colell, A.; Garcia-Ruiz, C.; Fernandez-Checa, J.C. Mitochondrial glutathione, a key survival antioxidant. *Antioxid. Redox Signal.* **2009**, *11*, 2685–2700. [CrossRef] [PubMed]
41. Michiels, C.; Raes, M.; Toussaint, O.; Remacle, J. Importance of Se-glutathione peroxidase, catalase, and Cu/Zn-SOD for cell survival against oxidative stress. *Free Radic. Biol. Med.* **1994**, *17*, 235–248. [CrossRef]
42. McCord, J.M.; Fridovich, I. Superoxide dismutase. An enzymic function for erythrocuprein (hemocuprein). *J. Biol. Chem.* **1969**, *244*, 6049–6055. [CrossRef]
43. Bosmann, M.; Ward, P.A. The inflammatory response in sepsis. *Trends Immunol.* **2013**, *34*, 129–136. [CrossRef]
44. Asgari, E.; Le Friec, G.; Yamamoto, H.; Perucha, E.; Sacks, S.S.; Kohl, J.; Cook, H.T.; Kemper, C. C3a modulates IL-1beta secretion in human monocytes by regulating ATP efflux and subsequent NLRP3 inflammasome activation. *Blood* **2013**, *122*, 3473–3481. [CrossRef] [PubMed]
45. Eder, C. Mechanisms of interleukin-1beta release. *Immunobiology* **2009**, *214*, 543–553. [CrossRef]
46. Fujino, S.; Andoh, A.; Bamba, S.; Ogawa, A.; Hata, K.; Araki, Y.; Bamba, T.; Fujiyama, Y. Increased expression of interleukin 17 in inflammatory bowel disease. *Gut* **2003**, *52*, 65–70. [CrossRef]
47. Fossiez, F.; Djossou, O.; Chomarat, P.; Flores-Romo, L.; Ait-Yahia, S.; Maat, C.; Pin, J.J.; Garrone, P.; Garcia, E.; Saeland, S.; et al. T cell interleukin-17 induces stromal cells to produce proinflammatory and hematopoietic cytokines. *J. Exp. Med.* **1996**, *183*, 2593–2603. [CrossRef] [PubMed]
48. Chabaud, M.; Fossiez, F.; Taupin, J.L.; Miossec, P. Enhancing effect of IL-17 on IL-1-induced IL-6 and leukemia inhibitory factor production by rheumatoid arthritis synoviocytes and its regulation by Th2 cytokines. *J. Immunol.* **1998**, *161*, 409–414.

49. Cai, X.Y.; Gommoll, C.P., Jr.; Justice, L.; Narula, S.K.; Fine, J.S. Regulation of granulocyte colony-stimulating factor gene expression by interleukin-17. *Immunol. Lett.* **1998**, *62*, 51–58. [CrossRef]
50. Katz, Y.; Nadiv, O.; Beer, Y. Interleukin-17 enhances tumor necrosis factor alpha-induced synthesis of interleukins 1,6, and 8 in skin and synovial fibroblasts: A possible role as a "fine-tuning cytokine" in inflammation processes. *Arthritis Rheum.* **2001**, *44*, 2176–2184. [CrossRef]
51. LeGrand, A.; Fermor, B.; Fink, C.; Pisetsky, D.S.; Weinberg, J.B.; Vail, T.P.; Guilak, F. Interleukin-1, tumor necrosis factor alpha, and interleukin-17 synergistically up-regulate nitric oxide and prostaglandin E2 production in explants of human osteoarthritic knee menisci. *Arthritis Rheum.* **2001**, *44*, 2078–2083. [CrossRef]
52. Veldhoen, M.; Hocking, R.J.; Flavell, R.A.; Stockinger, B. Signals mediated by transforming growth factor-beta initiate autoimmune encephalomyelitis, but chronic inflammation is needed to sustain disease. *Nat. Immunol.* **2006**, *7*, 1151–1156. [CrossRef] [PubMed]
53. Gill, R.; Tsung, A.; Billiar, T. Linking oxidative stress to inflammation: Toll-like receptors. *Free Radic. Biol. Med.* **2010**, *48*, 1121–1132. [CrossRef]
54. Cai, X.; Chen, Y.; Xie, X.; Yao, D.; Ding, C.; Chen, M. Astaxanthin prevents against lipopolysaccharide-induced acute lung injury and sepsis via inhibiting activation of MAPK/NF-kappaB. *Am. J. Transl. Res.* **2019**, *11*, 1884–1894.
55. Kensler, T.W.; Wakabayashi, N.; Biswal, S. Cell survival responses to environmental stresses via the Keap1-Nrf2-ARE pathway. *Annu. Rev. Pharmacol. Toxicol.* **2007**, *47*, 89–116. [CrossRef] [PubMed]
56. Mitsuishi, Y.; Motohashi, H.; Yamamoto, M. The Keap1-Nrf2 system in cancers: Stress response and anabolic metabolism. *Front. Oncol.* **2012**, *2*, 200. [CrossRef]
57. Alam, J.; Stewart, D.; Touchard, C.; Boinapally, S.; Choi, A.M.; Cook, J.L. Nrf2, a Cap'n'Collar transcription factor, regulates induction of the heme oxygenase-1 gene. *J. Biol. Chem.* **1999**, *274*, 26071–26078. [CrossRef] [PubMed]
58. Oh, G.S.; Pae, H.O.; Lee, B.S.; Kim, B.N.; Kim, J.M.; Kim, H.R.; Jeon, S.B.; Jeon, W.K.; Chae, H.J.; Chung, H.T. Hydrogen sulfide inhibits nitric oxide production and nuclear factor-kappaB via heme oxygenase-1 expression in RAW264.7 macrophages stimulated with lipopolysaccharide. *Free Radic. Biol. Med.* **2006**, *41*, 106–119. [CrossRef]
59. Kovac, S.; Angelova, P.R.; Holmstrom, K.M.; Zhang, Y.; Dinkova-Kostova, A.T.; Abramov, A.Y. Nrf2 regulates ROS production by mitochondria and NADPH oxidase. *Biochim. Biophys. Acta* **2015**, *1850*, 794–801. [CrossRef] [PubMed]
60. Zhang, H.; Liu, Y.Y.; Jiang, Q.; Li, K.R.; Zhao, Y.X.; Cao, C.; Yao, J. Salvianolic acid A protects RPE cells against oxidative stress through activation of Nrf2/HO-1 signaling. *Free Radic. Biol. Med.* **2014**, *69*, 219–228. [CrossRef] [PubMed]
61. Yin, Y.; Qin, T.; Wang, X.; Lin, J.; Yu, Q.; Yang, Q. CpG DNA assists the whole inactivated H9N2 influenza virus in crossing the intestinal epithelial barriers via transepithelial uptake of dendritic cell dendrites. *Mucosal Immunol.* **2015**, *8*, 799–814. [CrossRef]
62. D'Agostino, P.; Ferlazzo, V.; Milano, S.; La Rosa, M.; Di Bella, G.; Caruso, R.; Barbera, C.; Grimaudo, S.; Tolomeo, M.; Feo, S.; et al. Anti-inflammatory effects of chemically modified tetracyclines by the inhibition of nitric oxide and interleukin-12 synthesis in J774 cell line. *Int. Immunopharmacol.* **2001**, *1*, 1765–1776. [CrossRef]
63. Gawel, S.; Wardas, M.; Niedworok, E.; Wardas, P. Malondialdehyde (MDA) as a lipid peroxidation marker. *Wiad. Lek.* **2004**, *57*, 453–455. (In Polish) [PubMed]

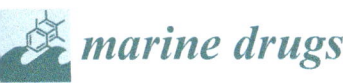

Article

A Comparative In Vitro Evaluation of the Anti-Inflammatory Effects of a *Tisochrysis lutea* Extract and Fucoxanthin

Elisabetta Bigagli [1], Mario D'Ambrosio [1], Lorenzo Cinci [1], Alberto Niccolai [2], Natascia Biondi [2], Liliana Rodolfi [2,3], Luana Beatriz Dos Santos Nascimiento [2], Mario R. Tredici [2,3] and Cristina Luceri [1,*]

[1] Department of NEUROFARBA, Section of Pharmacology and Toxicology, University of Florence, Viale Pieraccini 6, 50139 Florence, Italy; elisabetta.bigagli@unifi.it (E.B.); mario.dambrosio@unifi.it (M.D.); lorenzo.cinci@unifi.it (L.C.)

[2] Department of Agriculture, Food, Environment and Forestry (DAGRI), University of Florence, Piazzale delle Cascine 18, 50144 Florence, Italy; alberto.niccolai@unifi.it (A.N.); natascia.biondi@unifi.it (N.B.); liliana.rodolfi@unifi.it (L.R.); lulibia.17@gmail.com (L.B.D.S.N.); mario.tredici@unifi.it (M.R.T.)

[3] Fotosintetica Microbiologica S.r.l., Via di Santo Spirito, 14, 50125 Florence, Italy

* Correspondence: cristina.luceri@unifi.it; Tel.: +39-055-275-8305

Abstract: In this study, we compared the effects of a *Tisochrysis lutea* (T. lutea) F&M-M36 methanolic extract with those of fucoxanthin (FX) at equivalent concentration, on lipopolysaccharide (LPS)-stimulated RAW 264.7 macrophages. The T. lutea F&M-M36 methanolic extract contained 4.7 mg of FX and 6.22 mg of gallic acid equivalents of phenols per gram. HPLC analysis revealed the presence of simple phenolic acid derivatives. The T. lutea F&M-M36 extract exhibited a potent and concentration-dependent inhibitory activity against COX-2 dependent PGE2 production compared to FX alone. Compared to LPS, T. lutea F&M-M36 extract and FX reduced the expression of IL-6 and of Arg1 and enhanced that of IL-10 and of HO-1; T. lutea F&M-M36 extract also significantly abated the expression of NLRP3, enhanced mir-223 expression and reduced that of mir-146b, compared to LPS ($p < 0.05$). These findings indicate that T. lutea F&M-M36 methanolic extract has a peculiar anti-inflammatory activity against COX-2/PGE2 and NLRP3/mir-223 that might be attributable to the known anti-inflammatory effects of simple phenolic compounds found in the extract that may synergize with FX. Our data suggest that T. lutea F&M-M36 may serve as a source of anti-inflammatory compounds to be further evaluated in in vivo models of inflammation.

Keywords: microalgae; *Tisochrysis lutea*; fucoxanthin; inflammation; RAW 264.7; microRNA

Citation: Bigagli, E.; D'Ambrosio, M.; Cinci, L.; Niccolai, A.; Biondi, N.; Rodolfi, L.; Dos Santos Nascimiento, L.B.; Tredici, M.R.; Luceri, C. A Comparative In Vitro Evaluation of the Anti-Inflammatory Effects of a *Tisochrysis lutea* Extract and Fucoxanthin. *Mar. Drugs* **2021**, *19*, 334. https://doi.org/10.3390/md19060334

Academic Editor: Hitoshi Sashiwa

Received: 24 May 2021
Accepted: 8 June 2021
Published: 11 June 2021

Publisher's Note: MDPI stays neutral with regard to jurisdictional claims in published maps and institutional affiliations.

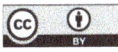

Copyright: © 2021 by the authors. Licensee MDPI, Basel, Switzerland. This article is an open access article distributed under the terms and conditions of the Creative Commons Attribution (CC BY) license (https://creativecommons.org/licenses/by/4.0/).

1. Introduction

Tisochrysis lutea (T. lutea) is a marine microalga belonging to Haptophyta, originally isolated from tropical seawater (Tahiti, French Polynesia), and currently used in aquaculture [1,2]. The presence of n-3 polyunsaturated fatty acids (PUFAs) such as docosahexaenoic acid (DHA) and eicosapentaenoic acid (EPA), vitamins, proteins, and xanthophylls such as fucoxanthin [3,4], makes this microalga an interesting source of compounds with anti-inflammatory and hypolipidemic activities [5–7]. Among the marine microalgae, *Tisochrysis* contains a high amount of the pigment fucoxanthin (FX) (1.8% w/w) [8]. In several in vitro and in vivo models, FX exerts anti-inflammatory effects by inhibiting pro-inflammatory cytokines and enzymes [9–12]. FX also attenuates alcohol-induced oxidative lesions and inflammatory responses [13]. However, *Tisochrysis* is also a source of phenolic compounds [14] which possess a high spectrum of biological activities including antioxidant, anti-aging, and anti-inflammatory effects [15–20]. Despite the anti-inflammatory and antioxidant effects of T. lutea that have been mostly attributed to FX, positive pharmacodynamic synergisms among various components, acting on different targets, cannot be excluded. Indeed, superior bioactivity of either the single component or the mixture was reported in studies on natural products [21].

The aim of this study was to perform a direct comparison between the anti-inflammatory activity of a methanolic extract of *T. lutea* F&M-M36 and FX at equivalent concentrations in order to explore potential interactions among the components and pharmacological mechanisms involved. Lipopolysaccharide (LPS)-stimulated RAW 264.7 mouse macrophages were used as an in vitro model of inflammation.

2. Results

2.1. Characterization of the T. lutea F&M-M36 Methanolic Extract

The amount of FX in the *T. lutea* F&M-M36 methanolic extract was 4.7 mg/g dry weight. The extract was also analyzed for the total soluble phenolic content, using gallic acid as a reference. The *T. lutea* F&M-M36 methanolic extract contained 6.22 ± 0.05 mg GAE/g dry weight.

HPLC characterization showed that the *T. lutea* F&M-M36 methanolic extract contains phenolic compounds (Figure 1), with maximum absorption at 255–280 nm which eluted early in the chromatogram (retention time between 4 and 20 min, Figure 1). The spectral absorption and chromatographic behavior of these compounds are typical of simple C6 or C6-C1 phenolic skeletons, such as derivatives of hydroxybenzoic and gallic acids, as well as some aromatic amino acids. The *T. lutea* F&M-M36 methanolic extract (Figure 1) showed a little variety of phenolics, with almost all compounds showing a similar UV spectrum, compatible with the structure of simple phenolics. The putative identification was conducted based on UV-vis absorption, retention time, in comparison with standards and literature data.

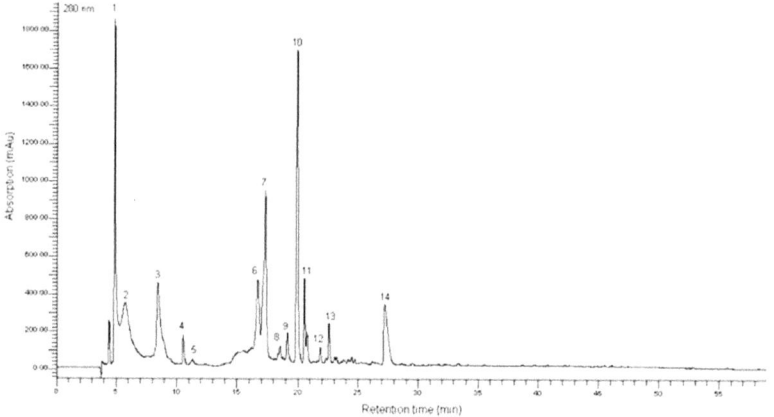

Figure 1. Chromatograms obtained by high-performance liquid chromatography coupled to a diode array detector—HPLC-DAD (280 nm) of methanolic extract of *T. lutea* F&M-M36. Peak 1–13: phenolic acid derivatives; pick 14: catechin derivative. The putative identification was conducted based on UV-vis absorption and retention time, in comparison with standards and literature data.

2.2. Effects of T. lutea F&M-M36 Methanolic Extract and FX on RAW 264.7 Macrophages Viability

In order to evaluate the effects of *T. lutea* F&M-M36 methanolic extracts on cell viability, preliminary experiments were carried out using the MTS test. Unstimulated RAW 264.7 cells macrophages were exposed to different extract concentrations for 24 h. *T. lutea* F&M-M36 extract caused a significant reduction of cell viability (about 40%) when treatments were performed at 1 mg/mL, but was not toxic at concentrations in the range of 1–100 µg/mL (data not shown). On the basis of these results, 100 µg/mL was selected as the highest non-toxic concentration of *T. lutea* F&M-M36 extract for further analyses. FX was tested at concentrations equivalent to those measured in the microalgal extract at the same dilution (4.7–470 ng/mL).

2.3. Comparative Effects of T. lutea F&M-M36 Extract and FX on Cell Morphology

Hematoxylin and eosin staining showed that unstimulated RAW 264.7 cells macrophages were almost all small and round, whereas those treated with LPS were flat and spindle-shaped and showed many dendritic-like structures typical of activated macrophages [22]. The treatment with *T. lutea* F&M-M36 extract, as well as with FX, significantly reduced the number of cells with dendritic structures ($p < 0.001$ and $p < 0.01$, respectively), an effect similar to that exerted by Celecoxib ($p < 0.001$). In particular, *T. lutea* F&M-M36 extract was more effective in counteracting this effect than FX ($p < 0.001$) (Figure 2).

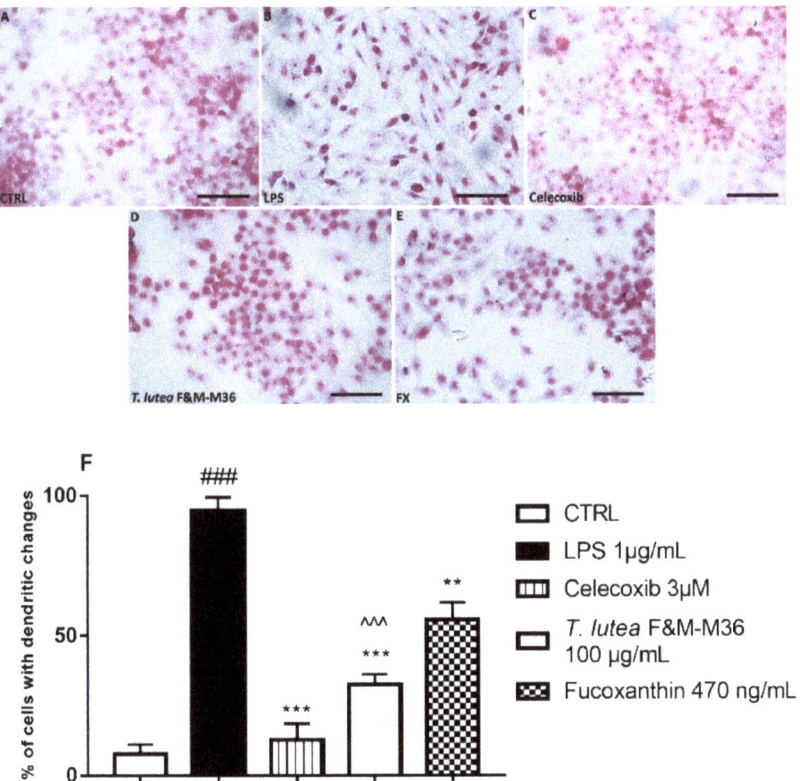

Figure 2. Morphology images of RAW 264.7 cells in different groups obtained by a light microscope. Hematoxylin and eosin staining of cells from different experimental groups: (**A**) Unstimulated RAW264.7 cells; (**B**) LPS-stimulated RAW264.7 cells; (**C**) LPS-stimulated RAW264.7 cells treated with Celecoxib 3 µM; (**D**) LPS-stimulated RAW264.7 cells treated with *T. lutea* F&M-M36 extract 100 µg/mL; (**E**) LPS-stimulated RAW264.7 cells treated with FX 470 ng/mL; (**F**) Percentage of cells with dendritic changes. ### $p < 0.001$ vs. unstimulated RAW 264.7 macrophages (CTRL); ** $p < 0.01$ and *** $p < 0.001$ vs. LPS ^^^ $p < 0.001$ vs. FX by ANOVA test and Dunnett's Multiple Comparison Test. Data are expressed as mean ± SEM of five replicates. Magnification = 400×; Scale bar = 20 µm.

2.4. Comparative Effects of T. lutea F&M-M36 Extract and FX on PGE2 Production and COX-2 Protein Expression

As shown in Figure 3, the methanolic extract of *T. lutea* F&M-M36 (1–100 µg/mL) significantly decreased the LPS-induced production of PGE2 in a concentration-dependent manner, whereas FX was significantly effective ($p < 0.05$) only at the highest concentration tested (470 ng/mL). When we compared directly the PGE2 levels measured in the media from cells treated with the methanolic extract and those of the cells treated with FX at equivalent concentrations, we observed a clear and significant reduction at all concentrations ($p < 0.001$).

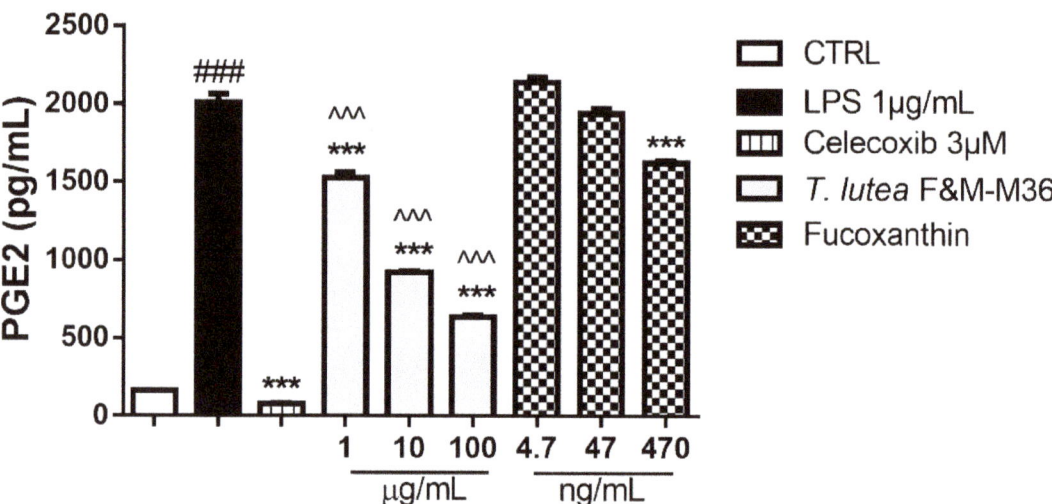

Figure 3. Effect of *T. lutea* F&M-M36 extract and FX on PGE2 production in RAW 264.7 stimulated with LPS for 18 h. ### $p < 0.001$ vs. unstimulated RAW 264.7 macrophages (CTRL); *** $p < 0.001$ vs. LPS ^^^ $p < 0.001$ vs. FX by ANOVA test and Dunnett's Multiple Comparison test. Data are expressed as the mean ± SEM of four replicates.

Immunofluorescent staining for COX-2 protein expression (Figure 4 Panels A–D) and dot blot analyses (Panel F) demonstrated that the methanolic extract from *T. lutea* F&M-M36 significantly counteracted LPS induced COX-2 protein expression ($p < 0.001$) as it did in FX alone, although to a lower extent ($p < 0.05$) (Figure 4 panel E). Similar to the results on PGE2, *T. lutea* F&M-M36 extract also significantly decreased COX-2 protein expression compared to FX alone ($p < 0.01$).

The effects on COX-2 were much more evident at the protein level than gene level, since COX-2 mRNA expression was not significantly decreased neither by *T. lutea* F&M-M36 extract nor by FX compared to LPS-treated cells; in this regard, however, it should be highlighted that when directly compared, the mRNA expression of COX-2 was significantly decreased by *T. lutea* F&M-M36 extract compared to FX ($p < 0.05$).

2.5. Comparative Effects of T. lutea F&M-M36 Extract and FX on the Expression of Pro-Inflammatory and Anti-Inflammatory Genes

As shown in Figure 5 and Table 1, both the *T. lutea* F&M-M36 extract and FX strongly reduced the expression of IL-6 ($p < 0.001$) and enhanced that of IL-10 ($p < 0.001$) compared to LPS, and the extent of these effects were similar to those exerted by Celecoxib 3 µM. *T. lutea* F&M-M36 extract, as well as FX also reduced the mRNA expression of Arg1 compared to LPS ($p < 0.001$) and slightly enhanced that of HO-1 ($p < 0.001$); moreover, the expression of Arg1 in cells treated with *T. lutea* F&M-M36 extract was significantly lower compared to cells treated with FX ($p < 0.001$). SOD2 expression was also reduced by both *T. lutea* F&M-M36 extract and FX, compared to LPS ($p < 0.001$). *T. lutea* F&M-M36 extract and FX were ineffective in reducing the expression of iNOS, IL-1β, and TNF-α. In addition, *T. lutea* F&M-M36 extract ($p < 0.001$) but not FX significantly abated the expression of NLRP3.

2.6. Comparative Effects of T. lutea F&M-M36 Extract and FX on mir-146b and mir-223 Expression

In RAW 264.7 macrophages stimulated with LPS, the expression of mir-146b was significantly enhanced compared to control cells (Figure 6 Panels B), whereas that of mir-223 was strongly reduced (Figure 6 Panels A); both of these effects were counteracted by Celecoxib 3 µM. *T. lutea* F&M-M36 extract, and FX showed similar effects in reducing the expression of mir-146b ($p < 0.05$). On the contrary, the expression of mir-223 was induced in cells treated with *T. lutea* F&M-M36 extract, but this difference did not reach statistical significance.

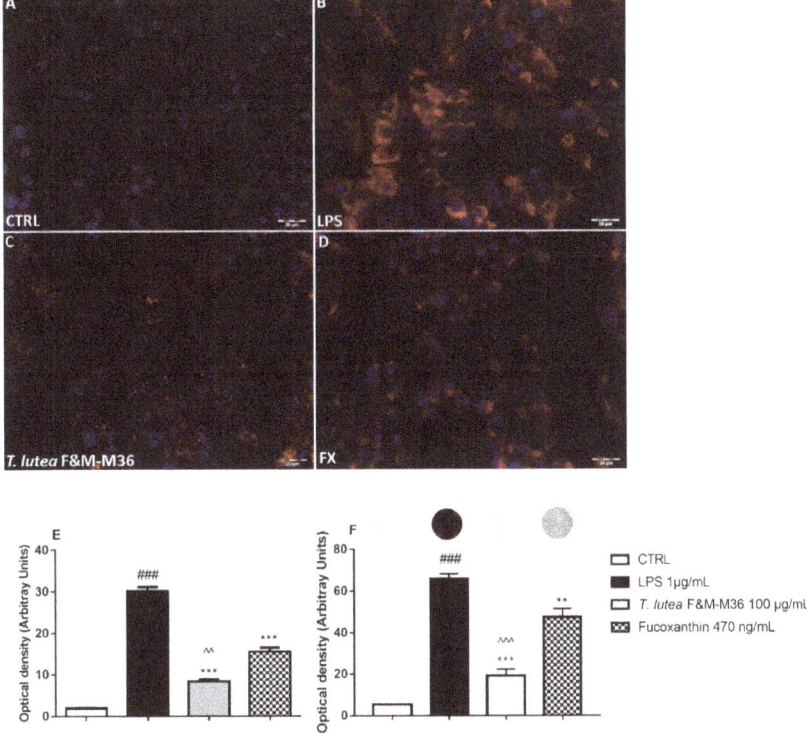

Figure 4. Effect of *T. lutea* F&M-M36 extract and FX on COX-2 protein expression in LPS-stimulated RAW 264.7 cells. Panels (**A**–**D**): COX-2 protein expression determined by immunocytochemistry with an anti-COX-2 antibody (red fluorescence). Nuclei were counterstained with DAPI (blue fluorescence); Magnification = 400×; Scale bar = 20 µm. Panel (**E**): Densitometric analysis of cells positive for COX-2. Panel (**F**): Densitometric analysis of dot blot results on COX-2 protein expression; above bars, representative dot blot images are shown. ### $p < 0.001$ vs. unstimulated RAW 264.7 macrophages (CTRL). ** $p < 0.01$ and *** $p < 0.001$ vs. LPS. ^^ $p < 0.01$ and ^^^ $p < 0.001$ vs. FX by ANOVA test and Dunnett's Multiple Comparison test. Data are expressed as means ± SEM of four replicates.

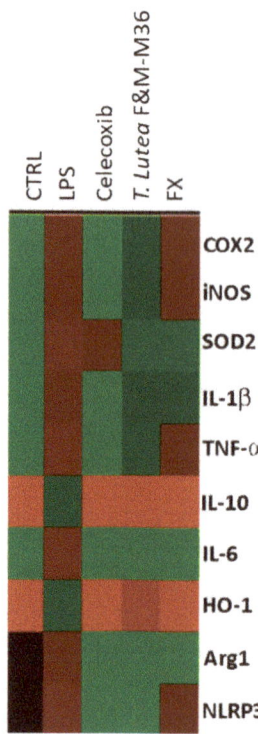

Figure 5. Gene expression profiles of unstimulated RAW 264.7 macrophages (CTRL), RAW 264.7 macrophages stimulated with LPS and those treated with LPS in the presence of *T. lutea* F&M-M36 extract at 100 µg/mL and FX at 470 ng/mL. Each column represents a different treatment and each row a different gene; the color code indicates down-regulation (green) or up-regulation (red) compared to LPS.

Table 1. Effect of *T. lutea* F&M-M36 extract at 100 µg/mL and FX at 470 ng/mL on COX-2, iNOS, SOD2, IL-1β, TNF-α, IL-10, IL-6, HO-1, Arg1, and NLRP3 mRNA expression in LPS-stimulated RAW 264.7 cells.

Gene	CTRL	LPS	Celecoxib	*T. lutea* F&M-M36 Extract	FX
COX-2	0.09 ± 0.01	0.86 ± 0.03 ###	0.37 ± 0.03 ***	0.81 ± 0.01 ^	0.91 ± 0.01
iNOS	0.02 ± 0.01	1.25 ± 0.03 ###	0.51 ± 0.02 ***	1.10 ± 0.06	1.20 ± 0.00
SOD2	0.04 ± 0.02	0.64 ± 0.00 ###	0.62 ± 0.01	0.44 ± 0.02 ***	0.44 ± 0.01 ***
IL-1b	0.36 ± 0.00	0.97 ± 0.02 ###	0.31 ± 0.01 ***	0.90 ± 0.01	0.92 ± 0.01
TNF-a	0.27 ± 0.03	0.76 ± 0.03 ###	0.20 ± 0.02 ***	0.69 ± 0.02	0.82 ± 0.01
IL-10	0.62 ± 0.03	0.16 ± 0.00 ###	0.71 ± 0.03 ***	0.61 ± 0.06 ***	0.62 ± 0.03 ***
IL-6	0.02 ± 0.01	0.74 ± 0.03 ###	0.06 ± 0.01 ***	0.04 ± 0.00 ***	0.07 ± 0.01 ***
HO-1	1.04 ± 0.00	0.25 ± 0.00 ###	0.95 ± 0.03 ***	0.38 ± 0.01 ***	0.46 ± 0.03 ***
Arg1	0.00 ± 0.00	1.71 ± 0.01 ###	0.06 ± 0.00 ***	0.61 ± 0.02 ***,^^^	0.91 ± 0.02 ***
NLRP3	0.00 ± 0.00	0.74 ± 0.02 ###	0.23 ± 0.02 ***	0.37 ± 0.03 ***,^^^	0.71 ± 0.05

Data are expressed as means ± SEM of four replicates; for each target gene, the relative amount of mRNA was calculated as the ratio to RPLP-1 mRNA [19]; ### $p < 0.001$ vs. CTRL; *** $p < 0.001$ vs. LPS; ^ $p < 0.05$ and ^^^ $p < 0.001$ vs. FX by one-way ANOVA and Dunnett's multiple comparisons test.

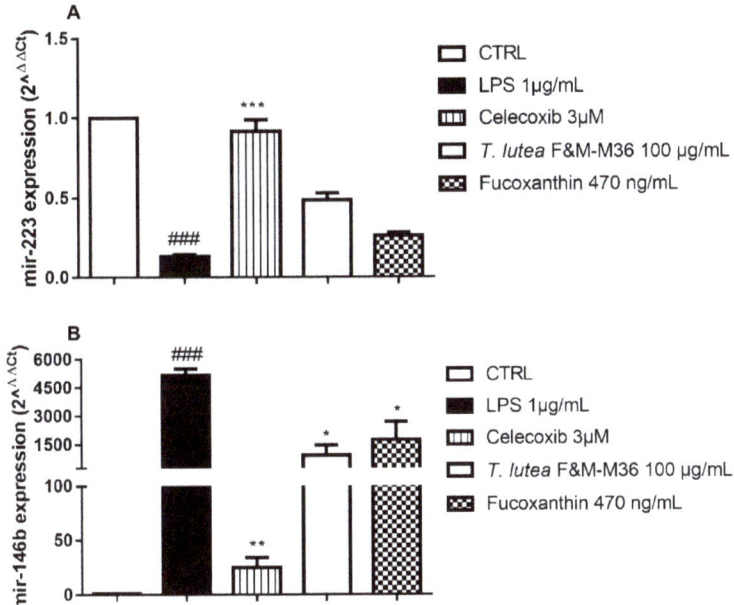

Figure 6. Effect of T. lutea F&M-M36 extract and FX on mir-223 (Panel **A**) and mir-146b (Panel **B**) expression in LPS-stimulated RAW 264.7 cells. ### $p < 0.001$ vs. CTRL; * $p < 0.05$, ** $p < 0.01$ and *** $p < 0.001$ vs. LPS by one-way ANOVA and Dunnett's Multiple Comparisons test.

3. Discussion

Inflammation is a key component of several chronic human diseases such as inflammatory bowel diseases, diabetes, cardiovascular diseases, neurodegeneration, and cancer [23]. The identification of new anti-inflammatory compounds is a great challenge for the scientific community, and in this context, the microalga *T. lutea* may represent an interesting source for the discovery of novel strategies for the prevention, and even control, of inflammation.

Overall, our results demonstrate that *T. lutea* F&M-M36 methanolic extract and FX, at equivalent concentrations, exert anti-inflammatory activities by regulating a number of pro-inflammatory mediators. It is interesting to highlight that the effects on the COX-2/PGE2 axis are concentration-dependent and therefore suggestive of a pharmacological mechanism of action of *T. lutea* F&M-M36 methanolic extract and FX; the prominent reduction of COX-2/PGE2 exerted by *T. lutea* F&M-M36 methanolic extract also suggests that compounds other than FX may exert additive or synergistic effects. This is also consistent with previous reports documenting the superior activities of botanical extracts compared to single components [24]. *T. lutea* F&M-M36 methanolic extract contains polyphenols equivalent to 6.22 mg of gallic acid/g dry weight, exhibiting a much lower content of total polyphenols compared to that reported for other species, as a polyphenolic content of 515 mg GAE per 100 g DW and of 13.4 mg GAE/g EW measured in an ethanolic extract from the closely related species *I. galbana* [14,24]. These differences may be ascribed to the extraction solvents used (methanol instead of ethanol), although differences in the analyzed species and in cultivation conditions may also have contributed [25].

Despite the presence of phenolic compounds in *T. lutea* being previously described, scarce information is available on their composition; our HPLC characterization showed that *T. lutea* F&M-M36 methanolic extract contains a number of simple phenolic acids which have characteristic UV spectra (maximum absorption in the 200–290 nm range [26,27].

Simple phenolic acids derivatives of hydroxybenzoic and gallic acids have been previously proved to exert anti-inflammatory activities; gallic acid exerted inhibitory effects on

LPS-stimulated PGE2 and IL-6 production and COX-2 expression in RAW 264.7 cells [27], and inhibited several NLRP3 inflammasome markers in an in vitro model of intestinal inflammation [28]. Moreover, we previously demonstrated that hydroxytyrosol, p-coumaric acid, or foods rich in simple phenols exhibited anti-inflammatory properties in in vitro and in vivo models of colon inflammation [18,20,29]. On the other hand, we cannot exclude the contribution of other, not characterized components of our methanolic extract. In particular, our *T. lutea* F&M-M36 biomass contains 4.1% of dry-weight polyunsaturated fatty acids (PUFAs) and 2.61% of total ω-3 [7] that are known to exert immunomodulatory and anti-inflammatory activities [30].

In addition, although FX is the main carotenoid found in *T. lutea*, other compounds such as diadinoxanthin, diatoxanthin, and β-carotene were found in an ethyl acetate extract from *T. lutea* containing a total amount of 132.8 mg of carotenoids/g of extract [31]. The anti-inflammatory activities of carotenoids such as β-carotene at relatively high concentrations (50–100 µM) have been reported in LPS-induced RAW264.7, showing effects on IL-1β, IL-6, and TNF-α; [32]. In the same model, other authors found significant effects of β-carotene 5 µM on IL-12, p40, and IL-1β expression [33]. MiRNAs are endogenous non-coding RNA molecules that silence target mRNA by binding to the 3′UTR of mRNA [34]. Several miRNAs are regulated during the inflammatory process [35]; mir-223 is emerging as an important regulator of the innate immune system, and its deficiency enhances pro-inflammatory macrophage activation [36,37]. mir-223 targets NLRP3 result in reduced inflammation [38,39]. Our results pointed out a peculiar superior effect of the *T. lutea* F&M-M36 methanolic extract toward the NLRP3/mir223 axis. For the first time, we showed that *T. lutea* F&M-M36 methanolic extract has the ability to enhance the secretion of mir-223 by LPS-stimulated RAW 264.7, although to a lesser extent than the selective COX-2 inhibitor Celecoxib, and that this effect may be attributable to the phenolic content of the extract, considering the negligible effects of FX alone.

The activity of *T. lutea* F&M-M36 methanolic extract was prominent over that of FX on the COX-2/PGE2 pathway and NLRP3/mir-223 axis, whereas similar effects were observed when other inflammatory mediators were investigated. The ability to simultaneously target different biological inflammatory networks certainly represents an added value of both the extract and FX.

Macrophages polarization between M1 and M2 phenotypes is an important regulatory mechanism for inflammation. M1 macrophages are classically activated by LPS and sustain inflammation, whereas M2 or M2-like phenotypes are associated with the resolution of inflammation [40]. M1 macrophages express pro-inflammatory cytokines such as TNF-α, COX-2, and IL-6, while M2 macrophages express IL-10 and Arg1, thus exhibiting anti-inflammatory properties [41].

T. lutea F&M-M36 methanolic extract and FX promoted some morphological and molecular characteristics of the M2 anti-inflammatory phenotype in RAW macrophages, such as increased expression of IL-10 and Arg1 and decreased expression of IL-6. The extent of these effects is almost completely attributable to the FX content.

Previous findings indicate that FX (100 µg/mL) inhibited the secretion of IL-1β and TNF-α and promoted that of IL-10 and IFN-γ in Caco-2 cells stimulated with LPS [8]. In LPS-induced RAW 264.7, FX 15-60 µM (corresponding to about 10–40 µg/mL) significantly inhibited NO, TNF-α, and IL-6 production but slightly reduced PGE2 production [10] and inhibited NF-κB activation and MAPK phosphorylation at 12–50 µM [11]. In the same model, the half-maximal inhibitory concentration (IC50) for IL-6 production was 2.19 µM [12]. In a recent report, Kim et al. (2021) [42] found that the pretreatment of RAW 264.7 with FX 5 µM also significantly decreased LPS-induced expression of IL-6, IL-1β, and TNF-α by activating the NRF2/PI3K/AKT pathway. It is worth highlighting that all these studies were conducted with FX concentrations largely greater than ours (470 ng/mL). From a pharmacological point of view, the smaller is the concentration at which the molecule is active, the greater is its potential application. Recently, in a model of metabolic syndrome, a high-fat diet, supplemented with 12% (w/w) of freeze-dried *T. lutea*, significantly reduced plasma TNF-α levels and increased IL-10 in abdominal adipose tissue [43].

In addition, for the first time, we reported the ability of *T. lutea* F&M-M36 methanolic extract to reduce the secretion of mir-146b, and this effect was almost completely attributable to FX [44]. Increased levels of mir-146b are associated with inflammatory disease: in particular, mir-146b is increased in the serum of patients with inflammatory bowel disease and decreases after treatment with infliximab [45]; moreover, circulating mir-146b correlates with endoscopic disease activity in patients with inflammatory bowel disease [46].

T. lutea is not approved for human consumption, and its safety has been evaluated only in short-term studies in animal models [2,47,48]. However, *T. lutea* is currently used in aquaculture [1], and our data suggest that it could be added to animal feed not only for its high nutritional value, but also as an anti-inflammatory additive.

Overall, our results demonstrate that *T. lutea* F&M-M36 methanolic extract exerts promising anti-inflammatory activity, even more pronounced than that of FX alone, thus providing the background for conducting studies on its long-term safety and efficacy in inflammatory disease models.

4. Materials and Methods

4.1. Microalgal Biomass

The biomass of *T. lutea* F&M-M36 strain belonging to the Fotosintetica & Microbiologica (F&M) S.r.l. Culture Collection (Florence, Italy) was produced at Archimede Ricerche S.r.l. (Camporosso, Imperia, Italy). *T. lutea* F&M-M36 was cultivated in F medium [49] in GWP®-II photobioreactors [50] in a semi-batch mode. The lyophilized biomass was stored at −20 °C until extraction.

4.2. Microalgal Extract Preparation

An aliquot of 250 mg of lyophilized *T. lutea* F&M-M36 biomass was extracted in 30 mL of methanol, overnight, at room temperature (RT). The mixture was then sonicated twice for 3 min at the maximum power. The solvent was separated from the biomass by filtration on paper. The residual biomass was extracted again with 15 mL of methanol at 37 °C for 4 h; then, the exhausted biomass was removed by filtration on paper, and the extract (30 + 15 = 45 mL) was evaporated under vacuum. The dry residue was solubilized in DMSO to obtain a final concentration of the extract of 65 mg/mL. Fucoxanthin (purity ≥ 95%) was purchased by Sigma Aldrich (Milan, Italy).

4.3. Sample Preparation and HPLC-DAD Analysis for Phenols Quantification and Characterization

The extract was dried under vacuum and resuspended in 9 mL of ethanol:water solution (75:25 *v/v* adjusted at pH 2 by formic acid addition) and partitioned with 5 mL of n-hexane in order to remove chlorophylls and other pigments, which could interfere in the analysis of phenolic compounds. The procedure was repeated three times. The last partition was carried out with chloroform instead of n-hexane. The polar phase was reduced to dryness, and the residue resuspended in 0.5 mL of methanol:water solution (50:50 *v/v* adjusted at pH 2.5 by formic acid addition).

Aliquots of the samples (15 µL) were injected into the Perkin® Elmer Flexar liquid chromatograph equipped with a quaternary 200Q/410 pump and an LC 200 diode array detector (DAD) (all from Perkin Elmer®, Bradford, CT, USA). The stationary phase was composed by a reverse-phase Agilent® Zorbax® SB-18 column (250 × 4.6 mm, 5 µm) (Agilent Technologies Inc., Santa Clara, CA, USA) kept at 30 °C. A gradient solvent system of solvent A (acidified water, 0.1% formic acid) and solvent B (acetonitrile, 0.1% formic acid), over a 59 min run in a flow rate of 0.6 mL/min was applied: 0–5 min (0% B), 5–8 min (0–3% B), 8–53 min (3–40% B), 53–58 min (40% B), 58–59 min (0% B).

The chromatograms were acquired at 280 and 350 nm, the most common wavelengths for the analysis of phenolic compounds. The putative identification of the phenolics detected was carried out based on the retention time, UV spectral characteristics, and comparison with standards, as well as based on literature data. A calibration curve of gallic acid ($R^2 = 0.99$) was used to quantify the compounds and the result of the total phenolic content was given in mg GAE/g dry weight. The analysis was conducted in triplicate.

4.4. Fucoxanthin Determination in the Methanolic Extract

FX content of *T. lutea* F&M-M36 extract was carried out by chromatographic analysis according to a modification of the method by Kim et al. [8]. FX separation was achieved with an HPLC 1050 (Hewlett Packard, Palo Alto, CA, USA) equipped with a C30 reverse-phase column (YCM Carotenoid, 4.6 mm × 250 mm, 5 µm particle size) (Waters, MA, USA), and a UV photodiode array detector 1050 (Hewlett Packard, Palo Alto, CA, USA). A gradient method with two eluents were used; eluent A: 81% Methyl Tert-Butyl Ether (MTBE), 10% methanol, and 9% deionized water, and eluent B: 93% MTBE and 7% methanol. The injection volume was 20 µL with a constant flow rate of 1 mL/min, at 25 °C temperature. The detection was performed at 450 nm. The quantification was performed by internal standard calibration. Commercial FX (Sigma-Aldrich, Milan, Italy) standard solutions (20, 40, 60, 80, 100, 120 µg/mL in methanol/MTBE 4:1), with β-apo-carotenal (50 µg/mL) and Sudan Red (90 µg/mL) were prepared. The rate between the area under the peaks of FX standard solutions and the area under the internal standard peak was plotted against FX standard solution concentrations (µg/mL) to obtain a calibration curve adopted to quantify the concentration of FX in the *T. lutea* F&M-M36 extract.

4.5. In Vitro Model of Inflammation and Anti-Inflammatory Assay

RAW 264.7 macrophages were purchased from the American Tissue Type Culture Collection (Manassas, VA, USA) and cultured in Dulbecco's modified Eagle's medium (Thermo Fisher Scientific, Milan, Italy) with 10% fetal bovine serum (FBS) (Thermo Fisher Scientific) and 100 U/mL penicillin-streptomycin (Thermo Fisher Scientific), in 5% CO_2 at 37 °C. The cytotoxicity of the extracts was first evaluated by MTS assay as previously described [18]. FX was dissolved in DMSO and diluted in a complete cell-culture medium in order to obtain the appropriate concentrations to be tested. The final concentrations of DMSO were below 0.1%, and the control cells were exposed only to DMSO 0.1%. The cultured cells were treated with lipopolysaccharide (LPS, 1 µg/mL Sigma-Aldrich, Milan, Italy) and with *T. lutea* F&M-M36 methanolic extract (1–100 µg/mL) or FX (4.7–470 ng/mL) (Sigma-Aldrich, Milan, Italy). After incubating for 18 h at 37 °C, the cells were harvested for RNA and protein extraction, and the cell medium was collected and stored at −20 °C for PGE2 determination [18,20].

4.6. Morphological Analysis: Hematoxylin and Eosin (H&E) Staining

RAW 264.7 were seeded in Poly-D-lysine-coated glass dishes for 24 h then treated with LPS and *T. lutea* F&M-M36 extract, FX, or Celecoxib as described above. After 18 h, cells were fixed with 4% (w/v) paraformaldehyde for 15 min at room temperature. Next, cells were washed in H_2O and then stained with hematoxylin for 2 min, differentiated in saturated lithium carbonate solution for 30 s, stained with eosin for 2 min, and dehydrated with ethanol series (50, 75, 96, and 100%), and finally xylene. Subsequently, glass dishes were mounted on microscope slides with a mounting medium and allowed to dry. Microscopic analysis was performed with ACT-2U software program (Nikon, Instruments Europe, Badhoevedorp, The Netherlands) connected via a camera to the microscope (Optiphot-2; Nikon). Five photomicrographs were randomly taken for each sample to evaluate cell morphology. The percentage of cells with dendritic changes (number of cells with clear morphological changes/total number of cells in the field × 100) were counted using ImageJ 1.33 image analysis software (http://rsb.info.nih.gov/ij (accessed on 22 April 2021)).

4.7. PGE2 Determination

PGE2 levels were measured in the RAW 264.7 cell media using an ELISA kit (Cayman Chemical, MI, USA) according to the manufacturer's specifications, and expressed as pg/mL. Celecoxib (Sigma-Aldrich, Milan, Italy) 3 µM (1.14 µg/mL), was used as a positive control.

4.8. RT-PCR

Total RNA was extracted from cell lysates using the Nucleo Spin® RNA kit (Macherey-Nagel, Bethlehem, PA, USA) according to the manufacturer's instructions. For first-strand cDNA synthesis, 1 µg of total RNA from each sample was reverse-transcribed. Primers were designed based on the mouse GenBank sequences for HO-1, IL-10, IL-6, IL1-β, COX-2, iNOS, TNF-α, SOD2, NLRP3, and Arg1, and are reported in Table 2. Ribosomal protein large P1 (RPLP-1) was co-amplified as the reference [18]. For each target gene, the relative amount of mRNA in the samples was calculated as the ratio to RPLP-1 mRNA [19].

Table 2. Primer sequences.

Gene	Primer Forward	Primer Reverse	Base Pair
RPLP-1	ATCTACTCCGCCCTCATCCT	CAGATGAGGCTCCCAATGTT	155
COX-2	TCCTCCTGGAACATGGACTC	CCCCAAAGATAGCATCTGGA	321
iNOS	CCCCAAAGATAGCATCTGGA	CCCCAAAGATAGCATCTGGA	305
SOD2	ACCCAAAGGAGAGTTGCTGGA	ATGTGGCCGTGAGTGAGGTT	354
HO-1	GGCTGCCCTGGAGCAGGACGT	AGGTCACCCAGGTAGCGG	165
TNFα	TAGCCCACGTCGTAGCAAAC	ACCCTGAGCCATAATCCCCT	566
NLRP3	TGGGTTCTGGTCAGACACGAG	GGGGCTTAGGTCCACACAGAA	176
ARG1	CATTGGCTTGCGAGACGTAG	CGGCCTTTTCTTCCTTCCCAG	151
IL-1β	CAGGCAGGCAGTATCACTCA	AGGCCACAGGTATTTTGTCG	350
IL-10	AGGCGCTGTCATCGATTTCTC	AGGAAGAACCCCTCCCATCA	489
IL-6	TCCTCTCTGCAAGAGACTTCC	TCCTCTCTGCAAGAGACTTCC	513

4.9. Real-Time PCR for mir-146b and mir-223 Expression Analysis

For miRNA expression analysis, the total RNA was extracted from cell culture media by using TRIzol (Invitrogen, Carlsbad, CA, USA). Reverse-transcription of RNA was performed using the miRCURY LNA RT Kit according to the manufacturer's instructions (Qiagen). qRT-PCR assays were carried out in a Rotor-Gene®Q PCR System (Qiagen) using a miRCURY LNA SYBR® Green PCR Kit and miRCURY LNA miRNA PCR Assay according to the manufacturer's instructions (Qiagen). Briefly, each reaction was performed in a final volume of 10 µL containing two µL of the cDNA, a master mix containing 5 µL of 2× miRCURY SYBR Green PCR Master Mix, 1 µL of miRCURY LNA miRNA PCR Assay, and RNase-free water. The amplification profile was: PCR initial heat activation at 95 °C for 2 min, followed by 40 cycles of denaturation at 95 °C for 10 s and combined annealing/extension at 56 °C for 60 s. The expression of mir-146b and mir-223 was normalized to RNU6B and calculated as $2^{-\Delta\Delta Ct}$.

4.10. Dot-Blotting for COX-2 Protein Expression

Cells were lysed in a 300 µL radioimmunoprecipitation assay buffer (RIPA) (Sigma-Aldrich, Milan, Italy). Total protein content was measured by using the Bio-Rad DC protein assay kit (Bio-Rad, Milan, Italy). Equal aliquots (30 µg) of proteins were applied to a nitrocellulose membrane (Millipore, Burlington, VT, USA) and allowed to dry for 30 min at RT. After blocking with 6% nonfat dry milk for 1 h at RT, the membranes were incubated overnight at RT with the Rabbit anti-COX-2 polyclonal antibody (1:200) (Cayman Chemical, MI, USA, catalog number 160126) followed by incubation with anti-rabbit IgG horseradish peroxidase-linked antibody (Cell Signaling, Danvers, MA, USA), 1:4000 for 1 h at RT. Chemiluminescence was developed by using the Immobilon Horseradish

Peroxidase Substrate (Merck Millipore, Darmstadt, Germany), and immunoreactive spots were quantified using Quantity-One software (Bio-Rad Laboratories S.r.l., Milan, Italy).

4.11. Immunocytochemistry for COX-2 Protein Expression

RAW 264.7 cells were grown in Poly-D-lysine-coated glass dishes for 24 h then treated with LPS and compounds and extracts tested as described above. After treatment, cells were fixed with cold 4% (*w/v*) paraformaldehyde for 20 min, washed in PBS, and then incubated for 15 min with 0.1% (*w/v*) TritonX-100 and 3% Bovine Serum Albumin (BSA). Thereafter, the cells were incubated with Rabbit anti-COX-2 polyclonal antibody (1:200) (Cayman, Ann Arbor, MI, USA, catalog number 160126) at 4 °C overnight, followed by the fluorescent secondary antibody: AlexaFluor 586 goat anti-rabbit (1:333) (Invitrogen, Carlsbad, CA, USA). Nuclei were also counterstained with DAPI dye (Sigma-Aldrich, Milan, Italy). Microscopic analysis was performed with an Olympus BX63 microscope equipped with a Metal Halide Lamp (Prior Scientific Instruments Ltd., Cambridge, UK) and a digital camera, Olympus XM 10 (Olympus, Milan, Italy).

4.12. Statistical Analysis

Data were analyzed by ANOVA test and Dunnett's Multiple Comparison test and expressed as the means ± standard error (SEM) of four independent experiments. All analyses were carried out using GraphPad Prism 7.0 (GraphPad Software, San Diego, CA, USA). p values less than 0.05 were considered significant.

Author Contributions: Conceptualization, all authors; methodology, E.B., M.D., L.C. and C.L.; validation, E.B., M.D. and L.C.; formal analysis, M.D., E.B. and C.L.; investigation, M.D., L.C., A.N. and L.B.D.S.N.; resources, C.L., M.R.T., N.B. and L.R.; writing—original draft preparation E.B., A.N. and C.L.; writing—review and editing, all authors; supervision, C.L.; funding acquisition, C.L. and M.R.T. All authors have read and agreed to the published version of the manuscript.

Funding: This research was co-funded by Ente Cassa di Risparmio Firenze grant numbers: 2015.0919 and 2018.1002 and by Regione Toscana (Italy) under Par-FAS 2007–2013 Projects (Centro di Competenza VALORE). A.N. holds a fellowship funded by the POR FSE 2014–2020—Progetto Strategico "STREAMING" sottoprogetto PhotoWING (grant number: UNIFI_FSE2017, Regione Toscana, Italy).

Institutional Review Board Statement: Not applicable.

Informed Consent Statement: Not applicable.

Data Availability Statement: The data that support the findings of this study are available on request from the corresponding author C.L. (cristina.luceri@unifi.it).

Acknowledgments: The authors wish to thank Massimo D'Ottavio for fucoxanthin determination.

Conflicts of Interest: *T. lutea* F&M-M36 belongs to the Culture Collection F&M S.r.l. culture collection, where M.R.T. and L.R. have a financial interest. The other authors have no conflicts of interest.

References

1. Bendif, E.; Probert, I.; Schroeder, D.C.; de Vargas, C. On the description of *Tisochrysis lutea* gen. nov., sp. nov. and *Isochrysis nuda* sp. nov. in the Isochrysidales, and the transfer of Dicrateria to the Prymnesiales (Haptophyta). *J. Appl. Phycol.* **2013**, *25*, 1763–1776. [CrossRef]
2. Camacho-Rodríguez, J.; Cerón-García, M.C.; González-López, C.V.; López-Rosales, L.; Contreras-Gómez, A.; Molina-Grima, E. Use of continuous culture to develop an economical medium for the mass production of *Isochrysis galbana* for aquaculture. *J. Appl. Phycol.* **2020**, *32*, 851–863. [CrossRef]
3. Custódio, L.; Soares, F.; Pereira, H.; Barreira, L.; Vizetto-Duarte, C.; Rodrigues, M.J.; Rauter, A.P.; Albericio, F.; Varela, J. Fatty acid composition and biological activities of *Isochrysis galbana* T-ISO, *Tetraselmis* sp. and *Scenedesmus* sp.: Possible application in the pharmaceutical and functional food industries. *J. Appl. Phycol.* **2014**, *26*, 151–161. [CrossRef]
4. Delbrut, A.; Albina, P.; Lapierre, T.; Pradelles, R.; Dubreucq, E. Fucoxanthin and Polyunsaturated Fatty Acids Co-Extraction by a Green Process. *Molecules* **2018**, *23*, 874. [CrossRef] [PubMed]
5. de los Reyes, C.; Ortega, M.J.; Rodríguez-Luna, A.; Talero, E.; Motilva, V.; Zubía, E. Molecular characterization and anti-inflammatory activity of galactosylglycerides and galactosylceramides from the microalga *Isochrysis galbana*. *J. Agric. Food Chem.* **2016**, *64*, 8783–8794. [CrossRef]

6. Hwang, P.A.; Phan, N.N.; Lu, W.J.; Ngoc Hieu, B.T.; Lin, Y.C. Low-molecular-weight fucoidan and high-stability fucoxanthin from brown seaweed exert prebiotics and anti-inflammatory activities in Caco-2 cells. *Food Nutr. Res.* **2016**, *60*, 32033. [CrossRef] [PubMed]
7. Bigagli, E.; Cinci, L.; Niccolai, A.; Biondi, N.; Rodolfi, L.; D'Ottavio, M.; D'Ambrosio, M.; Lodovici, M.; Tredici, M.R.; Luceri, C. Preliminary data on the dietary safety, tolerability and effects on lipid metabolism of the marine microalga *Tisochrysis lutea*. *Algal. Res.* **2018**, *34*, 244–249. [CrossRef]
8. Kim, S.M.; Kang, S.W.; Kwon, O.N.; Chung, D.; Pan, C.H. Fucoxanthin as a major carotenoid in *Isochrysis* aff. *galbana*: Characterization of extraction for commercial application. *J. Korean Soc. Appl. Biol. Chem.* **2012**, *55*, 477–483.
9. Heo, S.J.; Yoon, W.J.; Kim, K.N.; Ahn, G.N.; Kang, S.M.; Kang, D.H.; Affan, A.; Oh, C.; Jung, W.K.; Jeon, Y.J. Evaluation of anti-inflammatory effect of fucoxanthin isolated from brown algae in lipopolysaccharide-stimulated RAW 264.7 macrophages. *Food Chem. Toxicol.* **2010**, *48*, 2045–2051. [CrossRef]
10. Heo, S.J.; Yoon, W.J.; Kim, K.N.; Oh, C.; Choi, Y.U.; Yoon, K.T.; Kang, D.H.; Qian, Z.J.; Choi, I.W.; Jung, W.K. Anti-inflammatory effect of fucoxanthin derivatives isolated from *Sargassum siliquastrum* in lipopolysaccharide-stimulated RAW 264.7 macrophage. *Food Chem. Toxicol.* **2012**, *50*, 3336–3342. [CrossRef]
11. Kim, K.N.; Heo, S.J.; Yoon, W.J.; Kang, S.M.; Ahn, G.; Yi, T.H.; Jeon, Y.J. Fucoxanthin inhibits the inflammatory response by suppressing the activation of NF-jB and MAPKs in lipopolysaccharide-induced RAW 264.7 macrophages. *Eur. J. Pharmacol.* **2010**, *649*, 369–375. [CrossRef]
12. Su, J.; Guo, K.; Huang, M.; Liu, Y.; Zhang, J.; Sun, L.; Li, D.; Pang, K.L.; Wang, G.; Chen, L.; et al. Fucoxanthin, a Marine Xanthophyll Isolated From Conticribra weissflogii ND-8: Preventive Anti-Inflammatory Effect in a Mouse Model of Sepsis. *Front. Pharmacol.* **2019**, *10*, 906. [CrossRef]
13. Tan, C.P.; Hou, Y.H. First evidence for the anti-inflammatory activity of fucoxanthin in high-fat-diet-induced obesity in mice and the antioxidant functions in PC12 cells. *Inflammation* **2014**, *37*, 443–450. [CrossRef] [PubMed]
14. Matos, J.; Cardoso, C.; Gomes, A.; Campos, A.M.; Falé, P.; Afonso, C.; Bandarra, N.M. Bioprospection of Isochrysis galbana and its potential as a nutraceutical. *Food Funct.* **2019**, *10*, 7333–7342. [CrossRef] [PubMed]
15. Bigagli, E.; Cinci, L.; D'Ambrosio, M.; Luceri, C. Pharmacological activities of an eye drop containing *Matricaria chamomilla* and *Euphrasia officinalis* extracts in UVB-induced oxidative stress and inflammation of human corneal cells. *J. Photochem. Photobiol. B* **2017**, *173*, 618–625. [CrossRef]
16. Bigagli, E.; Cinci, L.; Paccosi, S.; Parenti, A.; D'Ambrosio, M.; Luceri, C. Nutritionally relevant concentrations of resveratrol and hydroxytyrosol mitigate oxidative burst of human granulocytes and monocytes and the production of pro-inflammatory mediators in LPS-stimulated RAW 264.7 macrophages. *Int. Immunopharmacol.* **2017**, *43*, 147–155. [CrossRef] [PubMed]
17. Bigagli, E.; Luceri, C.; Scartabelli, T.; Dolara, P.; Casamenti, F.; Pellegrini-Giampietro, D.E.; Giovannelli, L. Long-term Neuroglial Cocultures as a Brain Aging Model: Hallmarks of Senescence, MicroRNA Expression Profiles, and Comparison with In Vivo Models. *J. Gerontol. A Biol. Sci. Med. Sci.* **2016**, *71*, 50–60. [CrossRef] [PubMed]
18. Castagnini, C.; Luceri, C.; Toti, S.; Bigagli, E.; Caderni, G.; Femia, A.P.; Giovannelli, L.; Lodovici, M.; Pitozzi, V.; Salvadori, M.; et al. Reduction of colonic inflammation in HLA-B27 transgenic rats by feeding Marie Ménard apples, rich in polyphenols. *Br. J. Nutr.* **2009**, *102*, 1620–1628. [CrossRef] [PubMed]
19. Luceri, C.; Bigagli, E.; Pitozzi, V.; Giovannelli, L. A nutrigenomics approach for the study of anti-aging interventions: Olive oil phenols and the modulation of gene and microRNA expression profiles in mouse brain. *Eur. J. Nutr.* **2017**, *56*, 865–877. [CrossRef]
20. D'Ambrosio, M.; Bigagli, E.; Cinci, L.; Gori, A.; Brunetti, C.; Ferrini, F.; Luceri, C. Ethyl acetate extract from *Cistus x incanus* L. leaves enriched in myricetin and quercetin derivatives, inhibits inflammatory mediators and activates Nrf2/HO-1 pathway in LPS-stimulated RAW 264.7 macrophages. *Z. Naturforsch. C J. Biosci.* **2020**, *76*, 79–86. [CrossRef] [PubMed]
21. Yuan, H.; Ma, Q.; Cui, H.; Liu, G.; Zhao, X.; Li, W.; Piao, G. How Can Synergism of Traditional Medicines Benefit from Network Pharmacology? *Molecules* **2017**, *22*, 1135. [CrossRef]
22. Dunkhunthod, B.; Talabnin, C.; Murphy, M.; Thumanu, K.; Sittisart, P.; Hengpratom, T.; Eumkeb, G. Intracellular ROS Scavenging and Anti-Inflammatory Activities of *Oroxylum indicum* Kurz (L.) Extract in LPS plus IFN-γ-Activated RAW264.7 Macrophages. *Evid. Based. Complement. Alternat. Med.* **2020**, *27*, 2020. [CrossRef]
23. Sugimoto, M.A.; Sousa, L.P.; Pinho, V.; Perretti, M.; Teixeira, M.M. Resolution of Inflammation: What Controls Its Onset? *Front. Immunol.* **2016**, *26*, 160. [CrossRef]
24. Maadane, A.; Merghoub, N.; Ainane, T.; Arroussi, H.E.; Bennhima, R.; Amzazi, S.; Bakri, Y.; Wahby, I. Antioxidant activity of some Moroccan marine microalgae:Pufa profiles, carotenoids and phenolic content. *J. Biotechnol.* **2015**, *215*, 13–19. [CrossRef]
25. Robbins, R.J. Phenolic acids in foods: An overview of analytical methodology. *J. Agric. Food Chem.* **2003**, *51*, 2866–2887. [CrossRef]
26. Stalikas, C.D. Extraction, separation, and detection methods for phenolic acids and flavonoids. *J. Sep. Sci.* **2007**, *30*, 3268–3295. [CrossRef]
27. BenSaad, L.A.; Kim, K.H.; Quah, C.C.; Kim, W.R.; Shahimi, M. Anti-inflammatory potential of ellagic acid, gallic acid and punicalagin A&B isolated from *Punica granatum*. *BMC Complement. Altern. Med.* **2017**, *14*, 47.
28. Luzardo-Ocampo, I.; Loarca-Piña, G.; Gonzalez de Mejia, E. Gallic and butyric acids modulated NLRP3 inflammasome markers in a co-culture model of intestinal inflammation. *Food Chem. Toxicol.* **2020**, *146*, 111835. [CrossRef]
29. Luceri, C.; Guglielmi, F.; Lodovici, M.; Giannini, L.; Messerini, L.; Dolara, P. Plant phenolic 4-coumaric acid protects against intestinal inflammation in rats. *Scand. J. Gastroenterol.* **2004**, *11*, 1128–1133.

30. Gutiérrez, S.; Svahn, S.L.; Johansson, M.E. Effects of Omega-3 Fatty Acids on Immune Cells. *Int. J. Mol. Sci.* **2019**, *20*, 5028. [CrossRef]
31. Gallego, R.; Tardif, C.; Parreira, C.; Guerra, T.; Alves, M.J.; Ibáñez, E.; Herrero, M. Simultaneous extraction and purification of fucoxanthin from Tisochrysis lutea microalgae using compressed fluids. *J. Sep. Sci.* **2020**, *43*, 1967–1977. [CrossRef]
32. Li, R.; Hong, P.; Zheng, X. β-carotene attenuates lipopolysaccharide-induced inflamma-tion via inhibition of the NF-κB, JAK2/STAT3 and JNK/p38 MAPK signaling pathways in macrophages. *Anim. Sci. J.* **2019**, *90*, 140–148. [CrossRef]
33. Imamura, T.; Bando, N.; Yamanishi, R. Beta-carotene modulates the immunological function of RAW264, a murine macrophage cell line, by enhancing the level of intracellular glutathione. *Biosci. Biotechnol. Biochem.* **2006**, *70*, 2112–2120. [CrossRef]
34. Ambros, V. The functions of animal microRNAs. *Nature* **2004**, *431*, 350–355. [CrossRef]
35. Tahamtan, A.; Teymoori-Rad, M.; Nakstad, B.; Salimi, V. Anti-Inflammatory MicroRNAs and Their Potential for Inflammatory Diseases Treatment. *Front Immunol.* **2018**, *9*, 1377. [CrossRef]
36. Neudecker, V.; Haneklaus, M.; Jensen, O.; Khailova, L.; Masterson, J.C.; Tye, H.; Biette, K.; Jedlicka, P.; Brodsky, K.S.; Gerich, M.E.; et al. Myeloid-derived miR-223 regulates intestinal inflammation via repression of the NLRP3 inflammasome. *J. Exp. Med.* **2017**, *214*, 1737–1752. [CrossRef]
37. Zhang, N.; Fu, L.; Bu, Y.; Yao, Y.; Wang, Y. Downregulated expression of miR-223 promotes Toll-like receptor-activated inflammatory responses in macrophages by targeting RhoB. *Mol. Immunol.* **2017**, *91*, 42–48. [CrossRef]
38. Yuan, X.; Berg, N.; Lee, J.W.; Le, T.T.; Neudecker, V.; Jing, N.; Eltzschig, H. MicroRNA miR-223 as regulator of innate immunity. *J. Leukoc. Biol.* **2018**, *104*, 515–524. [CrossRef]
39. Bauernfeind, F.; Rieger, A.; Schildberg, F.A.; Knolle, P.A.; Schmid-Burgk, J.L.; Hornung, V. NLRP3 inflammasome activity is negatively controlled by miR-223. *J. Immunol.* **2012**, *189*, 4175–4181. [CrossRef]
40. Montana, G.; Lampiasi, N. Substance P Induces HO-1 Expression in RAW 264.7 Cells Promoting Switch towards M2-Like Macrophages. *PLoS ONE* **2016**, *11*, e0167420. [CrossRef]
41. Galvan-Pena, S.; O'Neill Luke, A.J. Metabolic reprogramming in macrophage polarization. *Front. Immunol.* **2014**, *2*, 420.
42. Kim, M.B.; Kang, H.; Li, Y.; Park, Y.K.; Lee, J.Y. Fucoxanthin inhibits lipopolysaccharide-induced inflammation and oxidative stress by activating nuclear factor E2-related factor 2 via the phosphatidylinositol 3-kinase/AKT pathway in macrophages. *Eur. J. Nutr.* **2021**, *60*, 1–10.
43. Mayer, C.; Richard, L.; Côme, M.; Ulmann, L.; Nazih, H.; Chénais, B.; Ouguerram, K.; Mimouni, V. The Marine Microalga, Tisochrysis lutea, Protects against Metabolic Disorders Associated with Metabolic Syndrome and Obesity. *Nutrients* **2021**, *3*, 430. [CrossRef]
44. O'Neill, L.A.; Sheedy, F.J.; McCoy, C.E. MicroRNAs: The fine-tuners of Toll-like receptor signalling. *Nat. Rev. Immunol.* **2011**, *11*, 163–175. [CrossRef]
45. Batra, S.K.; Heier, C.R.; Diaz-Calderon, L.; Tully, C.B.; Fiorillo, A.A.; van den Anker, J.; Conklin, L.S. Serum miRNAs Are Pharmacodynamic Biomarkers Associated with Therapeutic Response in Pediatric Inflammatory Bowel Disease. *Inflamm. Bowel. Dis.* **2020**, *26*, 1597–1606. [CrossRef] [PubMed]
46. Chen, P.; Li, Y.; Li, L.; Yu, Q.; Chao, K.; Zhou, G.; Qiu, Y.; Feng, R.; Huang, S.; He, Y.; et al. Circulating microRNA146b-5p is superior to C-reactive protein as a novel biomarker for monitoring inflammatory bowel disease. *Aliment. Pharmacol. Ther.* **2019**, *49*, 733–743. [CrossRef]
47. Nuño, K.; Villarruel-López, A.; Puebla-Pérez, A.M.; Romero-Velarde, E.; Puebla-Mora, A.G.; Ascencio, F. Effects of the marine microalgae Isochrysis galbana and Nannochloropsis oculata in diabetic rats. *J. Funct. Foods* **2013**, *5*, 106–115. [CrossRef]
48. Balakrishnan, J.; Dhavamani, S.; Sadasivam, S.G.; Arumugam, M.; Vellaikumar, S.; Ramalingam, J.; Shanmugam, K. Omega-3-rich Isochrysis sp. biomass enhances brain docosahexaenoic acid levels and improves serum lipid profile and antioxidant status in Wistar rats. *J. Sci. Food Agric.* **2019**, *99*, 6066–6075. [CrossRef]
49. Guillard, R.R.L.; Ryther, J.H. Studies of marine planktonic diatoms. I. Cyclotella nana Hustedt and Detonula confervacea Cleve. *Can. J. Microbiol.* **1962**, *8*, 229–239. [CrossRef] [PubMed]
50. Tredici, M.R.; Rodolfi, L.; Biondi, N.; Bassi, N.; Sampietro, G. Techno-economic analysis of microalgal biomass production in a 1-ha Green Wall Panel (GWP®) plant. *Algal. Res.* **2016**, *19*, 253–263. [CrossRef]

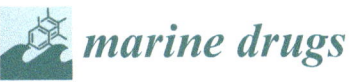

Article

Protective Effects of *Ulva lactuca* Polysaccharide Extract on Oxidative Stress and Kidney Injury Induced by D-Galactose in Mice

Qian Yang [1], Yanhui Jiang [2], Shan Fu [1], Zhaopeng Shen [3,*], Wenwen Zong [2], Zhongning Xia [4], Zhaoya Zhan [5] and Xiaolu Jiang [1,2,6,*]

[1] School of Food Science and Engineering, Ocean University of China, No. 5, Yushan Road, Qingdao 266003, China; 15205323877@163.com (Q.Y.); 21190731142@stu.ouc.edu.cn (S.F.)
[2] Marine Biomedical Research Institute of Qingdao, No. 23, Hong Kong Eastern Road, Qingdao 266071, China; jiangyanhui@ouc.edu.cn (Y.J.); 17864272822@163.com (W.Z.)
[3] School of Medicine and Pharmacy, Ocean University of China, No. 5, Yushan Road, Qingdao 266003, China
[4] Hainan Xin Kaiyuan Pharmaceutical Technology Co., Ltd., Hainan 570311, China; yundiao2009@163.com
[5] Fujian Blue Sea Food Technology Co., Ltd., Fujian 355200, China; yundiao2010@163.com
[6] State Key Laboratory of Bioactive Seaweed Substances, Qingdao Brightmoon Seaweed Group Co., Ltd., Qingdao 266400, China
* Correspondence: shenzp1987@ouc.edu.cn (Z.S.); jiangxl@ouc.edu.cn (X.J.)

Abstract: Reactive oxygen species (ROS) are the key factors that cause many diseases in the human body. Polysaccharides from seaweed have been shown to have significant antioxidant activity both in vivo and in vitro. The ameliorative effect of *Ulva lactuca* polysaccharide extract (UPE) on renal injury induced by oxidative stress was analyzed. As shown by hematoxylin–eosin staining results, UPE can significantly improve the kidney injury induced by D-galactose (D-gal). Additionally, the protective mechanism of UPE on the kidney was explored. The results showed that UPE could decrease the levels of serum creatinine (Scr), blood urea nitrogen (BUN), serum cystatin C (Cys-C), lipid peroxidation, protein carbonylation, and DNA oxidative damage (8-OHdG) and improve kidney glutathione content. Moreover, UPE significantly increased the activities of superoxide dismutase and glutathione peroxidase and total antioxidant activity in mice. UPE also decreased the levels of inflammatory cytokines TNF-α and IL-6. Further investigation into the expression of apoptotic protein caspase-3 showed that UPE decreased the expression of apoptotic protein caspase-3. These results indicate that UPE has a potential therapeutic effect on renal injury caused by oxidative stress, providing a new theoretical basis for the treatment of oxidative damage diseases in the future.

Keywords: *Ulva lactuca*; polysaccharide; D-galactose; oxidative stress; kidney

1. Introduction

Reactive oxygen species (ROS) are substances produced by human cells and tissues during normal physiological metabolism. Under normal circumstances, the body's antioxidant defense mechanisms play a role in the body's oxidative balance. However, when a large amount of ROS accumulates in the human body, it will cause oxidative imbalance and further aggravate the damage to the body [1]. The accumulation of ROS in the organism comes not only from the damage to the organism itself, but also from environmental pollution, radiation, and abuse of chemical products, which can cause the increase in ROS. Therefore, maintaining a balance of reactive oxygen species and antioxidant systems in the body is crucial to health. D-Galactose (D-gal) is a substance naturally occurring in the human body, but high concentrations of galactose will produce a large number of reactive oxygen species, leading to the aging of multiple tissues in the body and the occurrence of age-related immune decline; degenerative nervous system disorders; and damage to pancreas, kidney and other organs [2]. Therefore, the D-gal mouse model has become a widely used aging model.

Natural products with antioxidant activity have received extensive attention due to their good biological safety. With the attention to marine resources and the development of marine natural products, a variety of products that are raw materials with seaweed polysaccharides are gradually entering people's line of sight, and the antioxidant effect of algae polysaccharides has been confirmed [3]. It has been shown that fucoidans from brown algae can not only reduce the production of reactive oxygen species, but also increase the level of glutathione (GSH) and catalase (CAT) activity and reduce cytotoxicity [4,5]. *Ulva lactuca* is a kind of green algae in coastal areas of China. As a traditional Chinese medicine, it has good healthcare function. Ulvan is a water-soluble polysaccharide existing in the cell wall of *Ulva*, accounting for 8–29% of the dry weight [6]. It is a kind of sulfated heteropolysaccharide, which mainly includes sulfated rhamnose (Rha), xylose (Xyl), and uronic acid (glucuronic acid (GlcA) and iduronic acid (IdoA)); the structures of the main disaccharide repeating unit are [β-D-GlcpA-(1 → 4)-α-L-Rhap3s] and [α-L-IdopA-(1 → 4)-α-L-Rhap3s] [7]. Li et al. [8] found that the ulvan had a good scavenging ability against superoxide free radicals and DPPH free radicals in a concentration-dependent manner. Marlene Godardd et al. [9] reported that *U. lactuca* polysaccharide could significantly increase the activities of superoxide dismutase (SOD) and glutathione peroxidase (GSH-Px) and inhibit the production of lipid peroxidation and superoxide anion. In addition, ulvan with high sulfate content has obvious antioxidant ability and lipid-lowering activity [10]. Therefore, using ulvan as the raw material to develop medicine or food that can remove excess free radicals in the body is not only safe in composition but also effective and has a broad prospect.

In this study, *Ulva lactuca* polysaccharide extract (UPE) was obtained from *U. lactuca*, and D-gal was used to induce oxidative stress in mice to study the effects of UPE on oxidative stress and inflammation in mice. Hematoxylin and eosin staining and immunohistochemistry were used to explore the tissue damage and cell apoptosis in mice.

2. Results

2.1. Characterization of UPE

As shown in Table 1, the main component of UPE is carbohydrate, accounting for about 52.61% of the total composition; in addition, UPE contains uronic acid and sulfate group. By molecular weight analysis, the average molecular weight of UPE is about 891.25 kDa. According to the analysis of monosaccharide composition (Figure 1b,c), it is mainly composed of Rha, GlcA, glucose (Glc), and Xyl, and the content of Rha is the highest (45.33%). In addition, through FT-IR (Figure 1a), the signals at 1640, 1427, and 1054 cm^{-1} are respectively the absorption peaks of the stretching vibration of carbonyl group C=O, the absorption peaks of the stretching vibration of carboxyl group C-O, and the absorption peaks of the O-H angular vibration. These three absorption peaks are characteristic absorption peaks of uronic acids [11]. The absorption peaks of 1259 and 843 cm^{-1} are the characteristic absorption peaks of the sulfate group, where 1259 cm^{-1} is the absorption peak of S=O stretching vibration and 843 cm-1 is the absorption peak of C-O-S stretching vibration. According to the above results, it was proved that both sulfuric acid and uronic acid were present in UPE, which were the main characteristics of ulvan.

Table 1. Molecular weight, composition, and monosaccharide composition of UPE.

Molecular Weight (kDa)	Monosaccharide Composition (%)		Composition (%)	
891.25	Rha	45.33%	Total sugar	61.98
	GlcA	15.50%	Protein	2.39
	Glc	18.97%	Uronic acid	9.13
	Xyl	20.29%	Sulfate group	16.50

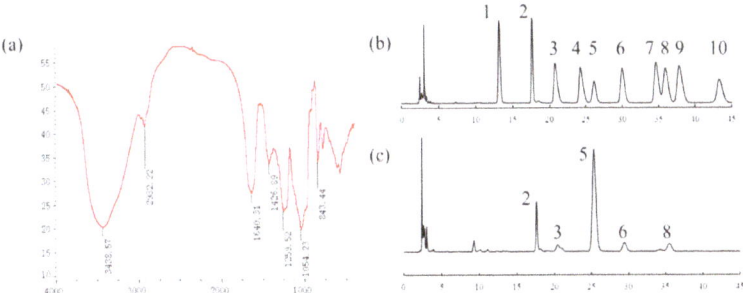

Figure 1. Structural characterization of UPE. (**a**) FT-IR. (**b**) Standard monosaccharide. 1-Man, 2-Rha, 3-GlcA, 4-GalA, 5-Lac (internal standard), 6-Glc, 7-Gal, 8-Xyl, 9-Ara, 10-Fuc. (**c**) Monosaccharide composition of UPE. 2-Rha, 3-GlcA, 5-Lac (internal standard), 6-Glc, 8-Xyl.

2.2. Effect of UPE on Organ Index

Organ index is the ratio of a certain organ to its body weight. After an animal's body is damaged, organ weight will change, and organ coefficient will also change. Therefore, the viscera ratio can intuitively judge the severity of body damage. The body weight and kidney weight of mice are shown in Table 2. The renal index of mice is shown in Figure 2a. The renal index of mice injected with D-gal decreased significantly ($p < 0.01$) when the initial body weight was basically the same. However, after UPE treatment, the renal index was significantly increased ($p < 0.01$), which indicated that UPE alleviated the phenomenon of renal atrophy to a certain extent and had a protective effect on the kidney.

Table 2. The different groups for body weights and kidney weights.

	BC	NC	PC	LD	HD
Body Weight (g)	28.125 ± 2.064	27.550 ± 2.263 *	29.300 ± 1.747 ##	29.171 ± 4.085 ##	27.85 ± 2.468
Kidney Weight (g)	0.306 ± 0.023	0.274 ± 0.019 **	0.307 ± 0.022 ##	0.307 ± 0.045 ##	0.304 ± 0.023 ##

* $p < 0.05$, ** $p < 0.01$ compared with BC group; ## $p < 0.01$ compared with NC group. BC: blank control, NC: negative control, PC: positive control, LD: low-dose UPE (50 mg/kg), HD: high-dose UPE (300 mg/kg).

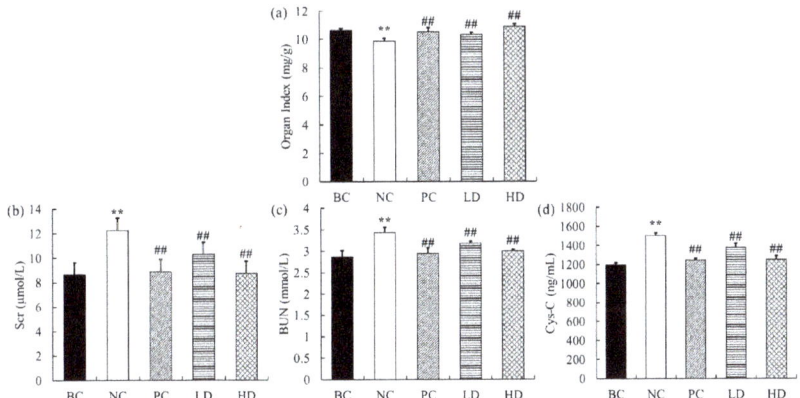

Figure 2. Effect of UPE on organ index and serum Scr, BUN, and Cys-C levels. (**a**) Organ index. (**b**) Scr content. (**c**) BUN content. (**d**) Cys-C content. The data are expressed as mean ± standard deviation ($n = 9$). ** $p < 0.01$ compared with BC group; ## $p < 0.01$ compared with NC group. BC: blank control, NC: negative control, PC: positive control, LD: low-dose UPE (50 mg/kg), HD: high-dose UPE (300 mg/kg).

2.3. Effects of UPE on Serum Indexes

The levels of Scr, BUN, and Cys-C in serum and kidney are shown in Figure 2b–d. Compared with the control mice, the contents of Scr, BUN, and Cys-C in serum of mice treated with D-gal were increased by 42.06%, 19.94%, and 25.43% ($p < 0.01$), respectively. When feeding low-dose UPE, the contents of Scr and Cys-C were significantly decreased (both $p < 0.01$) compared with the NC group, but there was no statistical significance in the change of BUN level. However, the contents of Scr, BUN, and Cys-C in the high-dose group were significantly decreased (28.76%, 12.65%, and 16.76%, respectively, $p < 0.01$), indicating that UPC had a protective effect on kidney injury induced by D-gal in mice.

2.4. Effects of UPE on Renal Oxidation and Antioxidant Indexes

The large amount of ROS produced by oxidative stress will cause oxidative damage to biological macromolecules such as proteins, lipids, and DNA and then cause damage to the body. The oxidant and antioxidant indexes of mice are shown in Figure 3. The contents of MDA, protein carbonyl, and 8-OHdG in mice in the D-gal group were significantly increased (52.46%, 31.48%, and 27.45%, respectively) compared with those in the BC group (all $p < 0.01$), and the content of GSH decreased significantly (23.16%, $p < 0.05$). Moreover, D-gal also led to a decrease in the activities of SOD (16.66%), GSH-Px (21.74%), and T-AOC (47.99%) in mice (all $p < 0.01$). After using low-dose UPE, the contents of MDA, protein carbonyl, and 8-OHdG in mice were reduced by 10.79%, 13.78%, and 9.72%, respectively ($p < 0.01$), and the activities of SOD, GSH-Px, and T-AOC were also significantly increased (10.51%, 46.65%, and 11.97%, respectively), but the change in GSH content was not statistically significant ($p > 0.05$). In contrast, in the high-dose group, MDA, protein carbonyl, and 8-OHdG were also significantly reduced (all $p < 0.01$); GSH content was significantly increased (43.18%, $p < 0.05$); and the activities of SOD, GSH-Px, and T-AOC were close to the level of normal mice. These results show that UPE can significantly reduce oxidative damage caused by D-gal and improve the antioxidant capacity of mice.

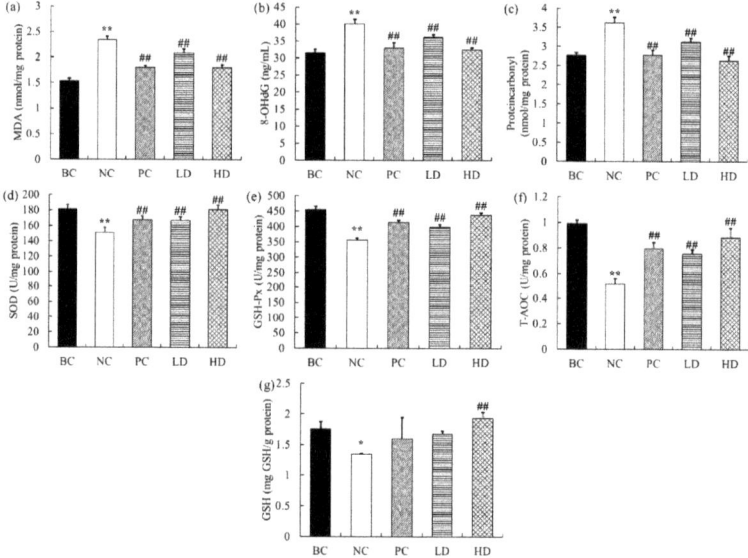

Figure 3. Levels of antioxidant indexes in the kidney of mice. (a) MDA content. (b) 8-OHdG concentration. (c) Protein carbonyl content. (d) SOD activity. (e) GSH-Px activity. (f) T-AOC activity. (g) GSH content. Data are presented as mean ± standard deviation ($n = 9$). * $p < 0.05$, ** $p < 0.01$ compared with BC group; ## $p < 0.01$ compared with NC group. BC: blank control, NC: negative control, PC: positive control, LD: low-dose UPE (50 mg/kg), HD: high-dose UPE (300 mg/kg).

2.5. Effects of UPE on Inflammatory Factors

The levels of inflammatory cytokines in mice are shown in Figure 4. Compared with the BC group, the levels of IL-6 and TNF-α in mice injected with D-gal were significantly increased ($p < 0.01$). The levels of IL-6 and TNF-α in mice in the low-dose group were slightly decreased, but there was no statistically significant difference ($p > 0.05$). The IL-6 level in the high-dose group showed no significant change, while the TNF-α level significantly decreased.

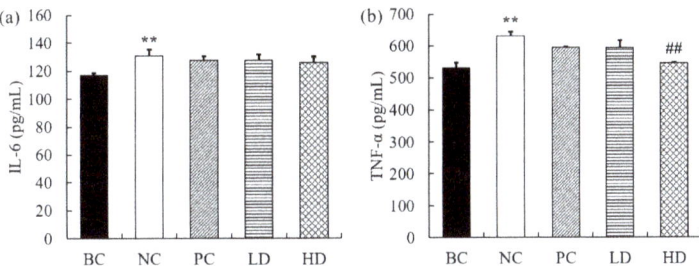

Figure 4. The levels of inflammatory factors in the kidneys of mice. (**a**) IL-6. (**b**) TNF-α. The data are expressed as mean ± standard deviation ($n = 9$). ** $p < 0.01$ compared with BC group; ## $p < 0.01$ compared with NC group. BC: blank control, NC: negative control, PC: positive control, LD: low-dose UPE (50 mg/kg), HD: high-dose UPE (300 mg/kg).

2.6. Histopathological Analysis

The most direct method to judge the pathological injury of the kidney is to observe the renal tissue morphology of mice by microscope. As shown in Figure 5, the glomeruli of mice in the normal group were round, with obvious renal cysts, and renal tubules were arranged neatly with obvious lumens, without pathological changes. However, D-gal-treated mice had irregular glomerulus shape, with some degree of atrophy, irregular renal capsule lumen, and fuzzy renal tubules. However, after UPE treatment, the glomeruli and renal lumen were normal, the margins of the lumen were clear, and the renal tubules and lumen were distinguishable. The histomorphological characteristics of renal sections stained with H&E showed that UPE had a protective effect on D-gal-induced renal injury.

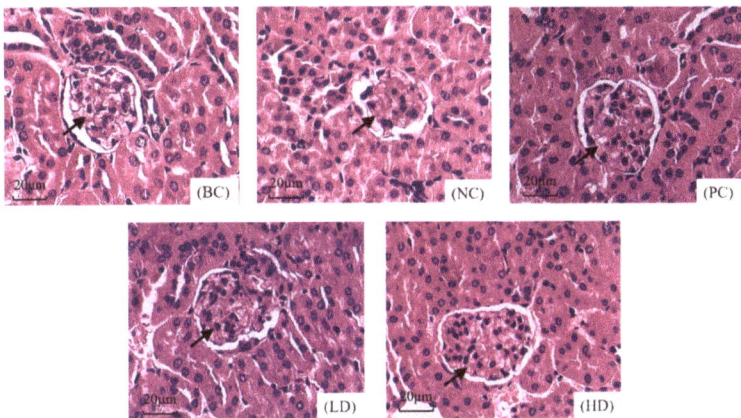

Figure 5. Effect of UPE on histopathological changes of the D-gal-treated kidney. The glomerulus is marked by the arrow. In the NC group, glomeruli are atrophic and deformed, and the renal sac is irregular. The LD and HD groups improved significantly (×400). BC: blank control, NC: negative control, PC: positive control, LD: low-dose UPE (50 mg/kg), HD: high-dose UPE (300 mg/kg).

2.7. Expression of Caspase-3 Protein in Kidney

During apoptosis, the caspase-3 protein was positively expressed, and the immunoreactive product was stained in renal tubules. The expression of the caspase-3 protein in the mouse kidney is shown in Figure 6. Apoptosis was observed in each group. Compared with the blank group, caspase-3 showed obvious positive expression in the NC group, and the positive cells were increasingly dense. The positive expression of UPE was significantly reduced in mice after UPE treatment, suggesting that UPE may have a protective effect on apoptosis. Image J software was used to analyze the staining situation, and it was found that compared with the BC group, the protein expression level of the NC group was significantly increased ($p < 0.05$), and the expression level of caspase-3 decreased significantly after treatment ($p < 0.05$), which further proved the improvement effect of UPE on apoptosis.

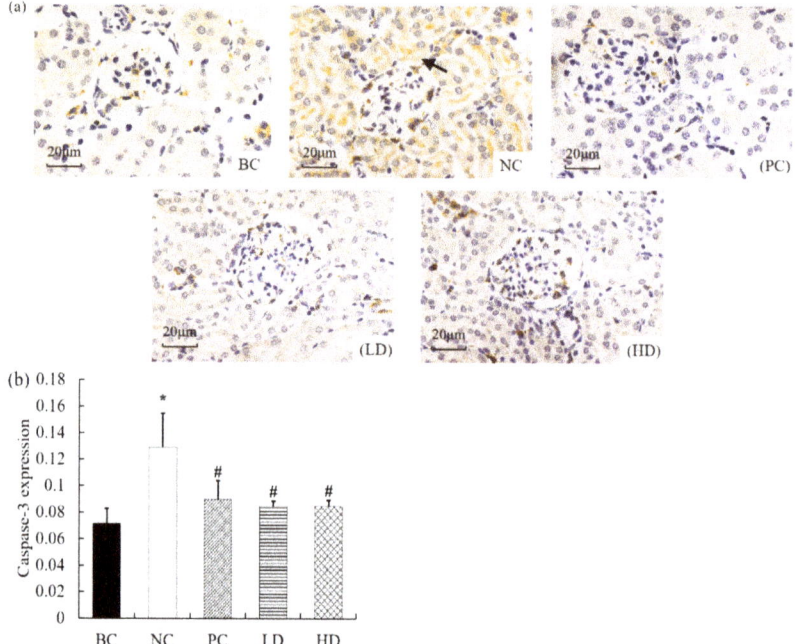

Figure 6. Effect of UPE on the expression of caspase-3 in kidney treated with D-gal. (**a**) The arrow in the image shows positive expression of caspase-3 protein and apoptosis (×400). (**b**) The expression of caspase-3. Data are presented as mean ± standard deviation ($n = 9$). * $p < 0.05$ compared with BC group; # $p < 0.05$ compared with NC group. BC: blank control, NC: negative control, PC: positive control, LD: low-dose UPE (50 mg/kg), HD: high-dose UPE (300 mg/kg).

3. Discussion

The kidney is an important organ in the human body. Through filtration, the kidney educts the excess waste in the human body through urine, so as to maintain the metabolism of the human body and ensure the stability of the internal environment of the body. It has been reported that the production of large amounts of reactive oxygen species is the key pathogenic factor for a variety of kidney diseases [12]. In the event of oxidative stress, both renal tubules and vascular cells produce large amounts of reactive oxygen species, which attack renal cells and tissues and further cause renal damage [13]. In this study, in order to investigate the antioxidant ability of ulvan in vivo, we established a model of oxidative stress induced by D-gal to study the protective effect of UPE on kidney injury induced by oxidative stress.

Previous studies have shown that D-gal can lead to decreased indexes of kidney, thymus, brain, and other organs [14,15]. The results showed that UPE significantly improved the kidney atrophy induced by D-gal, which proved the protective effect of UPE on kidneys to a certain extent. This result was also confirmed in the H&E observation. D-gal-induced oxidative stress can cause damage to various tissues and organs. In mice treated with D-gal, capillary congestion of glomeruli and renal tubules would occur, and renal tubules would degenerate and die, leading to renal injury [16]. In our study, changes in renal structure were observed in mice. Compared with D-gal-treated mouse kidneys, UPE improved the pathological phenomena of glomerular atrophy and renal lumen obscuration, suggesting that UPE had a certain therapeutic effect on mouse kidney injury induced by D-gal treatment.

Excessive production of reactive oxygen species can cause oxidative damage to biological macromolecules such as proteins, nucleic acids, lipids, and DNA [17]. Lipid is the most common target of oxidative stress, and its oxidation product MDA can cause serious damage to mitochondrial respiratory chain complex and cell membrane, and it is widely used as a marker of lipid peroxidation [18]. Although 8-OHDG is not a specific marker of oxidative damage, ROS and hydroxyl radicals can attack DNA to produce 8-OHDG, which is the most commonly used biomarker of oxidative damage of DNA [19]. The carbonyl group is a key marker of protein oxidation, which is formed because reactive oxygen species directly attack the free amino group in amino acid molecules [20]. GSH is an important antioxidant and free radical scavenger in the body, which can react with H_2O_2 under the catalysis of GSH-Px to form GSSH, and remove peroxides and hydroxyl radicals produced by cellular respiration metabolism [15]. As an important component of the body's antioxidant defense system, SOD is the primary material for scavenging free radicals in the body, which can convert superoxide free radicals into hydrogen peroxide. GSH-Px protects cells from damage by scavenging lipid and hydrogen peroxides [21]. T-AOC is an evaluation index of comprehensive antioxidant capacity. The changes of oxidation products (MDA, 8-OHdG, protein carbonyl group, and GSH) and antioxidant enzyme activities (SOD, GSH-Px, and T-AOC) can be used to determine the oxidation level in the body. Through our study, it was found that the levels of MDA, 8-OHdG, and protein carbonyl in mice after UPE treatment were significantly reduced, suggesting that UPE has a significant therapeutic effect on oxidative injury. At the same time, we also found that UPE could significantly increase the activities of SOD, GSH-Px, and T-AOC in mice, which was consistent with the study of Liu et al., which has shown that polysaccharide extracted from *U. lactuca* could improve the antioxidant capacity of SAMP8 mice and also reduce the contents of inflammatory factors such as TNF-α, IL-6, and IFN-γ in mice [22]. These results provide evidence that UPE can be used to treat oxidative stress.

Kidney damage is followed by problems with kidney function. Scr, BUN, and Cys-C are commonly used to measure kidney health, and their concentrations are increased by kidney injury or renal failure [23]. The creatinine and urea in the blood are filtered mainly in the glomerulus, part of which is filtered out of the blood and the rest of which is reabsorbed. Serum Cys-C has a better effect in marking glomerular filtration level and can therefore be used as a marker of glomerular filtration rate [24]. In this study, after acute kidney injury, Scr, BUN, and Cys-C levels were significantly increased, indicating a sharp decrease in renal tubular filtration rate, which was consistent with previous studies [25]. Based on these conclusions, the contents of serum creatinine, blood urea nitrogen, and Cys-C decreased significantly after treatment with UPE and approached the normal level with the increase in the concentration, indicating that the filtration ability of mouse kidneys gradually recovered. Studies have shown that alginate oligosaccharides have an obvious protective effect on kidney injury induced by D-gal in mice, and the levels of BUN and Scr are improved after 4 weeks of treatment [26]. Kelp polysaccharide can reduce the content of Scr and BUN. This protective effect may be related to the anti-inflammatory and antioxidant effects of sulfated polysaccharides [27]. Therefore, it was speculated that the protective effect of UPE on the kidney might be related to its antioxidant capacity.

Oxidative stress can activate a variety of transcription factors, such as NF-κB, AP-1, and P53, which lead to the expression of inflammatory cytokines, anti-inflammatory molecules, and other genes [28]. TNF-α is a major inflammatory cytokine that can kill target cells, promote cell apoptosis, and participate in local inflammation and activation of endothelial cells. IL-6 is a type of interleukin that acts as a proinflammatory cytokine and an anti-inflammatory myosin. In our study, the levels of IL-6 and TNF-α in mice in the BC group were significantly higher than those in the control group, indicating a severe inflammatory response in mice. It may be caused by the production of proinflammatory mediators stimulated by oxidative stress. Although the content of IL-6 in mice was decreased after using UPE, the effect was not obvious, but the level of TNF-α in mice was decreased significantly ($p < 0.05$). Some studies have shown that *U. lactuca* polysaccharide can significantly reduce the serum levels of TNF-α and NO in breast cancer mice, indicating that UPE can regulate inflammatory response and reduce the level of inflammatory cytokines [29]. It has also been reported that *Gracilaria* extract achieves anti-inflammatory effects by reducing the levels of NO, IL-6, and TNF-α [30]. Purified kelp polysaccharide can reduce inflammatory reactions by inhibiting the activation of the TGF-β1-mediated inflammatory cytokine signaling pathway, downregulating the levels of TNF-α and IL-1β, etc. [31]. It was suggested that UPE might regulate the expression of cytokines at the transcriptional level [32].

Apoptosis is closely related to oxidative stress induced by ROS. Oxidative stress can mediate apoptosis by stimulating the synthesis of inflammatory factor TNF-α. TNF-α can activate caspase-8 after binding to surface receptors and then shear and activate caspase-3, leading to the production of apoptosis [33]. In addition, excessive ROS will directly attack the mitochondrial membrane, change the ratio of proapoptotic protein Bax and anti-apoptotic protein Bcl-2, mediate the release of cytochrome C, activate apoptotic factor caspase-3, and cause cell apoptosis [34]. Cascade activation of the cysteine protease family is an essential procedure in apoptosis, in which caspase-3 plays a key role [35]. In this study, the renal tubular epithelial cells of mice treated with D-gal showed a strong positive reaction, the expression of caspase-3 was enhanced, and abnormal renal apoptosis occurred. However, after UPE treatment, the apoptosis of renal cells was significantly reduced, which indicated that UPE had a certain protective effect on the kidney. It has been reported that *Enteromorpha prolifera* polysaccharides can regulate the mitochondrial apoptosis pathway and reduce cell damage [36]. Astragalus polysaccharides can also protect acute kidney injury by regulating oxidative stress and improving mitochondrial apoptosis signals [37]. These results indicate that UPE has a good effect on apoptosis induced by D-gal and provide a direction for the development of UPE in the future.

4. Materials and Methods

4.1. Chemicals

D-gal and ascorbic acid (VC) were supplied by Sinopharm Chemical Reagent Co., Ltd. (Guangzhou, China). Assay kits for the measurements of superoxide dismutase (SOD), glutathione peroxidase (GSH-Px), glutathione (GSH), malondialdehyde (MDA), total antioxidant capability (T-AOC), serum creatinine (Scr), blood urea nitrogen (BUN), serum cystatin C (Cys-c), 8-hydroxylated deoxyguanosine (8-OHdG), and protein carbonyl were purchased from Jiancheng Bioengineering Institute (Nanjing, China). ELISA detection kits for IL-6 and TNF-α were obtained from Dakewe Biotech Corporation (Beijing, China).

4.2. Sample Preparation

U. lactuca was soaked in 80% alcohol for 18 h and heated at 70 °C for 4 h to remove pigment, protein, and some salt. The sample was centrifuged and dried. The polysaccharide was extracted by hot water extraction. The crude extract and water were dissolved in a ratio of 1:30 and reacted at 100 °C for 1 h. Ulvan crude extracts were filtered and centrifuged (4000 rpm, 10 min). The supernatants were collected and concentrated at reduced pressure. They were precipitated overnight at 4 °C with twice the volume of 95%

ethanol. The polysaccharide was obtained by freeze-drying after collecting the precipitation and named UPE.

4.3. Characterization of UPE

The content of total sugar in UPE was determined by phenol–sulfuric acid method, and glucose was taken as the standard [38]. Protein content was determined by Kjeldahl method [39]. The uronic acid content in UPE was calculated by m-hydroxybiphenyl method [40]. The sulfate radical content was evaluated by barium sulfate turbidimetry [41].

The molecular weight of UPE was analyzed by gel permeation chromatography (GPC). Agilent 1260 HPLC was used and equipped with a PL aquagel-OH 60 column (300 mm × 7.5 mm; Tosoh, Shiba, Tokyo, Japan) and refractive index detectors. The dried polysaccharide samples were ground and mixed with potassium bromide to make the tablets and scanned by Nexus 70 infrared spectrometer. The monosaccharide components of UPE were determined by reversed-phase HPLC method. After acidolysis with trifluoroacetic acid, PMP was used for derivation. Monosaccharide analysis was performed on a ZORBAX Eclipse XDB-C18 separation column (4.6 mm × 250 mm) at 245 nm.

4.4. Animals and Diet

Forty-five eight-week-old male Kunming mice were raised in an experimental environment and subjected to a light–dark cycle at 23 ± 1 °C for 12 h. During the week of domestication, the animals were given normal lab feed and free water. Mice were randomly divided into blank control group (BC), negative control group (NC), positive control group (PC) (VC, 100 mg/kg), low-dose group (LD) (UPE, dose of 50 mg/kg), and high-dose group (HD) (UPE, dose of 300 mg/kg), with 9 mice in each group. Mice in NC group, PC group, LD group, and HD group were subcutaneously injected with D-Gal at a dose of 400 mg/kg, and mice in BC group were injected with 0.9% normal saline for 10 weeks. Starting from week 7, the LD group and HD group were intragastrically given UPE at the corresponding dose, while the PC group was intragastrically given VC once a day for 4 consecutive weeks. The BC and NC groups were given the same volume of distilled water. The experiment design was approved by the Animal Care and Use Committee of Ocean University of China (certificate no. SYXK2012014).

4.5. Body Weight Measurement

The mice were weighed every 2 days. On the last day of the experimental period, after 8–12 h of fasting, the mice were sacrificed under ether narcotization. The kidney was isolated and weighed to calculate the organ coefficient, using the following formula:

$$\text{Coefficient (mg/g)} = \text{organ weight (mg)} / \text{body weight (g)}.$$

4.6. Serum Indexes Analysis

Blood samples were collected from the eye socket and centrifuged at 4 °C and 3000 rpm for 30 min, and the serum was stored at −80 °C. The contents of Scr, BUN, and Cys-c were determined.

4.7. Biochemical Analysis

Mice were sacrificed by cervical vertebrae removal. The kidneys were carefully removed, washed with 0.9% NaCl, frozen in liquid nitrogen, and stored at −80 °C for subsequent physical and chemical analysis. Kidney specimens were homogenized with tissue homogenizer in phosphate buffer pH 7.4, and the supernatant was collected centrifugally (3000 rpm, 10 min). The contents of MDA, SOD, GSH-Px, and T-AOC were measured according to the kit instructions, and the renal antioxidant enzyme activity was evaluated. The contents of protein carbonyl and 8-OHdG were determined to evaluate the oxidative damage level of protein and DNA. The levels of TNF-α and IL-6 in the kidney were determined by ELISA, and the levels of inflammatory factors were evaluated.

4.8. Hematoxylin and Eosin (H&E) Staining

Kidney specimens were fixed in 10% formaldehyde normal saline for 5–7 days, washed with clean water for 10 min, and dehydrated with alcohol classification (75%, 85%, 95%, 100%) in accordance with conventional sequence, and then they were treated with xylene to make them transparent. The specimen was then embedded in paraffin. The specimens were cut into 5 mm slices by a slicer. The tissues were stained with hematoxylin and observed under an optical microscope.

4.9. Immunohistochemical Analysis

The kidney slices were dewaxed and hydrated by SP immunohistochemical method, the antigens were repaired with citric acid buffer solution, catalase and nonspecific reaction sites were sealed with H_2O_2 and goat serum, and the slices were rinsed with PBS. According to the requirements of the kit, the expression of caspase-3 protein in renal tissue was detected. The images were observed with an optical microscope and analyzed with ImageJ software.

4.10. Statistical Analysis

Data are expressed as mean ± standard deviation. Statistical analysis was conducted through one-way ANOVA using SPSS 20.0 software (IBM, New York, NY, USA). All data are presented as the mean ± SD, and values of $p < 0.05$ and $p < 0.01$ were considered statistically significant.

5. Conclusions

In this study, we demonstrated the antioxidant activity and corresponding inflammatory response of ulvan against oxidative stress induced by D-gal in mice. The results showed that ulvan could significantly decrease the contents of Scr, BUN, and Cys-C in the kidney; increase the glomerular filtration rate; improve the activities of SOD and GSH-Px and total antioxidant capacity in mice; and reduce the damage to biomacromolecules caused by oxidative damage. In addition, it also significantly improved the changes in TNF-α and IL-6 caused by oxidative stress. In the aspect of apoptosis, ulvan could protect against the D-gal-induced apoptosis of renal tubule cells. These results confirm that ulvan has a protective effect on kidney injury caused by oxidative stress. It provides a basis for the development of antioxidants and the treatment of related diseases in the future.

Author Contributions: Conceptualization, Q.Y. and Z.S.; methodology, Q.Y. and S.F.; formal analysis, Q.Y., Y.J. and W.Z.; data curation, Q.Y., Y.J. and Z.S.; writing, Q.Y., Y.J. and Z.S.; visualization, Q.Y., Z.S. and X.J.; supervision, X.J. and Z.S.; project administration, Z.Z. and X.J.; funding acquisition, Z.X. All authors have read and agreed to the published version of the manuscript.

Funding: This work was funded by the Qingdao Marine Biological Medicine Science and Technology Innovation Center Construction Project (2017-CXZX01-4-6); the Key Project of New and Old Energy Transformation in Shandong Province; the University Co-construction Project—Marine Health Products, Qingdao, Shandong, China (grant number HYJK1907, 2019); and Fujian Provincial Regional Development Project, 2020N3016.

Institutional Review Board Statement: The study was conducted according to the guidelines of the Declaration of Helsinki, and approved by the Ethical Committee of Experimental Animal Care at Ocean University of China (certificate no. SYXK2012014).

Conflicts of Interest: The authors declare that they have no competing financial or nonfinancial conflict of interest.

References

1. Chen, J.; Huang, Z.; Wu, X.; Kang, J.; Ren, Y.; Gao, W.; Lu, X.; Wang, J.; Ding, W.; Nakabeppu, Y.; et al. Oxidative stress induces different tissue dependent effects on Mutyh-deficient mice. *Free Radic. Biol. Med.* **2019**, *143*, 482–493. [CrossRef]
2. Davalli, P.; Mitic, T.; Caporali, A.; Lauriola, A.; D'Arca, D. ROS, Cell Senescence, and Novel Molecular Mechanisms in Aging and Age-Related Diseases. *Oxid. Med. Cell. Longev.* **2016**, *2016*, 3565127. [CrossRef]

3. Díaz, R.T.A.; Arrojo, V.C.; Agudo, M.A.A.; Cárdenas, C.; Dobretsov, S.; Figueroa, F.L. Immunomodulatory and Antioxidant Activities of Sulfated Polysaccharides from *Laminaria ochroleuca*, *Porphyra umbilicalis*, and *Gelidium corneum*. *Mar. Biotechnol.* **2019**, *21*, 577–587. [CrossRef] [PubMed]
4. Castro, L.S.E.P.W.; Pinheiro, T.S.; Castro, A.J.G.; Dore, C.M.P.G.; da Silva, N.B.; das C. Faustino Alves, M.G.; Santos, M.S.N.; Leite, E.L. Fucose-containing sulfated polysaccharides from brown macroalgae *Lobophora variegata* with antioxidant, anti-inflammatory, and antitumoral effects. *J. Appl. Phycol.* **2014**, *26*, 1783–1790. [CrossRef]
5. Chale-Dzul, J.; Freile-Pelegrín, Y.; Robledo, D.; Moo-Puc, R. Protective effect of fucoidans from tropical seaweeds against oxidative stress in HepG2 cells. *J. Appl. Phycol.* **2017**, *29*, 2229–2238. [CrossRef]
6. Lahaye, M.; Robic, A. Structure and Functional Properties of Ulvan, a Polysaccharide from Green Seaweeds. *Biomacromolecules* **2007**, *8*, 1765–1774. [CrossRef] [PubMed]
7. Pengzhan, Y.; Quanbin, Z.; Ning, L.; Zuhong, X.; Yanmei, W. Polysaccharides from *Ulva pertusa* (Chlorophyta) and preliminary studies on their antihyperlipidemia activity. *J. Appl. Phycol.* **2003**, *15*, 21–27. [CrossRef]
8. Li, W.; Wang, K.; Jiang, N.; Liu, X.; Wan, M.; Chang, X.; Liu, D.; Qi, H. Antioxidant and antihyperlipidemic activities of purified polysaccharides from *Ulva pertusa*. *J. Appl. Phycol.* **2018**, *30*, 2619–2627. [CrossRef]
9. Godard, M.; Décordé, K.; Ventura, E.; Soteras, G.; Baccou, J.; Cristol, J.; Rouanet, J. Polysaccharides from the green alga *Ulva rigida* improve the antioxidant status and prevent fatty streak lesions in the high cholesterol fed hamster, an animal model of nutritionally-induced atherosclerosis. *Food Chem.* **2009**, *115*, 176–180. [CrossRef]
10. Li, B.; Xu, H.; Wang, X.; Wan, Y.; Jiang, N.; Qi, H.; Liu, X. Antioxidant and antihyperlipidemic activities of high sulfate content puri fi ed polysaccharide from *Ulva pertusa*. *Int. J. Biol. Macromol.* **2020**, *146*, 756–762. [CrossRef]
11. Chi, Y.; Zhang, M.; Wang, X.; Fu, X.; Guan, H.; Wang, P. Ulvan lyase assisted structural characterization of ulvan from *Ulva pertusa* and its antiviral activity against vesicular stomatitis virus. *Int. J. Biol. Macromol.* **2020**, *157*, 75–82. [CrossRef] [PubMed]
12. Sifuentes-Franco, S.; Padilla-Tejeda, D.E.; Carrillo-Ibarra, S.; Miranda-Díaz, A.G. Oxidative Stress, Apoptosis, and Mitochondrial Function in Diabetic Nephropathy. *Int. J. Endocrinol.* **2018**, *2018*, 1875870. [CrossRef]
13. Ratliff, B.B.; Abdulmahdi, W.; Pawar, R. Oxidant Mechanisms in Renal Injury and Disease 1,2 2 1. *Antioxid. Redox Signal.* **2016**, *25*, 119–146. [CrossRef]
14. Chen, P.; Chen, F.; Zhou, B. Antioxidative, anti-inflammatory and anti-apoptotic effects of ellagic acid in liver and brain of rats treated by D-galactose. *Sci. Rep.* **2018**, *8*, 1465. [CrossRef]
15. Wang, C.; Shen, Z.; Yu, J.; Yang, J.; Meng, F.; Jiang, X.; Zhu, C. Protective effects of enzyme degradation extract from Porphyra yezoensis against oxidative stress and brain injury in d -galactose-induced ageing mice. *Br. J. Nutr.* **2020**, *123*, 975–986. [CrossRef]
16. El-far, A.H.; Lebda, M.A.; Noreldin, A.E.; Atta, M.S.; Elewa, Y.H.A.; Elfeky, M.; Mousa, S.A. Quercetin attenuates pancreatic and renal d- galactose-induced aging-related oxidative alterations in rats. *Int. J. Mol. Sci.* **2020**, *21*, 4348. [CrossRef] [PubMed]
17. Xie, Z.X.; Xia, S.F.; Qiao, Y.; Shi, Y.H.; Le, G.W. Effect of GABA on oxidative stress in the skeletal muscles and plasma free amino acids in mice fed high-fat diet. *J. Anim. Physiol. Anim. Nutr.* **2015**, *99*, 492–500. [CrossRef] [PubMed]
18. Wang, J.; Sun, B.; Cao, Y.; Wang, C. Wheat bran feruloyl oligosaccharides enhance the antioxidant activity of rat plasma. *Food Chem.* **2010**, *123*, 472–476. [CrossRef]
19. Jiang, G.; Lei, A.; Chen, Y.; Yu, Q.; Xie, J.; Yang, Y.; Yuan, T.; Su, D. The protective effects of the: *Ganoderma atrum* polysaccharide against acrylamide-induced inflammation and oxidative damage in rats. *Food Funct.* **2021**, *12*, 397–407. [CrossRef]
20. Moretto, L.; Tonolo, F.; Folda, A.; Scalcon, V.; Bindoli, A.; Bellamio, M.; Feller, E.; Rigobello, M.P. Comparative analysis of the antioxidant capacity and lipid and protein oxidation of soy and oats beverages. *Food Prod. Process. Nutr.* **2021**, *3*, 1–10. [CrossRef]
21. Jnaneshwari, S.; Hemshekhar, M.; Santhosh, M.S.; Sunitha, K.; Thushara, R.; Thirunavukkarasu, C.; Kemparaju, K.; Girish, K.S. Crocin, a dietary colorant mitigates cyclophosphamide-induced organ toxicity by modulating antioxidant status and inflammatory cytokines. *J. Pharm. Pharmacol.* **2013**, *65*, 604–614. [CrossRef] [PubMed]
22. Liu, X.-y.; Liu, D.; Lin, G.-p.; Wu, Y.-j.; Gao, L.-y.; Ai, C.; Huang, Y.-f.; Wang, M.-f.; El-Seedi, H.R.; Chen, X.-h.; et al. Anti-ageing and antioxidant effects of sulfate oligosaccharides from green algae *Ulva lactuca* and *Enteromorpha prolifera* in SAMP8 mice. *Int. J. Biol. Macromol.* **2019**, *139*, 342–351. [CrossRef] [PubMed]
23. Hojs, R.; Bevc, S.; Ekart, R.; Gorenjak, M.; Puklavec, L. Serum Cystatin C as an Endogenous Marker of the Renal Function—A Review. *Ren. Fail.* **2008**, *30*, 181–186. [CrossRef] [PubMed]
24. Gowda, S.; Desai, P.B.; Kulkarni, S.S.; Hull, V.V.; Math, A.A.K.; Vernekar, S.N. Markers of renal function tests. *N. Am. J. Med. Sci.* **2010**, *2*, 170–173.
25. Feng, Y.; Yu, Y.H.; Wang, S.T.; Ren, J.; Camer, D.; Hua, Y.Z.; Zhang, Q.; Huang, J.; Xue, D.L.; Zhang, X.F.; et al. Chlorogenic acid protects D-galactose-induced liver and kidney injury via antioxidation and anti-inflammation effects in mice. *Pharm. Biol.* **2016**, *54*, 1027–1034. [CrossRef]
26. Pan, H.; Feng, W.; Chen, M.; Luan, H.; Hu, Y.; Zheng, X.; Wang, S.; Mao, Y. Alginate Oligosaccharide Ameliorates D-Galactose-Induced Kidney Aging in Mice through Activation of the Nrf2 Signaling Pathway. *BioMed Res. Int.* **2021**, *2021*, 6623328. [CrossRef]
27. Li, X.; Wang, J.; Zhang, H.; Zhang, Q. Renoprotective effect of low-molecular-weight sulfated polysaccharide from the seaweed *Laminaria japonica* on glycerol-induced acute kidney injury in rats. *Int. J. Biol. Macromol.* **2017**, *95*, 132–137. [CrossRef]
28. Reuter, S.; Gupta, S.C.; Chaturvedi, M.M.; Aggarwal, B.B. Oxidative stress, inflammation, and cancer: How are they linked? *Free Radic. Biol. Med.* **2010**, *49*, 1603–1616. [CrossRef]

29. Abd-Ellatef, G.E.F.; Ahmed, O.M.; Abdel-Reheim, E.S.; Abdel-Hamid, A.H.Z. *Ulva lactuca* polysaccharides prevent Wistar rat breast carcinogenesis through the augmentation of apoptosis, enhancement of antioxidant defense system, and suppression of inflammation. *Breast Cancer Targets Ther.* **2017**, *9*, 67–83. [CrossRef]
30. Hung, T.D.; Hye, J.L.; Eun, S.Y.; Shinde, P.B.; Yoon, M.L.; Hong, J.; Dong, K.K.; Jung, J.H. Anti-inflammatory constituents of the Red Alga *Gracilaria verrucosa* and their synthetic analogues. *J. Nat. Prod.* **2008**, *71*, 232–240. [CrossRef]
31. Li, X.Y.; Chen, H.R.; Zha, X.Q.; Chen, S.; Pan, L.H.; Li, Q.M.; Luo, J.P. Prevention and possible mechanism of a purified *Laminaria japonica* polysaccharide on adriamycin-induced acute kidney injury in mice. *Int. J. Biol. Macromol.* **2020**, *148*, 591–600. [CrossRef]
32. Liu, A.D.; Zheng, K.Y.; Miao, Q.F.; Ikejima, T.; Zhang, J.; Fei, X.F. Effect of polysaccharides from fruit body of *Ganoderma tsugae* on bidirectional regulation of proinflammatory cytokine production in THP-1 cells. *Chem. Res. Chin. Univ.* **2009**, *25*, 487–491.
33. Jiang, J.; Luo, Y.; Qin, W.; Ma, H.; Li, Q.; Zhan, J.; Zhang, Y. Electroacupuncture suppresses the NF-κB signaling pathway by upregulating cylindromatosis to alleviate inflammatory injury in cerebral ischemia/reperfusion rats. *Front. Mol. Neurosci.* **2017**, *10*, 363. [CrossRef] [PubMed]
34. Crow, M.T.; Mani, K.; Nam, Y.J.; Kitsis, R.N. The mitochondrial death pathway and cardiac myocyte apoptosis. *Circ. Res.* **2004**, *95*, 957–970. [CrossRef] [PubMed]
35. Jung, J.; Kim, H.Y.; Maeng, J.; Kim, M.; Shin, D.H.; Lee, K. Interaction of translationally controlled tumor protein with Apaf-1 is involved in the development of chemoresistance in HeLa cells. *BMC Cancer* **2014**, *14*, 165. [CrossRef] [PubMed]
36. Guo, Y.; Balasubramanian, B.; Zhao, Z.H.; Liu, W.C. Marine algal polysaccharides alleviate aflatoxin B1-induced bursa of Fabricius injury by regulating redox and apoptotic signaling pathway in broilers. *Poult. Sci.* **2021**, *100*, 844–857. [CrossRef]
37. Ma, Q.; Xu, Y.; Tang, L.; Yang, X.; Chen, Z.; Wei, Y.; Shao, X.; Shao, X.; Xin, Z.; Cai, B.; et al. Astragalus Polysaccharide Attenuates Cisplatin-Induced Acute Kidney Injury by Suppressing Oxidative Damage and Mitochondrial Dysfunction. *BioMed Res. Int.* **2020**, *2020*, 2851349. [CrossRef] [PubMed]
38. Nielsen, S.S. Phenol-sulfuric acid method for total carbohydrates. In *Food Analysis Laboratory Manual*; Springer: Boston, MA, USA, 2019; ISBN 9781441914620.
39. Bradstreet, R.B. Kjeldahl Method for Organic Nitrogen. *Anal. Chem.* **1954**, *26*, 185–187. [CrossRef]
40. Allen, J.; Brock, S.A. New method for quantitative determination of uronic acids. *Minn. Med.* **2000**, *83*, 45–48.
41. Sorbo, B. Sulfate: Turbidimetric and Nephelometric Methods. *Methods Enzymol.* **1987**, *143*, 3–6. [CrossRef]

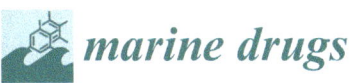

Review

Exploitation of Marine-Derived Robust Biological Molecules to Manage Inflammatory Bowel Disease

Muhammad Bilal [1,*], Leonardo Vieira Nunes [2], Marco Thúlio Saviatto Duarte [3], Luiz Fernando Romanholo Ferreira [4,5], Renato Nery Soriano [6] and Hafiz M. N. Iqbal [7,*]

1. School of Life Science and Food Engineering, Huaiyin Institute of Technology, Huaian 223003, China
2. Department of Medicine, Federal University of Juiz de Fora, Juiz de Fora-MG 36036-900, Brazil; leonardo.nunes@estudante.ufjf.br
3. Department of Medicine, Federal University of Juiz de Fora, Governador Valadares-MG 35010-180, Brazil; marco.saviatto@estudante.ufjf.br
4. Graduate Program in Process Engineering, Tiradentes University (UNIT), Av. Murilo Dantas, 300, Farolândia, Aracaju-Sergipe 49032-490, Brazil; luiz.fernando@souunit.com.br
5. Institute of Technology and Research (ITP), Tiradentes University (UNIT), Av. Murilo Dantas, 300, Farolândia, Aracaju-Sergipe 49032-490, Brazil
6. Division of Physiology and Biophysics, Department of Basic Life Sciences, Federal University of Juiz de Fora, Governador Valadares-MG 35010-180, Brazil; renato.soriano@ufjf.edu.br
7. School of Engineering and Sciences, Tecnologico de Monterrey, Monterrey 64849, Mexico
* Correspondence: bilaluaf@hyit.edu.cn or bilaluaf@hotmail.com (M.B.); hafiz.iqbal@tec.mx (H.M.N.I.)

Citation: Bilal, M.; Nunes, L.V.; Duarte, M.T.S.; Ferreira, L.F.R.; Soriano, R.N.; Iqbal, H.M.N. Exploitation of Marine-Derived Robust Biological Molecules to Manage Inflammatory Bowel Disease. *Mar. Drugs* **2021**, *19*, 196. https://doi.org/10.3390/md19040196

Academic Editors: Donatella Degl'Innocenti and Marzia Vasarri

Received: 6 March 2021
Accepted: 26 March 2021
Published: 30 March 2021

Publisher's Note: MDPI stays neutral with regard to jurisdictional claims in published maps and institutional affiliations.

Copyright: © 2021 by the authors. Licensee MDPI, Basel, Switzerland. This article is an open access article distributed under the terms and conditions of the Creative Commons Attribution (CC BY) license (https://creativecommons.org/licenses/by/4.0/).

Abstract: Naturally occurring biological entities with extractable and tunable structural and functional characteristics, along with therapeutic attributes, are of supreme interest for strengthening the twenty-first-century biomedical settings. Irrespective of ongoing technological and clinical advancement, traditional medicinal practices to address and manage inflammatory bowel disease (IBD) are inefficient and the effect of the administered therapeutic cues is limited. The reasonable immune response or invasion should also be circumvented for successful clinical translation of engineered cues as highly efficient and robust bioactive entities. In this context, research is underway worldwide, and researchers have redirected or regained their interests in valorizing the naturally occurring biological entities/resources, for example, algal biome so-called "treasure of untouched or underexploited sources". Algal biome from the marine environment is an immense source of excellence that has also been demonstrated as a source of bioactive compounds with unique chemical, structural, and functional features. Moreover, the molecular modeling and synthesis of new drugs based on marine-derived therapeutic and biological cues can show greater efficacy and specificity for the therapeutics. Herein, an effort has been made to cover the existing literature gap on the exploitation of naturally occurring biological entities/resources to address and efficiently manage IBD. Following a brief background study, a focus was given to design characteristics, performance evaluation of engineered cues, and point-of-care IBD therapeutics of diverse bioactive compounds from the algal biome. Noteworthy potentialities of marine-derived biologically active compounds have also been spotlighted to underlying the impact role of bio-active elements with the related pathways. The current review is also focused on the applied standpoint and clinical translation of marine-derived bioactive compounds. Furthermore, a detailed overview of clinical applications and future perspectives are also given in this review.

Keywords: algal biome; polysaccharides; bioactive entities; engineered cues; therapeutic attributes; inflammatory bowel disease

1. Introduction

Inflammatory bowel disease (IBD) is a chronic inflammation of the gastrointestinal tract (GIT) that occurs due to the dysregulation of the immune system. Although the explicit etiology and underlying remain uncertain, both environmental and genetic factors are involved in immune dysregulation. Historically, IBD has been categorized into Crohn's disease (CD) and ulcerative colitis (UC). Both diseases show heterogeneous pathological and clinical features and can be distinguished by their location, nature and characteristics of inflammation. More specifically, the laboratory analysis and careful stool evaluation are considered initial measures to diagnose the patient who is suspected to have IBD (Figure 1) [1]. Crohn's disease is a deeper transmural inflammation affecting any segment of the GI tract from the mouth to anus, whereas ulcerative colitis is a chronic inflammatory disease that attacks the colonic mucosa [1]. Approximately, 25% of UC patients require hospitalization for acute severe ulcerative colitis (ASUC) at any phase during this complication, leading to colectomy in 40% of patients [2,3].

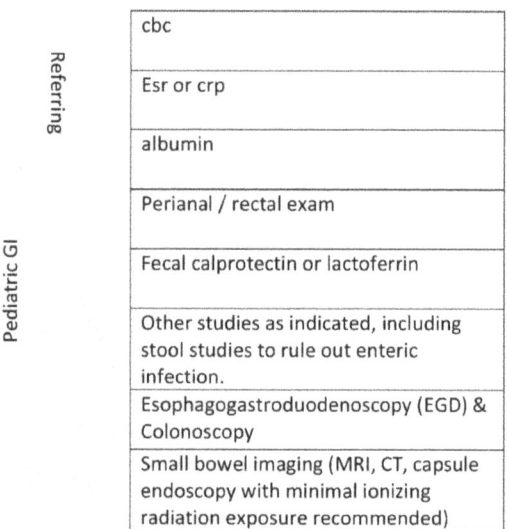

Figure 1. Initial workup of a patient suspected of having inflammatory bowel disease (IBD). The initial workup is ideally started by the referring physician, with the subspecialist performing anything missing plus endoscopies and small bowel assessment(s) [1]. License Number: 5022881429496. Abbreviations: CBC (Complete Blood Count), CRP (C-reactive protein), ESR (Erythrocyte Sedimentation Rate), MRI (Magnetic resonance imaging), and CT (computed tomography).

The origin and disease progression of UC and CD are significantly different from each other. The changes in microbial diversity of lumen, impaired barrier functions of mucus and epithelial layer through interrupting tight junctions are strongly associated with the UC pathogenesis. Figure 2 portrays a graphical representation of the pathophysiology of UC [4]. Though individuals with UC show a great percentage of Enterobacteriaceae Gammaproteobacteria [5], and sulfite-reducing bacteria [6], and minimum Firmicutes diversity, such changes are intestinal inflammation-mediated or vice versa remains debatable. In the case of CD, inflammation of the small bowel results in an increased concentration of pro-inflammatory cytokines, like IL-17A, and IFN-γ [7]. Furthermore, Th17 cell-derived IL-17 in turn favors the Th-1 response [8]. IL-6, IL-23, and TGF-β secreted by antigen-presenting and innate immune cells influence the IL-17 pathway (Figure 3) [4].

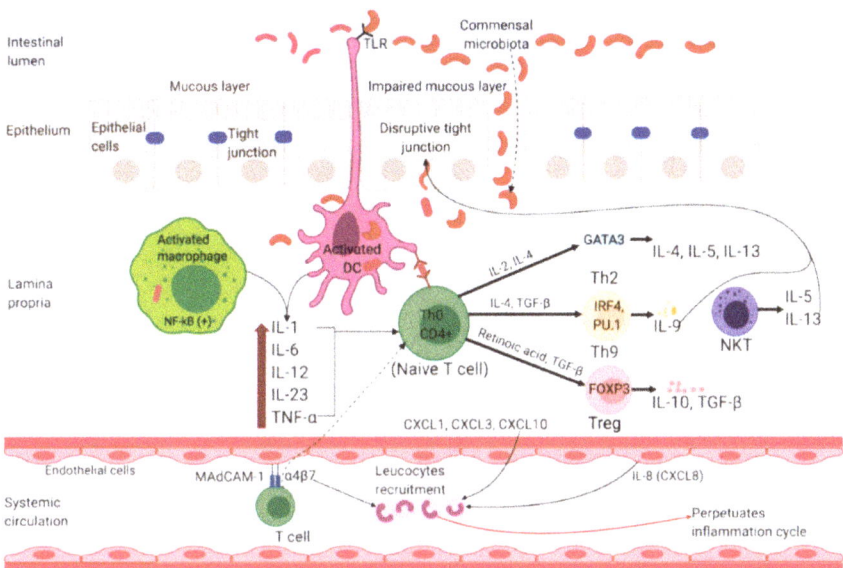

Figure 2. Pathophysiology of Ulcerative Colitis. Impairment of tight junctions and the mucous layer leads to increased permeability of the intestinal epithelium, resulting in more uptake of luminal antigens. Antigen presenting cells (APC) become activated upon recognizing non-pathogenic bacteria (commensal microbiota) through Toll-like receptors (TLRs). Activated APC initiate differentiation of naïve CD4+ T-cells into Th-2 effector cells (which produce pro-inflammatory cytokines such as TNF-α, IL-5, IL-6, and IL-13). TNF-α and IL-1 activate nuclear factor κB (NF-κB) pathway, which facilitate expression of pro-inflammatory and cell survival genes. Binding of integrin-α4β7 bearing T cells to the mucosal adhesion molecule MAdCAM-1 facilitate entry of more T cells into the lamina propria. Recruitment of circulating leucocytes due to the upregulation of inflammatory chemokines (chemokine ligands: CXCL1, CXCL3, CXCL8 and CXCL10) perpetuates the inflammatory cycle. MAdCAM-1, mucosal addressin cell adhesion molecule-1; IL, interleukin; TNF-α, tumor necrosis factor-alpha; TGF-β, transforming growth factor-beta; NKT, natural killer T; DC, dendritic cell; Th, T helper; GATA3, GATA binding protein 3; IRF4, interferon regulatory factor 4; PU.1, purine-rich PU-box binding protein; FOXP3, Forkhead box protein 3. Reprinted from Ref. [4] with permission under the Creative Commons Attribution (CC BY) license. Copyright © 2020 the authors. Licensee MDPI, Basel, Switzerland.

In 2017, about 6.8 million cases of IBD were documented worldwide [9]. Over 1.6 million, 85,000, 250,000 and 260,000 people are affected by IBD in Australia, the USA, the UK and China, respectively [10–12]. IBD remains dominant in western countries in the last few decades because of the higher prevalence and incidence rates than in the developing world. Nevertheless, the incidence of IBD has now intensified dramatically in several Asian countries [12] with a consistently increasing trend, mainly in China, Japan, Hong Kong, and Korea [13]. Due to lacking national registries in many African, Asian, and Latin American nations, there is very scarce information regarding the occurrence and prevalence of IBD.

IBD has been reported to occur at any age, however, the peak incidence appears in early adulthood and adolescence [14–16]. Symptoms associated with IBD can be unpredicted and highly variable. Children may exhibit inimitable physical examination findings along with several upper or lower GI manifestations. There might be only a few symptoms in some cases, with inexplicable weight loss and growth retardation. It is imperative to distinguish that IBD is not irritable bowel syndrome (IBS). Though both diseases may present identical symptoms, only IBD results in stunted height, growth retardation, ostomies, surgeries, and many other undesirable outcomes or risks. Besides the systemic symptoms, like fatigue, fever, mouth sores, uveitis, arthralgia, and nail clubbing, IBD is also related to a variety of extra-intestinal symptoms. These manifestations appear in approximately 25–35% of individuals with IBD particularly at a young age [17,18].

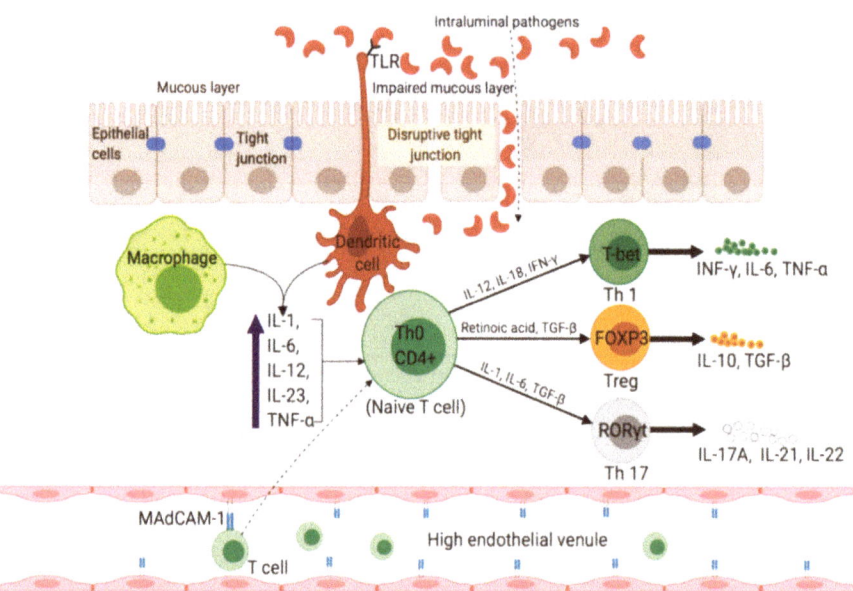

Figure 3. Pathophysiology in Crohn's disease. The uptake of luminal microflora stimulates APCs (e.g., dendritic cells and macrophages) which in turn produce proinflammatory cytokines such as TNF-α, IL-6, and IL-23. Activated APCs facilitate subsequent differentiation of naïve CD4⁺ T-cells into Th1 and Th17 via expression of master transcription factors. Inside the high endothelial venule, binding of α4β7-bearing lymphocytes to MAdCAM-1 causes entry of more T cells into the lamina propria. IFN-γ, interferon-gamma; FOXP3, Forkhead box protein 3; RORγt, retinoic acid receptor-related orphan nuclear receptor gamma. Reprinted from Ref. [4] with permission under the Creative Commons Attribution (CC BY) license. Copyright © 2020 the authors. Licensee MDPI, Basel, Switzerland.

The treatment protocols being practiced for the IBD involve either medication therapy or surgery [19]. The preferred choice of medication therapy in the case of IBD is the treatment with the use of anti-inflammatory drugs, such as aminosalicylates and corticosteroids. The second line medication for IBD encompasses using immunosuppressants to halt the immune response, responsible for un-regulated inflammation. In addition to immunosuppressants, tumor necrosis factor-α (TNF-α) inhibitors, or biologics works by neutralizing immune system protein. In Crohn's disease, where the infection is a concern, antibiotics can be used to reduce the chances of infection. On the other hand, surgery may be an option in severe cases when all these therapeutic options do not work. However, treatment protocols are also being practiced culminating devastating colorectal cancer, but no treatment is required for benevolent stage cancer. In the case of metastatic invasion, surgery can be opted to eradicate malignant tumors and lymph nodes [20].

The marine environment has been demonstrated as a prolific source of bio-active compounds with unique chemical, structural and functional features. Furthermore, the molecular modeling and synthesis of new drugs based on marine-derived therapeutic and biological cues might present greater efficacy and specificity for the therapeutics (Table 1). A vast number of compounds have been derived and identified from marine sources that exhibit a noteworthy role to circumvent the reactive oxygen species (ROS) generation, show anti-inflammatory effects, and hinder various metabolic pathways. The current review is focused on marine-derived bioactive compounds to treat and manage

IBD. Furthermore, a detailed overview of clinical applications and future perspectives are also given in this review.

Table 1. Marine-derived compounds and biological activities with therapeutic potential.

Marine-Derived Compound	Sources	Potential Applications and Benefits	References
Chondroitin Sulfate (CS)	Shark cartilage, octopus, salmon, zebrafish, ray, squid	Antiinflammatory, Immunomodulatory, Anticancer, Antiviral, Anticoagulant	[21–26]
Hyaluronic acid (HA)	Shark, stingray, eyeball, liver of swordfish, mollusk bivalves, tuna	Anti-inflammatory, Antioxidant, Anticoagulant	[27–31]
Chitosan	Arthropods (crustaceans), fungi	Anti-inflammatory, Antioxidant, Anticancer, Antimicrobial	[32–37]
Alginate	Brown seaweeds	Anti-inflammatory, Immunomodulatory, Antioxidant, Anticancer, Anticoagulant	[38–43]

2. Marine-Derived Bioactive Compounds against Inflammatory Bowel Diseases (IBD)

2.1. Chitosan-Structural Properties and Potential Therapy of IBD

Chitosan is a linear polysaccharide obtained from deacetylation of chitin, it has a cationic character because of its primary amino groups, which provides it with properties such as controlled drug release, mucoadhesion, in situ gelations, transfection and increased permeation [44,45]. It is an important constituent part of the exoskeleton of arthropods, fungi, and crustaceans, which are the main marine source [46,47]. Among its various properties and applications, those that stand out most are antimicrobial, antioxidant, anticancer and anti-inflammatory [32–37].

The mucoadhesive property of chitosan has been a key point of its application in the treatment of IBD (Table 2) and has also been indicated in a study with patients with IBD [48,49]. For rectal use, this characteristic allows a prolonged local retention time of the drugs. In line with this idea, a chitosan-based hydrogel was able to enhance the efficacy of rectal administration of sulfasalazine (SSZ) in a mice model of ulcerative colitis. The mucoadhesive drug delivery system was more therapeutic than the conventional oral treatment and reduced the plasma concentration of a potentially toxic by-product of the drug [50]. Besides its excellent mucosa adhesion, chitosan polymers are widely employed in targeted drug delivery systems, providing better efficacy results in oral treatments. Pillay et al. were able to develop Stimuli-Synchronized-Matrix (SSM) for colonic delivery, defined by the space, of mesalamine (5-amino-salicylic acid or 5-ASA), the therapeutic metabolite of SSZ, employing chitosan in a polysaccharide matrix coated with an alloy layer [51]. Their SSM was both time and pH-independent, while provided a responsive release of the chemical in the presence of colonic enzymes. These characteristics also allowed the minimization of variations of the plasma concentration and reduced the systemic presence of 5-ASA. A similar approach was used in bioadhesive chitosan pallets and coated beads to increase the topical delivery of 5-ASA [52–54]. Mesalamine has also been loaded in N-succinyl-chitosan microparticles, improving its therapeutic results [54].

Table 2. Applications of Chitosan in drug delivery systems for IBD treatment.

Strategy	Drug Delivered	References
Hydrogel	Sulfasalazine	[50]
Coated matrix	5-amino-salicylic acid (5-ASA)	[51]
Coated beads	5-amino-salicylic acid (5-ASA)	[53,54]
Microparticles	5-amino-salicylic acid (5-ASA)	[54]
Coated bioadhesive pellets	5-amino-salicylic acid (5-ASA)	[52]
Microgel	5-amino-salicylic acid (5-ASA)	[55]
Matrix tablets	5-amino-salicylic acid (5-ASA)	[56]
Coated tablets	5-amino-salicylic acid (5-ASA)	[57]
Coated microparticles	5-amino-salicylic acid (5-ASA) and curcumin	[58]
Lipid nanoparticles	Dexamethasone	[59]
Beads	Azathioprine	[60]
Microcrystals	Dexamethasone	[61]
Beads and microparticles	Prednisolone and inulin	[62]
swellable hydrogel	pentosan polysulphate (PP)	[63]
Hydrogel	Resveratrol	[64]
Hydrogel	Curcumin	[65]
Hydrogel	6-shogaol	[66]
Hydrogel	siCD98	[67]
Hydrogel	PS-ATNF-α	[68]
Colloidal particles	NK007	[69]
Coated microparticles	AvrA nanoparticles	[70]
Coated pellets	Rutin	[71]
Microspheres	Icariin	[72]
Coated microparticle tablets	Quercetin	[73]
Coated liposomes	Quercetin	[74]
Monolithic tablet	Diamide oxidase and catalase	[75]
Polymer-enzyme cojugate	Superoxide dismutase	[76]
Nanoparticles	Berberine	[77]
Coated nanoemulsion	Curcumin	[78]
Coated agglomerates of nanoparticles	Diclofenac sodium	[79]
Nanoparticle	SIGIRR gene	[80]
Microspheres	Ketoprofen and ascorbic acid	[81]

Additional research has been conducted to ameliorate the pharmacokinetics of the conventional treatment for IBD. A microgel based on oxidized sodium alginate and water-soluble chitosan demonstrated in vitro potential application as a carrier for mesalamine [55]. A different formulation of chitosan and alginate composite microparticles associated with an enteric coat was capable of effectively delivering 5-ASA and curcumin in a colitis rat model [58]. Another preparation combined a cellulose-derived polymer with pectin and chitosan in matrix tablets of 5-ASA to provide desirable changes in its physicochemical characteristics and drug release profiles [56]. An additional antibacterial effect was reached by preparing mesalamine tablets with a chitosan-ethylenediaminediacetic acid disodium (CH-EDTA) conjugate coating [57]. Research has also been conducted to improve the pharmacokinetics of immunosuppressive drugs. Some strategies, such as loading chitosan modified lipid nanoparticles (NPs) with dexamethasone and preparing azathioprine-loaded chitosan beads have shown promising results in targeted and sensitive drug delivery at the colitis site [59,60]. Dexamethasone microcrystals coated with chitosan, alginate, and an enteric coat multilayers also exhibited significant therapeutic effects in mice [61]. Another corticoid, prednisolone, was loaded with inulin, a naturally occurring polysaccharide, in beads and microparticles coated with calcium (Ca)-alginate core and a chitosan coating. The resulting formulations were tested in vitro and were deemed suitable to be used to deliver substances to the colon [62].

The possibility of producing hydrogels with chitosan to obtain a sustained release of a drug in the intestine is another relevant aspect for its application in the treatment of

IBD. A biodegradable and reversible polyelectrolyte complex (PEC) of poly acrylic-acid (PAA) and chitosan was engineered to be used as a swellable hydrogel colonic delivery system for topical treatment of IBD with pentosan polysulfate (PP). However, an enteric coat was still needed to protect the proposed formulation from the gastric environment [63]. Resveratrol, a polyphenol present in red wine with anti-inflammatory properties, was also successfully loaded in nanostructured chitosan-based hydrogel and had its pharmacokinetics improved [64]. Two similar studies demonstrated the use of a chitosan and alginate hydrogel to encapsulate nanoparticles loaded with curcumin and 6-shogaol, a biologic compound found in ginger. The formulations significantly alleviated the colitis symptoms and quickened wound repair in mice (Figure 4) [65,66]. Interesting use of other chitosan hydrogel was in the design of an antibody functionalized nanoparticles-releasing hydrogel. The authors developed nanoparticles prepared with single-chain CD98 antibodies on their surface, for carrying inside of it CD98 small interfering RNAs (siCD98). It was already known that the overexpression of CD98 in the colonic epithelial cells and macrophages was associated with the development and progression of IBD. By using this strategy, the authors were able to downregulate CD98 and efficiently diminished the manifestations of IBD in vitro and in vivo [67]. This idea of using oligonucleotides to inhibit the synthesis of pro-inflammatory molecules has been recently employed to reduce TNF-α production in a mice colitis model. Xu et al. [68] loaded a chitosan-alginate hydrogel with phosphorothioated antisense oligodeoxyribonucleotide of TNF-α (PS-ATNF-α) and reportedly inhibited the molecule at both the protein and mRNA levels [68].

A different approach for targeted delivery of anti-inflammatory substances to macrophages was reported by Chen et al. [69]. The researchers used chitosan associated with alginate and tripolyphosphate (TPP) to form colloidal particles with the drug tylophorine malate (NK007) and to incorporate it inside glucan mannan particles (GMPs). The formulation was capable of specifically delivering the drug to macrophages and effectively cured colitis in the mice model after being administered orally [69]. Chitosan was also used in association with alginate to form gastroprotective microparticles capable of releasing in the small intestine and colon nanoparticles of AvrA, an anti-inflammatory and anti-apoptotic bacterial protein. The authors reported that the formulation diminished clinical and histological scores of inflammations in a colitis model. The encapsulation with alginate and chitosan allowed the drug to be administered orally, instead of transrectally, which was undesired and restricted the delivery to the distal portion of the colon [70]. This association was also applied to develop alginate/chitosan-coated pellets intended for the colon delivery of rutin, a flavonoid with antioxidant and anti-inflammatory effects. The results were promising dissolution profiles and great stability for rutin, which could be a valuable alternative for mild-to-moderate IBD therapy [71].

An analogous approach was applied to the development of chitosan-alginate microspheres as a carrier for icariin, a type of flavonoid, to reduce colonic injury and inflammatory response in rats [72]. Chitosan-alginate microspheres have also been employed to colon deliver a combination of ketoprofen and ascorbic acid, bringing together anti-inflammatory and antioxidant properties [81]. Quercetin, a flavonoid, has been incorporated in a chitosan-xanthan microparticle coated tablet, allowing a sustained and targeted delivery to the target [73]. Alike, a hybrid system made liposomes coated with cross-linked chitosan was proposed to deliver quercetin to the intestine [74]. Another strategy to protect a drug against the gastric environment and control its release within the intestine was the development of carboxymethyl starch (CMS)—chitosan monolithic tablets. A study has employed these tablets as a carrier for diamine oxidase and catalase, two enzymes possibly capable of reducing bowel inflammation [75]. A chitosan-derived polymer-enzyme conjugate was developed as a promising option in the treatment of IBD with superoxide dismutase, an antioxidant enzyme [76]. Also for oral delivery, a nanocarrier based on chitosan and fucoidan was loaded with berberine, an alkaloid capable of promoting tightness of the intestinal epithelial tight junction, and revealed promising results [77].

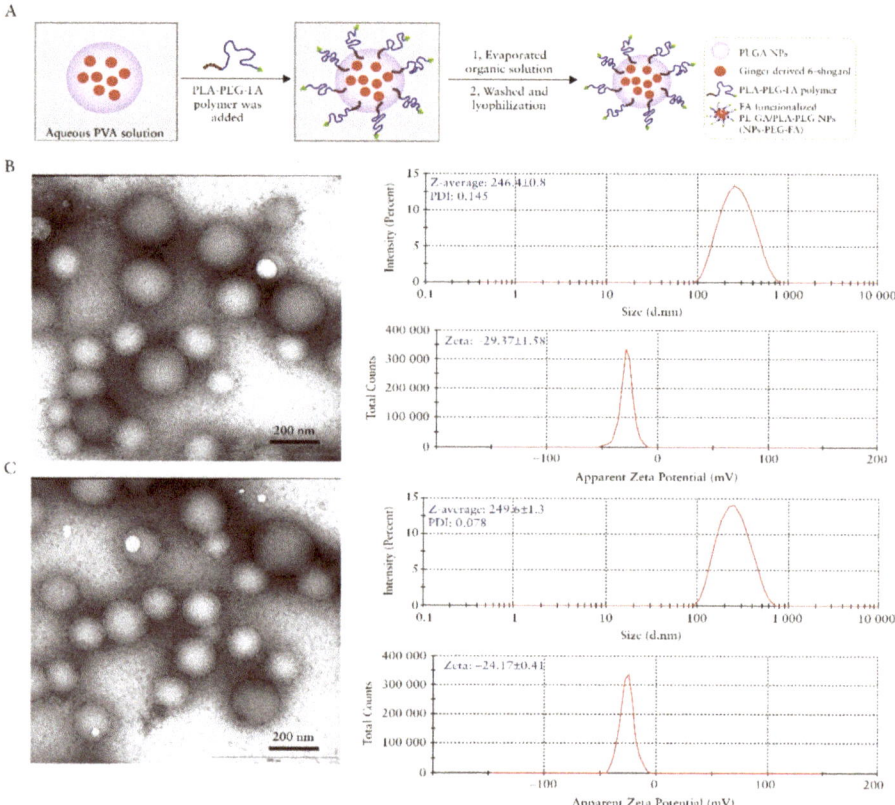

Figure 4. Preparation and characterization of 6-shogaol loaded polymeric nanoparticles, (**A**) Schematic illustration of process through which PLGA/PLA-PEG-FA nanoparticles [NPs-PEG-FA] were fabricated using a versatile single-step surface-functionalising technique, (**B**) The morphology of PLGA/PLA-PEG nanoparticles [NPs-PEG] was characterised by transmission electron microscopy [TEM], and their size and zeta potential were measured by dynamic light scattering [DLS] using a Malvern Zetasizer Nano ZS90 Apparatus, and (**C**) The morphology, size, and zeta potential of PLGA/PLA-PEG-FA [NPs-PEG-FA] were characterized. Reprinted from Ref. [66] with permission from Oxford University Press. Copyright © 2017, Oxford University Press. License Number: 5022890402536. Abbreviations: PVA (Polyvinyl alcohol), PLGA (poly(lactic-co-glycolic acid)), PLA (Polylactic acid), PEG (Polyethylene glycol), FA (Folic acid), and NPs (Nanoparticles).

A different design proposed an oil-in-water nanoemulsion coated with a chitosan-based polysaccharide layer film as a nanocarrier for curcumin, an agent with anti-inflammatory and antioxidant properties but lipophilic and unstable in aqueous solutions. The in vitro tests demonstrated that the formulation was capable of protecting the drug from degradation, evidencing its promising use for oral delivery of similar agents (Figure 5) [78]. A multiple stepwise spinning disk processing (SDP) technique was developed to fabricate a drug delivery system based on a composite diclofenac sodium-chitosan-poly(methyl acrylates) nanoparticulate. This approach allowed scale-up manufacturing of the nanoparticulate. Additionally, the drug uptake noticed was three times higher than the control drug solution, with no evident toxicity [79].

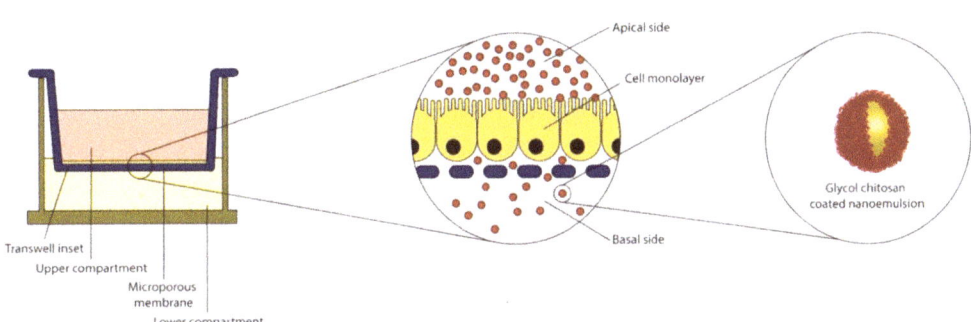

Figure 5. Schematic representation of air liquid interface of human colon carcinoma cell line (CaCo-2) equivalent epithelium in Transwell system. In the central insert, an enlarged view of the cell monolayer grown on the microporous membrane. On the right, the oral nano-delivery system consisting of oil-in-water (O/W) nanoemulsion coated with a thiolated glycol chitosan. Reprinted from Ref. [78] with permission from Elsevier. Copyright © 2018 Elsevier B.V. License Number: 5022890619360.

A more complex approach employed chitosan nanoparticles as a delivery vector for gene therapy in a colitis mice model. The authors developed a very cost-effective way of constructing a carrier for a plasmid of Single Ig-domain containing IL-1 receptor-related molecule (SIGIRR), a subtype of the IL-1R family, capable of attenuate colonic tissue inflammation as a result of the inhibition of TLR4/NF-κB overactivation. The study suggested a possible new gene therapy for IBD [80]. Along with the possibility of improving the pharmacokinetics of other compounds, Chitosan oligosaccharide (COS), the major degradation product of chitosan, has also been shown biological activity [82]. For this reason, it has been pointed out as a potential compound to be used in colitis-associated colorectal cancer (CRC) chemoprevention, due to its activation of AMP-activated protein kinase (AMPK) and inhibition of the NF-κB and mTOR signaling pathways in intestinal epithelial cells (IEC) [83–86].

Another relevant application of chitosan is in tissue engineering. Its antimicrobial effect and biodegradability have made it possible for the compound to be used as a bioscaffold for colorectal tissue engineering. A study has shown that a 3-layer chitosan hydrogel patch revealed good wound healing, effective regulation of the inflammation, and an integral regeneration of the colonic wall, along with the smooth cell layer. The latter was achievable due to the soft gel layers on each side, which ensured the colonization of cells and the formation of neo-tissue [87]. In a different approach, an association of chitosan-based hydrogel and stromal vascular fraction from adipose tissue has successfully replaced a circular colonic wall section [88]. Chitosan grafts could be useful for severe cases of IBD that require surgical intervention, such as those on which cancer develops.

2.2. Hyaluronic Acid-Physicochemical Attributes and Potential Therapy of IBD

Hyaluronic acid (HA) is the only GAG that is not sulfated and not bound to proteins and it's formed by units of disaccharides N-acetyl-D-glucosamine (GalNAc) and D-glucuronic acid (GlcA) [89,90]. HA is a crucial component of the extracellular matrix and performs several functions like cell signaling mediation, morphogenesis, damage repair, and matrix organization [91,92]. HA is found in almost all tissue in humans and also in other vertebrates, can be extracted from marine sources like a shark, stingray, eyeball, liver of swordfish, mollusk bivalves, and tuna [93–96]. It has numerous applications in biotechnology, regenerative medicine, drug delivery vehicles, development of new biomaterials, and other biomedicals and pharmaceutical applications by cause of their properties as biocompatibility, viscoelasticity, lubricity, and immunostimulatory [93,97,98]. HA has been studied as a potential therapeutic agent against several diseases due to its antioxidant, anti-inflammatory, and anticoagulant biological activities [27–31].

HA has potentially useful biological activities against IBD, and studies have shown that sodium hyaluronate, a derivative of HA, has beneficial effects in the treatment for IBD. To investigate whether supplementation of the lining of the colon mucosa with sodium hyaluronate may be a possible and effective alternative treatment for IBD, a clinical study recruited 21 individuals with distal UC and applied 60 mL of sodium hyaluronate gel (IBD98E) once a day for 28 days. 38.1% of patients achieved clinical remission and 47.6% achieved endoscopic remission, showing that the local application of IBD98E enhances endoscopic and clinical outcomes in subjects with active distal UC [99]. However, this study did not have a placebo-controlled group, therefore, the results need to be analyzed with caution. Another study demonstrated the improvement of mucosal healing by quickening intestinal epithelial repair with HA therapy in vitro and in vivo [100]. HA can also be an option to improve the effectiveness of conventional treatments like mesalamine (5-ASA), combined therapy with HA and 5-ASA was capable to accelerate wound repair and diminish inflammatory reaction in rat colitis [101].

Another potential application of HA was reported in a novel study based on the synthesis of methylcellulose (MC) and HA-coated thermo-responsive hydrogel for successful targeted rectal delivery against IBD [102]. The gelling behavior of the hydrogel was improved due to the in situ gelling capability of HA [103]. Moreover, other remarkable features of HA like the slow and prolonged controlled release, non-toxic, stability, and entero-protection were also observed in the mice intestinal model via applicating final formulated hydrogel. It was evident that the HA-MC hydrogel can be employed in safe and inexpensive systems for rectal delivery of substances in IBD [104]. IBD is a risk factor for the development of colorectal cancer and some studies also pointed out applications of HA in these cancer treatments [105–108]. In the last years, nanoparticles (NPs) have been identified with promising strategies for the diagnosis and treatment of many diseases. In comparison to more traditional approaches, they offer advantages such as nanometer-scale dimension, controlled drug release, targeted drug delivery capacity, lower plasma concentrations, and lessen adverse effects [109–111]. Several pieces of research with NPs have been conducted to try to overcome the biggest problems with oral drug administration such as loss of stability in GIT, systemic absorption, risk of side effects, difficulty in transporting sufficient quantities of active drugs, and transporting them to specific target sites [111,112]. In this regard, NPs have been an innovative approach for IBD treatment, and the results have shown that they are much more effective than traditional drug formulation (Figure 6) [111].

Lysine-proline-valine (KPV) is a tripeptide with anti-inflammatory properties, Xiao et al. [113] loaded KPV into HA-functionalized polymeric nanoparticles (HANPs), resulting in an NPs called HA-KPV-NPs. The authors encapsulated the HA-KPV-NPs in a hydrogel (chitosan/alginate) for oral administration against UC in a mouse model and used a group control without HA. The results show that HA-KPV-NPs/Hydrogel system exhibited a much stronger capacity to prevent mucosa injury and downregulate TNF-α compared with group control. Therefore, this study reveals the important role of the HA in the NPs, which was able to penetrate the colitis tissue and allow the KPV to be internalized in the target cells, thereby alleviate UC [113]. In another study that also used a model of UC in mice, HANPs was used to deliver the siRNA of the CD98 transmembrane protein involved in the colon's innate immune responses, siCD98, in association with a robust anti-inflammatory agent, curcumin. The results of the analyzes showed that cell uptake of drugs in groups treated with HANPs was much higher than those treated with NPs without HA, demonstrating that HANPs could be a good alternative for UC-target therapy [114]. The same group reported in previous studies that surface functionalization with HA increases the cellular uptake efficiency of NPs as a consequence of interactions mediated by receptor [67], which seems to be related to the fact that HA is a ligand of CD44, a membrane glycoprotein, that in UC has increased expression on the surfaces of colon epithelial cells and macrophages [115–117]. Accordingly, Vafaei et al. [118] used HANPs to release budesonide in an in vitro model of inflamed CACO-2 cells, the anti-inflammatory effect with HAMPs was much greater compared to cells that received the free drug [118]. Similar to HANPs, Li et al. [119] use HA functionalized porous silicon nanoparticles to unite enzyme-responsive hydrogel and pH-responsive polymer to develop a hierarchical structured and programmable responsive AP@PSi-HA@HPMCAS carrier for efficient local delivery of drugs to sites of inflammation in the intestine in IBD treatment via oral administrations. The vehicle with HA exhibited superior therapeutic efficacy and significantly diminished systemic drug exposure [119]. No clinical studies have been found using HANPs to treat IBD, however, due to wide marine availability and the promising results of experimental studies they have great potential for the developing of alternative therapies capable of overcoming the limitations of traditional oral drug formulation.

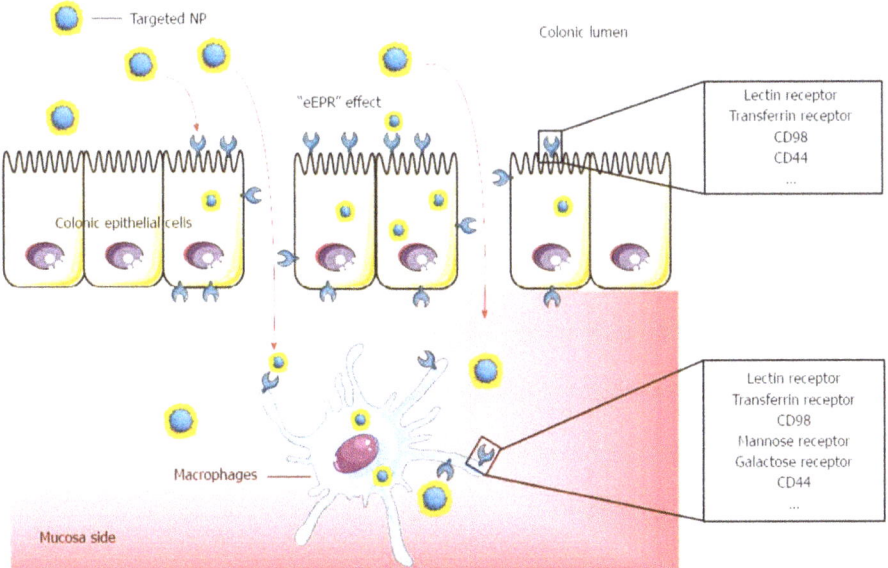

Figure 6. Schematic illustration of orally administered cell-specific nanotherapeutics for IBD. Reprinted from Ref. [111] with permission under the Creative Commons Attribution Non Commercial (CC BY-NC 4.0) license. Copyright ©The Author(s) 2016. Published by Baishideng Publishing Group Inc.

2.3. Chondroitin Sulfate-Physicochemical Traits and Potential Therapy of IBD

Chondroitin Sulfate (CS) is a sulfated glycosaminoglycan (GAG) found on cell surfaces and inside the pericellular matrix in the form of proteoglycans from different organisms and is involved with several physiological events [120,121]. CS is a linear polysaccharide formed by the repetition of disaccharide units N-acetyl-D-galactosamine (GalNAc) and D-glucuronic acid (GlcA), which have sulfate groups added by several sulfotransferases in various positions, forming diverse structures with heterogenous characteristics [122,123]. Commercially, the main marine source of CS is shark cartilage but it can also be extracted from octopus, salmon, zebrafish, ray, and squid [96]. CS has biological activity as an immunomodulator, anti-inflammatory, anticancer, antiviral, and anticoagulant [21–26]. It has been highly employed in the treatment of osteoarthritis and tissue engineering, as CS hydrogels proved to accelerate wound healing [21,96] and several studies have investigated its use in the management of IBD.

Similar to chitosan, research has been conducted to employ CS to obtain a controlled release of drugs already in use to treat IBD. Cesar et al. [124] successfully synthesized a polymeric conjugate of 5-ASA and CS capable of improving the biodistribution of the drug and of providing it with a mucoadhesive profile (Figure 7) [124]. The authors suggested that the pharmaceutical could be considered as an alternative therapy for ulcerative colitis [124]. Prednisolone has also been conjugated with CS to improve its delivery to the lower intestines. The result was a nanogel that had its ability to target areas affected by colitis confirmed in vivo [125]. Furthermore, the multi-bioresponsive drug, curcumin, has been used in association with CS. Two studies described the development of curcumin-loaded nanoparticles with their surfaces functionalized with CS. This modification yielded prominently targeted drug delivery to macrophages and was considered a promising therapeutic platform for IBD [65,126]. Additionally, a prospective, observational, follow-up study indicated that IBD patients in remission under CS treatment for osteoarthritis could have a lower incidence of relapses than generally reported in the literature. Although the study had a small sample, it suggested that CS could be applied as a candidate for the treatment of IBD due to its good safety profile and capability of alleviating osteoarthritis-related pain in these patients [127].

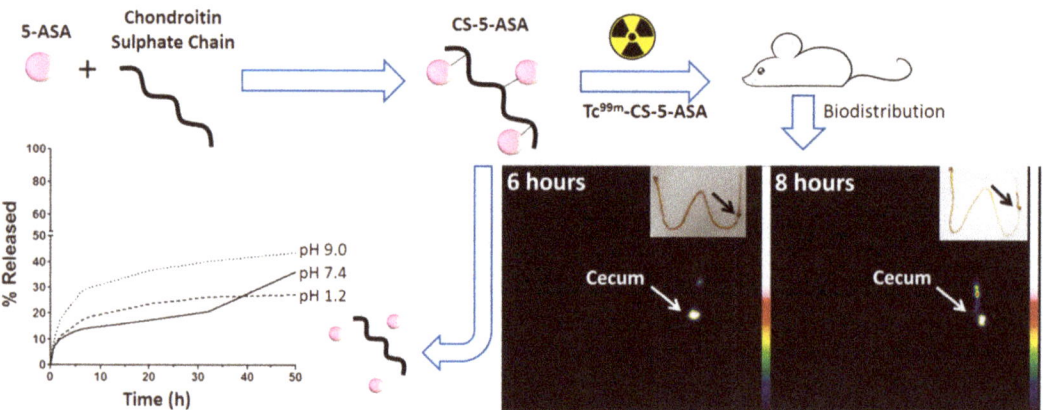

Figure 7. Mesalamine polymeric conjugate for controlled release. Reprinted from Ref. [124] with permission from Elsevier. Copyright © 2017 Elsevier B.V. License Number: 5022891040345.

2.4. Alginate-Physicochemical Attributes and Therapeutic Option for IBD

Alginates are a natural biopolymer composed of 1,4-linked (-L-guluronic acid) (G) and (-D-mannuronic acid) (M) residues to form GG, GM, and MM blocks [128]. *Ascophyllum nodosum, Laminaria hyperborea, Saccharina japonica, Macrocystis pyrifera, Laminaria digitata*, and other species of brown seaweeds are the main source extraction with 17 to 45% of the dry weight composed of alginate [129,130]. It is widely available, biocompatible, non-toxic, low cost a has wide application in food processing, biotechnology, and biomedical industry [131,132]. Some studies have pointed out the biological activities of alginates as an antioxidant, anti-inflammatory, immunomodulating, anticoagulant, and anticancer [38–43].

Alginate has non-toxic, non-immunogenic, biocompatible and biodegradable properties [131,133,134], which make it a versatile material for biomedical application as in microspheres, microcapsules, gel beads, hydrogel, film, nanoparticles, pellets, and tablets for drug delivery [133,135]. Several alginate formulations with other marine compounds have been studied in treatments against IBD and some of them were described previously with chitosan. The main applications are in the engineering of drug delivery systems specifically for the colon, which allows its use in the treatment of IBD in a different way than relying solely on pH sensitivity [136]. In this regard, alginate offers a range of microencapsulation through a series of techniques, Samak et al. [137] analyzed alginate microparticles loaded with hydrocortisone hemisuccinate and fabricated via aerosolization and homogenization methods. In vitro experiments were carried out to verify whether the microparticles by each of the techniques were able to suppress the release of the drug in the simulated gastric fluid and promote the release correctly in the simulated intestinal fluid.

The results indicated that both methods show potential for producing alginate hydrogel microparticles suitable for colon-specific drug delivery in IBD treatment [137]. A subsequent study confirmed the potential of these techniques for delivering *Nigella sativa* extract using the same in vitro tests [138]. Other studies have investigated alginate formulations to see if they can improve the delivery and effectiveness of drugs used in conventional IBD treatments like corticosteroids) [139,140].

3. Concluding Remarks and Outlook

Inflammatory bowel disease continues to result in substantial productivity loss and extensive morbidity worldwide. The devastating consequence of inflammatory bowel disease urgently calls for proper treatments, and thus implicate a considerable financial and economic burden to individuals and the entire health care structure, particularly in emerging countries. Marine-derived bioproducts attract incredible interest and appear a revolutionary therapy for IBD due to their health beneficial properties that are ascribed to the presence of characteristic biologically active functional constituents. This review presents some naturally occurring biological entities/compounds derived from different marine species for the efficient management of IBD. Particular focus has been devoted to characteristic attributes, performance evaluation of engineered cues, and point-of-care IBD therapeutics of diverse bioactive compounds from the algal biome. Although the ratio of early surgery is reduced in IBD-associated patient by introducing biological active substances based therapeutic modalities, many challenges remain. Hence, additional research efforts are required to inspect their bioavailability and efficiency in human and animal models. The exploration of marine-derived bioactive compounds will continue to increase in the future depending on new extraction strategies and novel modes of action. Ideally, intensive future research and new research opportunities for marine bioproducts would lead to a more efficacious and safer way for preventing and management of inflammatory bowel disease.

Author Contributions: Conceptualization, M.B. and H.M.N.I.; data curation, M.B.; L.V.N.; M.T.S.D.; L.F.R.F. and R.N.S. writing—original draft preparation, M.B.; L.V.N.; M.T.S.D.; L.F.R.F. and R.N.S. writing—review and editing, M.B. and H.M.N.I.; funding acquisition, H.M.N.I. All authors have read and agreed to the published version of the manuscript.

Funding: This research received no external funding.

Institutional Review Board Statement: Not applicable.

Informed Consent Statement: Not applicable.

Data Availability Statement: Not applicable.

Acknowledgments: Consejo Nacional de Ciencia y Tecnología (CONACYT) is thankfully acknowledged for partially supporting this work under Sistema Nacional de Investigadores (SNI) program awarded to Hafiz M.N. Iqbal (CVU: 735340).

Conflicts of Interest: The authors declare no conflict of interest.

References

1. Sandberg, K.; Yarger, E.; Saeed, S. Updates in diagnosis and management of inflammatory bowel disease. *Curr. Probl. Pediatr. Adolesc. Health Care* **2020**, *50*, 100785. [CrossRef]
2. Dinesen, L.C.; Walsh, A.J.; Protic, M.N.; Heap, G.; Cummings, F.; Warren, B.F.; George, B.; Mortensen, N.J.M.; Travis, S.P.L. The pattern and outcome of acute severe colitis. *J. Crohn's Colitis* **2010**, *4*, 431–437. [CrossRef]
3. Kaur, M.; Dalal, R.L.; Shaffer, S.; Schwartz, D.A.; Rubin, D.T. Inpatient Management of Inflammatory Bowel Disease-Related Complications. *Clin. Gastroenterol. Hepatol.* **2020**, *18*, 1346–1355. [CrossRef] [PubMed]
4. Yeshi, K.; Ruscher, R.; Hunter, L.; Daly, N.L.; Loukas, A.; Wangchuk, P. Revisiting Inflammatory Bowel Disease: Pathology, Treatments, Challenges and Emerging Therapeutics Including Drug Leads from Natural Products. *J. Clin. Med.* **2020**, *9*, 1273. [CrossRef] [PubMed]

5. Frank, D.N.; St Amand, A.L.; Feldman, R.A.; Boedeker, E.C.; Harpaz, N.; Pace, N.R. Molecular-phylogenetic characterization of microbial community imbalances in human inflammatory bowel diseases. *Proc. Natl. Acad. Sci. USA* **2007**, *104*, 13780–13785. [CrossRef]
6. Roediger, W.E.W.; Moore, J.; Babidge, W. Colonic sulfide in pathogenesis and treatment of ulcerative colitis. *Dig. Dis. Sci.* **1997**, *42*, 1571–1579. [CrossRef]
7. Fuss, I.J.; Neurath, M.; Boirivant, M.; Klein, J.S.; de la Motte, C.; Strong, S.A.; Fiocchi, C.; Strober, W. Disparate CD4+ lamina propria (LP) lymphokine secretion profiles in inflammatory bowel disease. Crohn's disease LP cells manifest increased secretion of IFN-gamma, whereas ulcerative colitis LP cells manifest increased secretion of IL-5. *J. Immunol.* **1996**, *157*, 1261–1270.
8. Kolls, J.K.; Lindén, A. Interleukin-17 family members and inflammation. *Immunity* **2004**, *21*, 467–476. [CrossRef]
9. Alatab, S.; Sepanlou, S.G.; Ikuta, K.; Vahedi, H.; Bisignano, C.; Safiri, S.; Sadeghi, A.; Nixon, M.R.; Abdoli, A.; Abolhassani, H.; et al. The global, regional, and national burden of inflammatory bowel disease in 195 countries and territories, 1990–2017: A systematic analysis for the Global Burden of Disease Study 2017. *Lancet Gastroenterol. Hepatol.* **2020**, *5*, 17–30. [CrossRef]
10. Kaplan, G.G.; Ng, S.C. Globalisation of inflammatory bowel disease: Perspectives from the evolution of inflammatory bowel disease in the UK and China. *Lancet Gastroenterol. Hepatol.* **2016**, *1*, 307–316. [CrossRef]
11. Aniwan, S.; Tremaine, W.J.; Raffals, L.E.; Kane, S.V.; Loftus, E.V., Jr. Antibiotic Use and New-Onset Inflammatory Bowel Disease in Olmsted County, Minnesota: A Population-Based Case-Control Study. *J. Crohn's Colitis* **2018**, *12*, 137–144. [CrossRef] [PubMed]
12. Ng, S.C.; Tang, W.; Ching, J.Y.; Wong, M.; Chow, C.M.; Hui, A.J.; Wong, T.C.; Leung, V.K.; Tsang, S.W.; Yu, H.H.; et al. Incidence and phenotype of inflammatory bowel disease based on results from the Asia-Pacific Crohn's and colitis epidemiology study. *Gastroenterology* **2013**, *145*, 158–165.e2. [CrossRef]
13. Yang, Y.; Owyang, C.; Wu, G.D. East Meets West: The Increasing Incidence of Inflammatory Bowel Disease in Asia as a Paradigm for Environmental Effects on the Pathogenesis of Immune-Mediated Disease. *Gastroenterology* **2016**, *151*, e1–e5. [CrossRef]
14. Vernier-Massouille, G.; Balde, M.; Salleron, J.; Turck, D.; Dupas, J.L.; Mouterde, O.; Merle, V.; Salomez, J.L.; Branche, J.; Marti, R.; et al. Natural History of Pediatric Crohn's Disease: A Population-Based Cohort Study. *Gastroenterology* **2008**, *135*, 1106–1113. [CrossRef]
15. Lehtinen, P.; Pasanen, K.; Kolho, K.-L.; Auvinen, A. Incidence of Pediatric Inflammatory Bowel Disease in Finland. *J. Pediatr. Gastroenterol. Nutr.* **2016**, *63*, 65–70. [CrossRef] [PubMed]
16. Lopez, R.N.; Appleton, L.; Gearry, R.B.; Day, A.S. Rising Incidence of Paediatric Inflammatory Bowel Disease in Canterbury, New Zealand, 1996–2015. *J. Pediatr. Gastroenterol. Nutr.* **2018**, *66*, e45–e50. [CrossRef]
17. Jose, F.A.; Garnett, E.A.; Vittinghoff, E.; Ferry, G.D.; Winter, H.S.; Baldassano, R.N.; Kirschner, B.S.; Cohen, S.A.; Gold, B.D.; Abramson, O.; et al. Development of extraintestinal manifestations in pediatric patients with inflammatory bowel disease. *Inflamm. Bowel Dis.* **2009**, *15*, 63–68. [CrossRef]
18. Dotson, J.L.; Hyams, J.S.; Markowitz, J.; LeLeiko, N.S.; Mack, D.R.; Evans, J.S.; Pfefferkorn, M.D.; Griffiths, A.M.; Otley, A.R.; Bousvaros, A.; et al. Extraintestinal Manifestations of Pediatric Inflammatory Bowel Disease and Their Relation to Disease Type and Severity. *J. Pediatr. Gastroenterol. Nutr.* **2010**, *51*, 140–145. [CrossRef] [PubMed]
19. Jimenez, K.M.; Gasche, C. Management of Iron Deficiency Anaemia in Inflammatory Bowel Disease. *Acta Haematol.* **2019**, *142*, 30–36. [CrossRef]
20. Hashiguchi, Y.; Muro, K.; Saito, Y.; Ito, Y.; Ajioka, Y.; Hamaguchi, T.; Hasegawa, K.; Hotta, K.; Ishida, H.; Ishiguro, M.; et al. Japanese Society for Cancer of the Colon and Rectum (JSCCR) guidelines 2019 for the treatment of colorectal cancer. *Int. J. Clin. Oncol.* **2020**, *25*, 1–42. [CrossRef]
21. Bishnoi, M.; Jain, A.; Hurkat, P.; Jain, S.K. Chondroitin sulphate: A focus on osteoarthritis. *Glycoconj. J.* **2016**, *33*, 693–705. [CrossRef]
22. Volpi, N. Anti-inflammatory activity of chondroitin sulphate: New functions from an old natural macromolecule. *Inflammopharmacology* **2011**, *19*, 299–306. [CrossRef]
23. Du Souich, P.; García, A.G.; Vergés, J.; Montell, E. Immunomodulatory and anti-inflammatory effects of chondroitin sulphate. *J. Cell. Mol. Med.* **2009**, *13*, 1451–1463. [CrossRef] [PubMed]
24. Pumphrey, C.Y.; Theus, A.M.; Li, S.; Parrish, R.S.; Sanderson, R.D. Neoglycans, Carbodiimide-modified Glycosaminoglycans. *Cancer Res.* **2002**, *62*, 3722–3728. [PubMed]
25. Borsig, L.; Wang, L.; Cavalcante, M.C.M.; Cardilo-Reis, L.; Ferreira, P.L.; Mourão, P.A.S.; Esko, J.D.; Pavão, M.S.G. Selectin blocking activity of a fucosylated chondroitin sulfate glycosaminoglycan from sea cucumber: Effect on tumor metastasis and neutrophil recruitment. *J. Biol. Chem.* **2007**, *282*, 14984–14991. [CrossRef] [PubMed]
26. Bergefall, K.; Trybala, E.; Johansson, M.; Uyama, T.; Naito, S.; Yamada, S.; Kitagawa, H.; Sugahara, K.; Bergström, T. Chondroitin sulfate characterized by the E-disaccharide unit is a potent inhibitor of herpes simplex virus infectivity and provides the virus binding sites on gro2C cells. *J. Biol. Chem.* **2005**, *280*, 32193–32199. [CrossRef] [PubMed]
27. Kanchana, S.; Arumugam, M.; Giji, S.; Balasubramanian, T. Isolation, characterization and antioxidant activity of hyaluronic acid from marine bivalve mollusc Amussium pleuronectus (Linnaeus, 1758). *Bioact. Carbohydr. Diet. Fibre* **2013**, *2*, 1–7. [CrossRef]
28. Moseley, R.; Walker, M.; Waddington, R.J.; Chen, W.Y.J. Comparison of the antioxidant properties of wound dressing materials-carboxymethylcellulose, hyaluronan benzyl ester and hyaluronan, towards polymorphonuclear leukocyte-derived reactive oxygen species. *Biomaterials* **2003**, *24*, 1549–1557. [CrossRef]

29. Šoltés, L.; Mendichi, R.; Kogan, G.; Schiller, J.; Stankovská, M.; Arnhold, J. Degradative action of reactive oxygen species on hyaluronan. *Biomacromolecules* **2006**, *7*, 659–668. [CrossRef]
30. Greenberg, D.D.; Stoker, A.; Kane, S.; Cockrell, M.; Cook, J.L. Biochemical effects of two different hyaluronic acid products in a co-culture model of osteoarthritis. *Osteoarthr. Cartil.* **2006**, *14*, 814–822. [CrossRef]
31. Petrey, A.C.; de la Motte, C.A. Hyaluronan in inflammatory bowel disease: Cross-linking inflammation and coagulation. *Matrix Biol.* **2019**, *78–79*, 314–323. [CrossRef] [PubMed]
32. Shah, H.; Patel, R. Statistical modeling of zaltoprofen loaded biopolymeric nanoparticles: Characterization and anti-inflammatory activity of nanoparticles loaded gel. *Int. J. Pharm. Investig.* **2015**, *5*, 20. [CrossRef]
33. Kim, K.W.; Thomas, R.L. Antioxidative activity of chitosans with varying molecular weights. *Food Chem.* **2007**, *101*, 308–313. [CrossRef]
34. Kamil, J.Y.V.A.; Jeon, Y.J.; Shahidi, F. Antioxidative activity of chitosans of different viscosity in cooked comminuted flesh of herring (*Clupea harengus*). *Food Chem.* **2002**, *79*, 69–77. [CrossRef]
35. Hajji, S.; Younes, I.; Rinaudo, M.; Jellouli, K.; Nasri, M. Characterization and In Vitro Evaluation of Cytotoxicity, Antimicrobial and Antioxidant Activities of Chitosans Extracted from Three Different Marine Sources. *Appl. Biochem. Biotechnol.* **2015**, *177*, 18–35. [CrossRef] [PubMed]
36. Azuma, K.; Osaki, T.; Minami, S.; Okamoto, Y. Anticancer and Anti-Inflammatory Properties of Chitin and Chitosan Oligosaccharides. *J. Funct. Biomater.* **2015**, *6*, 33–49. [CrossRef] [PubMed]
37. Raafat, D.; Sahl, H.G. Chitosan and its antimicrobial potential—A critical literature survey. *Microb. Biotechnol.* **2009**, *2*, 186–201. [CrossRef]
38. Hajiali, H.; Summa, M.; Russo, D.; Armirotti, A.; Brunetti, V.; Bertorelli, R.; Athanassiou, A.; Mele, E. Alginate-lavender nanofibers with antibacterial and anti-inflammatory activity to effectively promote burn healing. *J. Mater. Chem. B* **2016**, *4*, 1686–1695. [CrossRef]
39. Iizima-Mizui, N. Antitumor activity of polysaccharide fractions from the brown seaweed Sargassum kjelimanianum. *Kitasato Arch. Exp. Med.* **1985**, *58*, 59–71.
40. Jeong, H.-J.; Lee, S.-A.; Moon, P.-D.; Na, H.-J.; Park, R.-K.; Um, J.-Y.; Kim, H.-M.; Hong, S.-H. Alginic acid has anti-anaphylactic effects and inhibits inflammatory cytokine expression via suppression of nuclear factor-κB activation. *Clin. Exp. Allergy* **2006**, *36*, 785–794. [CrossRef]
41. Tomida, H.; Yasufuku, T.; Fujii, T.; Kondo, Y.; Kai, T.; Anraku, M. Polysaccharides as potential antioxidative compounds for extended-release matrix tablets. *Carbohydr. Res.* **2010**, *345*, 82–86. [CrossRef]
42. Wang, P.; Jiang, X.; Jiang, Y.; Hu, X.; Mou, H.; Li, M.; Guan, H. In vitro antioxidative activities of three marine oligosaccharides. *Nat. Prod. Res.* **2007**, *21*, 646–654. [CrossRef] [PubMed]
43. Yoshida, T.; Hirano, A.; Wada, H.; Takahashi, K.; Hattori, M. Alginic Acid Oligosaccharide Suppresses Th2 Development and IgE Production by Inducing IL-12 Production. *Int. Arch. Allergy Immunol.* **2004**, *133*, 239–247. [CrossRef] [PubMed]
44. Younes, I.; Rinaudo, M. Chitin and chitosan preparation from marine sources. Structure, properties and applications. *Mar. Drugs* **2015**, *13*, 1133–1174. [CrossRef] [PubMed]
45. Bernkop-Schnürch, A.; Dünnhaupt, S. Chitosan-based drug delivery systems. *Eur. J. Pharm. Biopharm.* **2012**, *81*, 463–469. [CrossRef]
46. Leung, T.C.Y.; Wong, C.K.; Xie, Y. Green synthesis of silver nanoparticles using biopolymers, carboxymethylated-curdlan and fucoidan. *Mater. Chem. Phys.* **2010**, *121*, 402–405. [CrossRef]
47. Jayakumar, R.; Menon, D.; Manzoor, K.; Nair, S.V.; Tamura, H. Biomedical applications of chitin and chitosan based nanomaterials—A short review. *Carbohydr. Polym.* **2010**, *82*, 227–232. [CrossRef]
48. Lautenschläger, C.; Schmidt, C.; Lehr, C.M.; Fischer, D.; Stallmach, A. PEG-functionalized microparticles selectively target inflamed mucosa in inflammatory bowel disease. *Eur. J. Pharm. Biopharm.* **2013**, *85*, 578–586. [CrossRef] [PubMed]
49. Kootala, S.; Filho, L.; Srivastava, V.; Linderberg, V.; Moussa, A.; David, L.; Trombotto, S.; Crouzier, T. Reinforcing Mucus Barrier Properties with Low Molar Mass Chitosans. *Biomacromolecules* **2018**, *19*, 872–882. [CrossRef]
50. Xu, J.; Tam, M.; Samaei, S.; Lerouge, S.; Barralet, J.; Stevenson, M.M.; Cerruti, M. Mucoadhesive chitosan hydrogels as rectal drug delivery vessels to treat ulcerative colitis. *Acta Biomater.* **2017**, *48*, 247–257. [CrossRef]
51. Bawa, P.; Choonara, Y.E.; Du Toit, L.C.; Kumar, P.; Ndesendo, V.M.K.; Meyer, L.C.R.; Pillay, V. A novel stimuli-synchronized alloy-treated matrix for space-defined gastrointestinal delivery of mesalamine in the Large White pig model. *J. Control. Release* **2013**, *166*, 234–245. [CrossRef] [PubMed]
52. Bautzová, T.; Rabišková, M.; Béduneau, A.; Pellequer, Y.; Lamprecht, A. Bioadhesive pellets increase local 5-aminosalicylic acid concentration in experimental colitis. *Eur. J. Pharm. Biopharm.* **2012**, *81*, 379–385. [CrossRef] [PubMed]
53. Ribeiro, L.N.M.; Alcântara, A.C.S.; Darder, M.; Aranda, P.; Araújo-Moreira, F.M.; Ruiz-Hitzky, E. Pectin-coated chitosan-LDH bionanocomposite beads as potential systems for colon-targeted drug delivery. *Int. J. Pharm.* **2014**, *463*, 1–9. [CrossRef] [PubMed]
54. Mura, P.; Nácher, A.; Merino, V.; Merino-Sanjuan, M.; Carda, C.; Ruiz, A.; Manconi, M.; Loy, G.; Fadda, A.M.; Diez-Sales, O. N-Succinyl-chitosan systems for 5-aminosalicylic acid colon delivery: In vivo study with TNBS-induced colitis model in rats. *Int. J. Pharm.* **2011**, *416*, 145–154. [CrossRef]
55. Chen, C.; Liu, M.; Lii, S.; Gao, C.; Chen, J. In Vitro Degradation and Drug-Release Properties of Water-Soluble Chitosan Cross-Linked Oxidized Sodium Alginate Core–Shell Microgels. *J. Biomater. Sci. Polym. Ed.* **2012**, *23*, 2007–2024. [CrossRef]

56. Newton, A.M.J.; Lakshmanan, P. Effect of HPMC—E15 LV premium Polymer on Release Profile and Compression Characteristics of Chitosan/ Pectin Colon Targeted Mesalamine Matrix Tablets and in vitro Study on Effect of pH Impact on the Drug Release Profile. *Recent Pat. Drug Deliv. Formul.* **2014**, *8*, 46–62. [CrossRef]
57. Singh, K.; Suri, R.; Tiwary, A.K.; Rana, V. Exploiting the synergistic effect of chitosan-EDTA conjugate with MSA for the early recovery from colitis. *Int. J. Biol. Macromol.* **2013**, *54*, 186–196. [CrossRef]
58. Duan, H.; Lü, S.; Gao, C.; Bai, X.; Qin, H.; Wei, Y.; Wu, X.; Liu, M. Mucoadhesive microparticulates based on polysaccharide for target dual drug delivery of 5-aminosalicylic acid and curcumin to inflamed colon. *Colloids Surf. B Biointerfaces* **2016**, *145*, 510–519. [CrossRef]
59. Chen, S.-Q.; Song, Y.-Q.; Wang, C.; Tao, S.; Yu, F.-Y.; Lou, H.-Y.; Hu, F.-Q.; Yuan, H. Chitosan-modified lipid nanodrug delivery system for the targeted and responsive treatment of ulcerative colitis. *Carbohydr. Polym.* **2020**, *230*, 115613. [CrossRef]
60. Helmy, A.M.; Elsabahy, M.; Soliman, G.M.; Mahmoud, M.A.; Ibrahim, E.A. Development and in vivo evaluation of chitosan beads for the colonic delivery of azathioprine for treatment of inflammatory bowel disease. *Eur. J. Pharm. Sci.* **2017**, *109*, 269–279. [CrossRef]
61. Oshi, M.A.; Naeem, M.; Bae, J.; Kim, J.; Lee, J.; Hasan, N.; Kim, W.; Im, E.; Jung, Y.; Yoo, J.W. Colon-targeted dexamethasone microcrystals with pH-sensitive chitosan/alginate/Eudragit S multilayers for the treatment of inflammatory bowel disease. *Carbohydr. Polym.* **2018**, *198*, 434–442. [CrossRef]
62. Araujo, V.; Gamboa, A.; Caro, N.; Abugoch, L.; Gotteland, M.; Valenzuela, F.; Merchant, H.A.; Basit, A.W.; Tapia, C. Release of prednisolone and inulin from a new calcium-alginate chitosan-coated matrix system for colonic delivery. *J. Pharm. Sci.* **2013**, *102*. [CrossRef]
63. Shah, H.K.; Conkie, J.A.; Tait, R.C.; Johnson, J.R.; Wilson, C.G. A novel, biodegradable and reversible polyelectrolyte platform for topical-colonic delivery of pentosan polysulphate. *Int. J. Pharm.* **2011**, *404*, 124–132. [CrossRef]
64. Iglesias, N.; Galbis, E.; Díaz-Blanco, M.J.; Lucas, R.; Benito, E.; De-Paz, M.V. Nanostructured Chitosan-based biomaterials for sustained and colon-specific resveratrol release. *Int. J. Mol. Sci.* **2019**, *20*, 398. [CrossRef]
65. Zhang, X.; Ma, Y.; Ma, L.; Zu, M.; Song, H.; Xiao, B. Oral administration of chondroitin sulfate-functionalized nanoparticles for colonic macrophage-targeted drug delivery. *Carbohydr. Polym.* **2019**, *223*, 1–9. [CrossRef]
66. Zhang, M.; Xu, C.; Liu, D.; Han, M.K.; Wang, L.; Merlin, D. Oral Delivery of Nanoparticles Loaded With Ginger Active Compound, 6-Shogaol, Attenuates Ulcerative Colitis and Promotes Wound Healing in a Murine Model of Ulcerative Colitis. *J. Crohn's Colitis* **2018**, *12*, 217–229. [CrossRef]
67. Xiao, B.; Laroui, H.; Viennois, E.; Ayyadurai, S.; Charania, M.A.; Zhang, Y.; Zhang, Z.; Baker, M.T.; Zhang, B.; Gewirtz, A.T.; et al. Nanoparticles with surface antibody against CD98 and carrying CD98 small interfering RNA reduce colitis in mice. *Gastroenterology* **2014**, *146*, 1289–1300.e19. [CrossRef] [PubMed]
68. Duan, B.; Li, M.; Sun, Y.; Zou, S.; Xu, X. Orally Delivered Antisense Oligodeoxyribonucleotides of TNF-α via Polysaccharide-Based Nanocomposites Targeting Intestinal Inflammation. *Adv. Healthc. Mater.* **2019**, *8*, 1801389. [CrossRef] [PubMed]
69. Chen, S.; Wang, J.; Cheng, H.; Guo, W.; Yu, M.; Zhao, Q.; Wu, Z.; Zhao, L.; Yin, Z.; Hong, Z. Targeted Delivery of NK007 to Macrophages to Treat Colitis. *J. Pharm. Sci.* **2015**, *104*, 2276–2284. [CrossRef] [PubMed]
70. Ling, K.; Wu, H.; Neish, A.S.; Champion, J.A. Alginate/chitosan microparticles for gastric passage and intestinal release of therapeutic protein nanoparticles. *J. Control. Release* **2019**, *295*, 174–186. [CrossRef]
71. Rabišková, M.; Bautzová, T.; Gajdziok, J.; Dvořáčková, K.; Lamprecht, A.; Pellequer, Y.; Spilková, J. Coated chitosan pellets containing rutin intended for the treatment of inflammatory bowel disease: In vitro characteristics and in vivo evaluation. *Int. J. Pharm.* **2012**, *422*, 151–159. [CrossRef]
72. Wang, Q.S.; Wang, G.F.; Zhou, J.; Gao, L.N.; Cui, Y.L. Colon targeted oral drug delivery system based on alginate-chitosan microspheres loaded with icariin in the treatment of ulcerative colitis. *Int. J. Pharm.* **2016**, *515*, 176–185. [CrossRef]
73. Caddeo, C.; Nácher, A.; Díez-Sales, O.; Merino-Sanjuán, M.; Fadda, A.M.; Manconi, M. Chitosan-xanthan gum microparticle-based oral tablet for colon-targeted and sustained delivery of quercetin. *J. Microencapsul.* **2014**, *31*, 694–699. [CrossRef] [PubMed]
74. Caddeo, C.; Díez-Sales, O.; Pons, R.; Carbone, C.; Ennas, G.; Puglisi, G.; Fadda, A.M.; Manconi, M. Cross-linked chitosan/liposome hybrid system for the intestinal delivery of quercetin. *J. Colloid Interface Sci.* **2016**, *461*, 69–78. [CrossRef] [PubMed]
75. Calinescu, C.; Mondovi, B.; Federico, R.; Ispas-Szabo, P.; Mateescu, M.A. Carboxymethyl starch: Chitosan monolithic matrices containing diamine oxidase and catalase for intestinal delivery. *Int. J. Pharm.* **2012**, *428*, 48–56. [CrossRef]
76. Zhao, N.; Feng, Z.; Shao, M.; Cao, J.; Wang, F.; Liu, C. Stability profiles and therapeutic effect of cu/zn superoxide dismutase chemically coupled to o-quaternary chitosan derivatives against dextran sodium sulfate-induced colitis. *Int. J. Mol. Sci.* **2017**, *18*, 1121. [CrossRef] [PubMed]
77. Wu, S.J.; Don, T.M.; Lin, C.W.; Mi, F.L. Delivery of berberine using chitosan/fucoidan-taurine conjugate nanoparticles for treatment of defective intestinal epithelial tight junction barrier. *Mar. Drugs* **2014**, *12*, 5677–5697. [CrossRef] [PubMed]
78. Langella, A.; Calcagno, V.; De Gregorio, V.; Urciuolo, F.; Imparato, G.; Vecchione, R.; Netti, P.A. In vitro study of intestinal epithelial interaction with engineered oil in water nanoemulsions conveying curcumin. *Colloids Surf. B Biointerfaces* **2018**, *164*, 232–239. [CrossRef] [PubMed]
79. Huanbutta, K.; Sriamornsak, P.; Luangtana-Anan, M.; Limmatvapirat, S.; Puttipipatkhachorn, S.; Lim, L.Y.; Terada, K.; Nunthanid, J. Application of multiple stepwise spinning disk processing for the synthesis of poly(methyl acrylates) coated chitosan-diclofenac sodium nanoparticles for colonic drug delivery. *Eur. J. Pharm. Sci.* **2013**, *50*, 303–311. [CrossRef]

80. Liu, J.; Chen, Y.; Liu, D.; Liu, W.; Hu, S.; Zhou, N.; Xie, Y. Ectopic expression of SIGIRR in the colon ameliorates colitis in mice by downregulating TLR4/NF-κB overactivation. *Immunol. Lett.* **2017**, *183*, 52–61. [CrossRef]
81. Maestrelli, F.; Zerrouk, N.; Cirri, M.; Mura, P. Comparative evaluation of polymeric and waxy microspheres for combined colon delivery of ascorbic acid and ketoprofen. *Int. J. Pharm.* **2015**, *485*, 365–373. [CrossRef] [PubMed]
82. Naveed, M.; Phil, L.; Sohail, M.; Hasnat, M.; Baig, M.M.F.A.; Ihsan, A.U.; Shumzaid, M.; Kakar, M.U.; Mehmood Khan, T.; Akabar, M.D.; et al. Chitosan oligosaccharide (COS): An overview. *Int. J. Biol. Macromol.* **2019**, *129*, 827–843. [CrossRef] [PubMed]
83. Muanprasat, C.; Wongkrasant, P.; Satitsri, S.; Moonwiriyakit, A.; Pongkorpsakol, P.; Mattaveewong, T.; Pichyangkura, R.; Chatsudthipong, V. Activation of AMPK by chitosan oligosaccharide in intestinal epithelial cells: Mechanism of action and potential applications in intestinal disorders. *Biochem. Pharmacol.* **2015**, *96*, 225–236. [CrossRef]
84. Huang, B.; Xiao, D.; Tan, B.; Xiao, H.; Wang, J.; Yin, J.; Duan, J.; Huang, R.; Yang, C.; Yin, Y. Chitosan Oligosaccharide Reduces Intestinal Inflammation That Involves Calcium-Sensing Receptor (CaSR) Activation in Lipopolysaccharide (LPS)-Challenged Piglets. *J. Agric. Food Chem.* **2016**, *64*, 245–252. [CrossRef] [PubMed]
85. Mattaveewong, T.; Wongkrasant, P.; Chanchai, S.; Pichyangkura, R.; Chatsudthipong, V.; Muanprasat, C. Chitosan oligosaccharide suppresses tumor progression in a mouse model of colitis-associated colorectal cancer through AMPK activation and suppression of NF-κB and mTOR signaling. *Carbohydr. Polym.* **2016**, *145*, 30–36. [CrossRef] [PubMed]
86. Yang, J.W.; Tian, G.; Chen, D.W.; Yao, Y.; He, J.; Zheng, P.; Mao, X.B.; Yu, J.; Huang, Z.Q.; Yu, B. Involvement of PKA signalling in anti-inflammatory effects of chitosan oligosaccharides in IPEC-J2 porcine epithelial cells. *J. Anim. Physiol. Anim. Nutr.* **2018**, *102*, 252–259. [CrossRef]
87. Denost, Q.; Adam, J.P.; Pontallier, A.; Montembault, A.; Bareille, R.; Siadous, R.; Delmond, S.; Rullier, E.; David, L.; Bordenave, L. Colorectal tissue engineering: A comparative study between porcine small intestinal submucosa (SIS) and chitosan hydrogel patches. *Surgery* **2015**, *158*, 1714–1723. [CrossRef]
88. Quentin, D.; Arnaud, P.; Etienne, B.; Reine, B.; Robin, S.; Marlene, D.; Samantha, D.; Laurent, D.; Laurence, B. Colorectal wall regeneration resulting from the association of chitosan hydrogel and stromal vascular fraction from adipose tissue. *J. Biomed. Mater. Res. Part A* **2017**, *106*, 460–467.
89. Fraser, J.R.E.; Laurent, T.C.; Laurent, U.B.G. Hyaluronan: Its nature, distribution, functions and turnover. *J. Intern. Med.* **1997**, *242*, 27–33. [CrossRef] [PubMed]
90. Lindahl, U.; Couchman, J.; Kimata, K.; Esko, J.D. *Proteoglycans and Sulfated Glycosaminoglycans*; Cold Spring Harbor: New York, NY, USA, 2015; ISBN 9780879697709.
91. Burdick, J.A.; Prestwich, G.D. Hyaluronic acid hydrogels for biomedical applications. *Adv. Mater.* **2011**, *23*. [CrossRef] [PubMed]
92. Toole, B.P. Hyaluronan in morphogenesis. *Semin. Cell Dev. Biol.* **2001**, *12*, 79–87. [CrossRef]
93. Kogan, G.; Šoltés, L.; Stern, R.; Gemeiner, P. Hyaluronic acid: A natural biopolymer with a broad range of biomedical and industrial applications. *Biotechnol. Lett.* **2007**, *29*, 17–25. [CrossRef]
94. Giji, S.; Arumugam, M. Isolation and characterization of hyaluronic acid from marine organisms. In *Advances in Food and Nutrition Research*; Academic Press Inc.: Cambridge, MA, USA, 2014; Volume 72, pp. 61–77.
95. Vázquez, J.A.; Rodríguez-Amado, I.; Montemayor, M.I.; Fraguas, J.; Del González, M.P.; Murado, M.A. Chondroitin sulfate, hyaluronic acid and chitin/chitosan production using marine waste sources: Characteristics, applications and eco-friendly processes: A review. *Mar. Drugs* **2013**, *11*, 747–774. [CrossRef]
96. Abdallah, M.M.; Fernández, N.; Matias, A.A.; do Rosario Bronze, M. Hyaluronic acid and Chondroitin sulfate from marine and terrestrial sources: Extraction and purification methods. *Carbohydr. Polym.* **2020**, *243*, 116441. [CrossRef] [PubMed]
97. Collins, M.N.; Birkinshaw, C. Hyaluronic acid based scaffolds for tissue engineering—A review. *Carbohydr. Polym.* **2013**, *92*, 1262–1279. [CrossRef] [PubMed]
98. Passi, A.; Vigetti, D. Hyaluronan as tunable drug delivery system. *Adv. Drug Deliv. Rev.* **2019**, *146*, 83–96. [CrossRef]
99. Fiorino, G.; Gilardi, D.; Naccarato, P.; Sociale, O.R.; Danese, S. Safety and efficacy of sodium hyaluronate (IBD98E) in the induction of clinical and endoscopic remission in subjects with distal ulcerative colitis. *Dig. Liver Dis.* **2014**, *46*, 330–334. [CrossRef]
100. Sammarco, G.; Shalaby, M.; Elangovan, S.; Petti, L.; Roda, G.; Restelli, S.; Arena, V.; Ungaro, F.; Fiorino, G.; Day, A.J.; et al. Hyaluronan Accelerates Intestinal Mucosal Healing through Interaction with TSG-6. *Cells* **2019**, *8*, 1074. [CrossRef]
101. Chiu, C.-T.; Kuo, S.-N.; Hung, S.-W.; Yang, C.-Y. Combined Treatment with Hyaluronic Acid and Mesalamine Protects Rats from Inflammatory Bowel Disease Induced by Intracolonic Administration of Trinitrobenzenesulfonic Acid. *Molecules* **2017**, *22*, 904. [CrossRef] [PubMed]
102. Narayanaswamy, R.; Torchilin, V.P. Hydrogels and Their Applications in Targeted Drug Delivery. *Molecules* **2019**, *24*, 603. [CrossRef] [PubMed]
103. Luo, J.W.; Liu, C.; Wu, J.H.; Lin, L.X.; Fan, H.M.; Zhao, D.H.; Zhuang, Y.Q.; Sun, Y.L. In situ injectable hyaluronic acid/gelatin hydrogel for hemorrhage control. *Mater. Sci. Eng. C* **2019**, *98*, 628–634. [CrossRef]
104. Aprodu, A.; Mantaj, J.; Raimi-Abraham, B.; Vllasaliu, D. Evaluation of a Methylcellulose and Hyaluronic Acid Hydrogel as a Vehicle for Rectal Delivery of Biologics. *Pharmaceutics* **2019**, *11*, 127. [CrossRef]
105. Fattahi, F.S.; Khoddami, A.; Avinc, O. *Sustainable, Renewable, and Biodegradable Poly(Lactic Acid) Fibers and Their Latest Developments in the Last Decade*; Springer: Cham, Switzerland, 2020; pp. 173–194.
106. Makkar, S.K.; Riehl, T.E.; Stenson, W.F. Blocking Hyaluronic Acid Binding to TLR4 Results in Decreased Growth of Colon Cancer and Increased Sensitivity to Radiation. *Gastroenterology* **2017**, *152*, S641. [CrossRef]

107. Mármol, I.; Sánchez-de-Diego, C.; Pradilla Dieste, A.; Cerrada, E.; Rodriguez Yoldi, M. Colorectal Carcinoma: A General Overview and Future Perspectives in Colorectal Cancer. *Int. J. Mol. Sci.* **2017**, *18*, 197. [CrossRef]
108. Qu, D.; Wang, L.; Huo, M.; Song, W.; Lau, C.-W.; Xu, J.; Xu, A.; Yao, X.; Chiu, J.-J.; Tian, X.Y.; et al. Focal TLR4 activation mediates disturbed flow-induced endothelial inflammation. *Cardiovasc. Res.* **2020**, *116*, 226–236. [CrossRef] [PubMed]
109. Wachsmann, P.; Lamprecht, A. Polymeric nanoparticles for the selective therapy of inflammatory bowel disease. In *Methods in Enzymology*; Academic Press Inc.: Cambridge, MA, USA, 2012; Volume 508, pp. 377–397.
110. Xiao, B.; Han, M.K.; Viennois, E.; Wang, L.; Zhang, M.; Si, X.; Merlin, D. Hyaluronic acid-functionalized polymeric nanoparticles for colon cancer-targeted combination chemotherapy. *Nanoscale* **2015**, *7*, 17745–17755. [CrossRef] [PubMed]
111. Si, X.Y.; Merlin, D.; Xiao, B. Recent advances in orally administered cell-specific nanotherapeutics for inflammatory bowel disease. *World J. Gastroenterol.* **2016**, *22*, 7718–7726. [CrossRef] [PubMed]
112. Lautenschläger, C.; Schmidt, C.; Lange, K.; Stallmach, A. Drug-Delivery-Strategien zur gezielten Behandlung von chronisch-entzündlichen Darmerkrankungen. *Z. Gastroenterol.* **2015**, *53*, 226–234. [CrossRef]
113. Xiao, B.; Xu, Z.; Viennois, E.; Zhang, Y.; Zhang, Z.; Zhang, M.; Han, M.K.; Kang, Y.; Merlin, D. Orally Targeted Delivery of Tripeptide KPV via Hyaluronic Acid-Functionalized Nanoparticles Efficiently Alleviates Ulcerative Colitis. *Mol. Ther.* **2017**, *25*, 1628–1640. [CrossRef]
114. Xiao, B.; Zhang, Z.; Viennois, E.; Kang, Y.; Zhang, M.; Han, M.K.; Chen, J.; Merlin, D. Combination Therapy for Ulcerative Colitis: Orally Targeted Nanoparticles Prevent Mucosal Damage and Relieve Inflammation. *Theranostics* **2016**, *6*, 2250–2266. [CrossRef] [PubMed]
115. Farkas, S.; Hornung, M.; Sattler, C.; Anthuber, M.; Gunthert, U.; Herfarth, H.; Schlitt, H.J.; Geissler, E.K.; Wittig, B.M. Short-term treatment with anti-CD44v7 antibody, but not CD44v4, restores the gut mucosa in established chronic dextran sulphate sodium (DSS)-induced colitis in mice. *Clin. Exp. Immunol.* **2005**, *142*, 260–267. [CrossRef]
116. Hankard, G.F.; Cezard, J.P.; Aigrain, Y.; Navarro, J.; Peuchmaur, M. CD44 variant expression in inflammatory colonic mucosa is not disease specific but associated with increased crypt cell proliferation. *Histopathology* **1998**, *32*, 317–321. [CrossRef]
117. Dreaden, E.C.; Morton, S.W.; Shopsowitz, K.E.; Choi, J.H.; Deng, Z.J.; Cho, N.J.; Hammond, P.T. Bimodal tumor-targeting from microenvironment responsive hyaluronan layer-by-layer (LbL) nanoparticles. *ACS Nano* **2014**, *8*, 8374–8382. [CrossRef] [PubMed]
118. Vafaei, S.Y.; Esmaeili, M.; Amini, M.; Atyabi, F.; Ostad, S.N.; Dinarvand, R. Self assembled hyaluronic acid nanoparticles as a potential carrier for targeting the inflamed intestinal mucosa. *Carbohydr. Polym.* **2016**, *144*, 371–381. [CrossRef]
119. Li, W.; Li, Y.; Liu, Z.; Kerdsakundee, N.; Zhang, M.; Zhang, F.; Liu, X.; Bauleth-Ramos, T.; Lian, W.; Mäkilä, E.; et al. Hierarchical structured and programmed vehicles deliver drugs locally to inflamed sites of intestine. *Biomaterials* **2018**, *185*, 322–332. [CrossRef]
120. Sugahara, K.; Kitagawa, H. Recent advances in the study of the biosynthesis and functions of sulfated glycosaminoglycans. *Curr. Opin. Struct. Biol.* **2000**, *10*, 518–527. [CrossRef]
121. Sugahara, K.; Mikami, T.; Uyama, T.; Mizuguchi, S.; Nomura, K.; Kitagawa, H. Recent advances in the structural biology of chondroitin sulfate and dermatan sulfate. *Curr. Opin. Struct. Biol.* **2003**, *13*, 612–620. [CrossRef] [PubMed]
122. Kusche-Gullberg, M.; Kjellén, L. Sulfotransferases in glycosaminoglycan biosynthesis. *Curr. Opin. Struct. Biol.* **2003**, *13*, 605–611. [CrossRef] [PubMed]
123. Malavaki, C.; Mizumoto, S.; Karamanos, N.; Sugahara, K. Recent advances in the structural study of functional chondroitin sulfate and dermatan sulfate in health and disease. *Connect. Tissue Res.* **2008**, *49*, 133–139. [CrossRef] [PubMed]
124. Cesar, A.L.A.; Abrantes, F.A.; Farah, L.; Castilho, R.O.; Cardoso, V.; Fernandes, S.O.; Araújo, I.D.; Faraco, A.A.G. New mesalamine polymeric conjugate for controlled release: Preparation, characterization and biodistribution study. *Eur. J. Pharm. Sci.* **2018**, *111*, 57–64. [CrossRef] [PubMed]
125. Onishi, H.; Ikeuchi-Takahashi, Y.; Kawano, K.; Hattori, Y. Preparation of chondroitin sulfate-glycyl-prednisolone conjugate nanogel and its efficacy in rats with ulcerative colitis. *Biol. Pharm. Bull.* **2019**, *42*, 1155–1163. [CrossRef]
126. Gou, S.; Huang, Y.; Wan, Y.; Ma, Y.; Zhou, X.; Tong, X.; Huang, J.; Kang, Y.; Pan, G.; Dai, F.; et al. Multi-bioresponsive silk fibroin-based nanoparticles with on-demand cytoplasmic drug release capacity for CD44-targeted alleviation of ulcerative colitis. *Biomaterials* **2019**, *212*, 39–54. [CrossRef]
127. Linares, P.M.; Chaparro, M.; Algaba, A.; Román, M.; Moreno Arza, I.; Abad Santos, F.; Ochoa, D.; Guerra, I.; Bermejo, F.; Gisbert, J.P. Effect of Chondroitin Sulphate on Pro-Inflammatory Mediators and Disease Activity in Patients with Inflammatory Bowel Disease. *Digestion* **2015**, *92*, 203–210. [CrossRef]
128. Ching, S.H.; Bansal, N.; Bhandari, B. Alginate gel particles–A review of production techniques and physical properties. *Crit. Rev. Food Sci. Nutr.* **2017**, *57*, 1133–1152. [CrossRef]
129. Vera, J.; Castro, J.; Gonzalez, A.; Moenne, A. Seaweed Polysaccharides and Derived Oligosaccharides Stimulate Defense Responses and Protection Against Pathogens in Plants. *Mar. Drugs* **2011**, *9*, 2514–2525. [CrossRef]
130. Aderibigbe, B.A.; Buyana, B. Alginate in Wound Dressings. *Pharmaceutics* **2018**, *10*, 42. [CrossRef] [PubMed]
131. Lee, K.Y.; Mooney, D.J. Alginate: Properties and biomedical applications. *Prog. Polym. Sci.* **2012**, *37*, 106–126. [CrossRef] [PubMed]
132. García-Ríos, V.; Ríos-Leal, E.; Robledo, D.; Freile-Pelegrin, Y. Polysaccharides composition from tropical brown seaweeds. *Phycol. Res.* **2012**, *60*, 305–315. [CrossRef]
133. Paques, J.P.; van der Linden, E.; van Rijn, C.J.M.; Sagis, L.M.C. Preparation methods of alginate nanoparticles. *Adv. Colloid Interface Sci.* **2014**, *209*, 163–171. [CrossRef]

134. Pawar, S.N.; Edgar, K.J. Alginate derivatization: A review of chemistry, properties and applications. *Biomaterials* **2012**, *33*, 3279–3305. [CrossRef] [PubMed]
135. Wong, T.W. Alginate graft copolymers and alginate-co-excipient physical mixture in oral drug delivery. *J. Pharm. Pharm.* **2011**, *63*, 1497–1512. [CrossRef]
136. Krishnaiah, Y.S.R.; Khan, M.A. Strategies of targeting oral drug delivery systems to the colon and their potential use for the treatment of colorectal cancer. *Pharm. Dev. Technol.* **2012**, *17*, 521–540. [CrossRef]
137. Samak, Y.O.; El Massik, M.; Coombes, A.G.A. A Comparison of Aerosolization and Homogenization Techniques for Production of Alginate Microparticles for Delivery of Corticosteroids to the Colon. *J. Pharm. Sci.* **2017**, *106*, 208–216. [CrossRef]
138. Samak, Y.O.; Santhanes, D.; El-Massik, M.A.; Coombes, A.G.A. Formulation strategies for achieving high delivery efficiency of thymoquinone-containing Nigella sativa extract to the colon based on oral alginate microcapsules for treatment of inflammatory bowel disease. *J. Microencapsul.* **2019**, *36*, 204–214. [CrossRef] [PubMed]
139. You, Y.C.; Dong, L.Y.; Dong, K.; Xu, W.; Yan, Y.; Zhang, L.; Wang, K.; Xing, F.J. In vitro and in vivo application of pH-sensitive colon-targeting polysaccharide hydrogel used for ulcerative colitis therapy. *Carbohydr. Polym.* **2015**, *130*, 243–253. [CrossRef] [PubMed]
140. Md Ramli, S.H.; Wong, T.W.; Naharudin, I.; Bose, A. Coatless alginate pellets as sustained-release drug carrier for inflammatory bowel disease treatment. *Carbohydr. Polym.* **2016**, *152*, 370–381. [CrossRef] [PubMed]

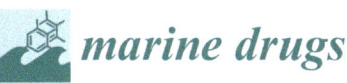

Article

First Report of OvoA Gene in Marine Arthropods: A New Candidate Stress Biomarker in Copepods

Vittoria Roncalli [1,*], Chiara Lauritano [2,†] and Ylenia Carotenuto [1,†]

1. Integrative Marine Ecology Department, Stazione Zoologica Anton Dohrn, Villa Comunale, 80121 Napoli, Italy; ylenia.carotenuto@szn.it
2. Marine Biotechnology Department, Stazione Zoologica Anton Dohrn, Villa Comunale, 80121 Napoli, Italy; chiara.lauritano@szn.it
* Correspondence: vittoria.roncalli@szn.it
† These authors equally contributed to the work.

Abstract: Ovothiol is one of the most powerful antioxidants acting in marine organisms as a defense against oxidative stress during development and in response to environmental cues. The gene involved in the ovothiol biosynthesis, OvoA, is found in almost all metazoans, but open questions existed on its presence among arthropods. Here, using an in silico workflow, we report a single OvoA gene in marine arthropods including copepods, decapods, and amphipods. Phylogenetic analyses indicated that OvoA from marine arthropods separated from the other marine phyla (e.g., Porifera, Mollusca) and divided into two separate branches, suggesting a possible divergence through evolution. In the copepod *Calanus finmarchicus*, we suggest that OvoA has a defense role in oxidative stress as shown by its high expression in response to a toxic diet and during the copepodite stage, a developmental stage that includes significant morphological changes. Overall, the results of our study open possibilities for the use of OvoA as a biomarker of stress in copepods and possibly also for other marine holozooplankters. The finding of OvoA in copepods is also promising for the drug discovery field, suggesting the possibility of using copepods as a new source of bioactive compounds to be tested in the marine biotechnological sector.

Keywords: zooplankton; natural products; antioxidant; transcriptome mining

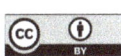

1. Introduction

Ovothiols are low molecular weight thiol-containing methylated amino acids with unique antioxidant properties that are broadly distributed among invertebrates, microalgae, protozoans, and bacteria [1]. Playing a key role in the maintenance of cellular redox homeostasis, ovothiols allow the organism to overcome environmental stress conditions. In marine organisms, ovothiols play a key role also during development as suggested by their antioxidant activity during oxidative stress at fertilization and larval development in the sea urchin [2], and during gametogenesis in the mollusc *Mytilus galloprovincialis* collected from polluted sites [3]. Ovothiols also act as a defense against the immune system of host cells during parasite infections [4,5], and as a protective compound in the mucus of Polychaeta [6]. These molecules have also been suggested as signaling molecules released in the urine of cephalopods [6], in pathways induced by light in microalgae [7,8], and as pheromones in marine worms and cone snails [9].

Recent studies showed new ovothiol bioactivities, highlighting interesting possible applications of this antioxidant in the pharmaceutical sector. Ovothiol A isolated from the sea urchin *Paracentrotus lividus* oocytes, reduced the cell viability of the human liver carcinoma cell line (Hep-G2) by activating autophagy [10]. Additional possible ovothiol A antiatherogenic activities have been found by cell-based assays suggesting its application for cardiovascular diseases associated with oxidative and inflammatory stress, as well as endothelial dysfunction [11]. In addition, in an in vivo study in mice ovothiol A showed activity against liver fibrosis progression [12].

The ovothiol biosynthetic pathway includes three enzymatic steps in which OvoA is the key enzyme with a bifunctional role. First, the OvoA enzyme, 5-histidylcysteine sulfoxide synthase, catalyzes the addition of the cysteine sulfur group into histidine to produce an intermediate; subsequently the intermediate is cleaved by sulfoxide b-lyase (OvoB) into thiohistidine that is finally methylated to ovothiol (π-N-methyl-5-thiohistidine) by OvoA. This final step is specific of the S-adenosylmethionine (SAM) methyltransferase domain situated in the C-terminal of the enzyme. OvoA also contains an N-terminal DNA damage-inducible (DinB) superfamily domain and a formylglycine-generating sulfatase (FGE-sulfatase) domain that contains the recognition/binding sites for the substrates (cysteine and histidine) [13] (Figure 1). The methyltransferases that can methylate the a-amino group of ovothiol A to form ovothiol B and C are not yet known.

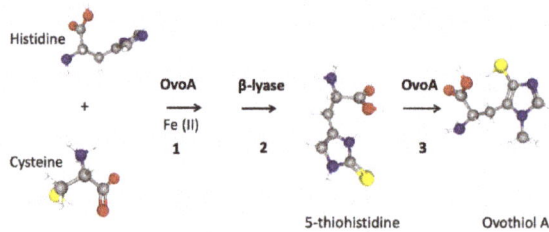

Figure 1. Ovothiol A biosynthetic pathway. Schematic representation of Ovothiol A pathway which consists of three steps (1–3) catalyzed by two enzymes (in bold). (1) OvoA enzyme (5-histidylcysteine sulfoxide synthase) catalyzes the addition of the cysteine sulfur group into histidine to produce an intermediate (not shown); (2) The intermediate (not shown) is cleaved by sulfoxide β lyase (OvoB) into thiohistidine which is then (3) methylated by OvoA to ovothiol (π-N-methyl-5-thiohistidine). Chemical structures were downloaded from the National Center for Biotechnology Information (NCBI) PubChem database. Histidine: PubChem Identifier CID: 6274, https://pubchem.ncbi.nlm.nih.gov/compound/Histidine, accessed on the 3 November 2021; Cysteine: PubChem Identifier CID: 6419722, https://pubchem.ncbi.nlm.nih.gov/compound/Cysteine, accessed on the 3 November 2021; OvothiolA: PubChem Identifier CID: 130131 https://pubchem.ncbi.nlm.nih.gov/compound/Ovothiol-A, accessed on the 3 November 2021.

Braunshausen and Seebeck [14] were the first to characterize the OvoA gene from the bacterium *Erwinia tasmaniensis* and the protozoan *Trypanosoma cruzi*. They also found homologous OvoA enzymes in more than 80 genomes ranging from proteobacteria to uni- and multicellular eukaryotes [14]. From a phylogenetic point of view, OvoA has been reported in many metazoans including Porifera, Emichordata, and Placozoa. Through evolution, the gene was lost twice, once in the common ancestor of nematodes and arthropods and once in the ancestor of Osteichthyes fish [15]. In freshwater fish, ovothiol A has been identified in the metabolites of the lens and other tissues as well as in the eggs, suggesting that these organisms might not have the gene, but are able to acquire the metabolite through their diet [16,17]. In contrast, still little is known of arthropods; it has been suggested that the lack of OvoA in most terrestrial species (e.g., insects) could be related to a specific role of ovothiol in the transition from the aquatic to the terrestrial environment [1,15]. Recently, Brancaccio and coauthors [18] conducted a genomic and metagenomics data mining to investigate the distribution and diversification of the enzymes involved in ovothiol biosynthesis in bacteria. They observed a horizontal gene transfer event of OvoB from Bacteroidetes living in symbiosis with Hydrozoa and suggested that the evolution of ovothiol biosynthesis may have involved symbiosis processes [18]. Overall, from all these studies, it is clear that ovothiol A is an important antioxidant as it is conserved in many metazoans; however, the studies highlight the need to better investigate the presence of OvoA gene in other phyla.

Gene expression changes of OvoA have been reported in *P. lividus* during development and when exposed to stress conditions. Relative expression of OvoA was high in eggs and decreased immediately after fertilization, remaining low in the early developmental stages (early and the swimming blastula) with a final significant increase in the last larval stage (pluteus) [2]. A significant increase in the expression of OvoA has also been reported in larvae exposed algae and to the metals Cd and Mn [2,19]. Overall, these results suggested that in *P. lividus* ovothiol may act as a protective compound against environmental stressors, and/or as a regulation factor during development.

The aim of this study was to explore the occurrence and diversity of the OvoA gene in marine arthropods. Since the OvoB gene has not been identified in metazoan genomes or transcriptomes, except hydrozoans [1,18], we focused our investigation on OvoA. Using a well-established in silico workflow we mined the new publicly available transcriptomic resources for copepods, expanding the searches also to malacostraca. Copepods are an important component in most trophic marine food webs [20–22]. As part of zooplankton, those tiny crustaceans live in highly variable environments and are constantly subject to natural and anthropogenic-related stressful conditions that might compromise their cellular redox homeostasis [23–27]. However, in these herbivorous consumers, still little is known on which genes are activated during detoxification and which genes are responsible of antioxidant production. Given the high antioxidant properties of ovothiol in many marine organisms, we decided to examine the occurrence of OvoA gene in copepods. Using an in silico workflow, we identified OvoA transcripts in copepods but also in other marine arthropods. The identified OvoA transcripts were used in a phylogenetic analysis to support their annotation and to investigate their relationship to other marine metazoans. Lastly, using previous RNA-Seq-based studies, the expression of OvoA across development and after feeding on toxic phytoplankton species was investigated in two crustacean copepods, to evaluate the potential role of ovothiol as protective antioxidant in these holozooplankters.

2. Results

2.1. Identification of OvoA Encoding Transcripts in Marine Arthropods

In this study we report for the first time that marine arthropods also possess OvoA, a key player gene of ovothiol biosynthesis. By mining the publicly available transcriptome database (TSA) limiting to Arthropoda, we identified a single transcript encoding OvoA in 19 copepods and nine malacostracans (Table 1, Table S1). Within the copepod subphylum, OvoA was identified in 11 Calanoids, three Cyclopoids, three Harpacticoids and two Siphonostomatoids. The Calanoida order, with the highest number, included mostly individuals from the Calanidae family such as *Calanus finmarchicus*, *C. helgolandicus* and *Neocalanus flemingeri*. Among the malacrustacans, OvoA were found in seven decapods and two amphipods (e.g., *Gammarus pulex*, *G. fossarum*) (Table 1, Table S1). Reciprocal blast confirmed that all transcripts were annotated as protein OvoA with 70% encoding for full length proteins. Structural domain analysis confirmed the presence of the three expected functional domains, the DNA damage-inducible (DinB), the formylglycine-generating sulfatase (FGE-sulfatase), and the S-adenosylmethionine (SAM) methyltransferase) domains, as shown in the copepods *C. finmarchicus* and *C. helgolandicus* (Figure 2).

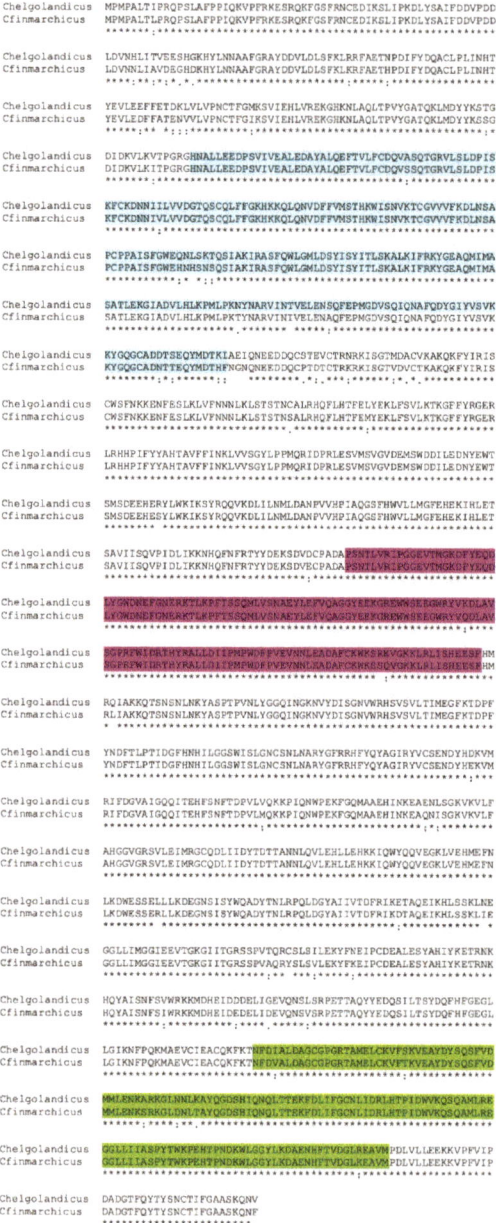

Figure 2. OvoA alignment in the copepods *Calanus finmarchicus* and *C. helgolandicus*. Protein alignment of the deduced OvoA sequenecs for the copepod *C. finmarhcicus* and *C. helgolandius*; "*" beneath the alignment indicates residues that are identical in the two sequences while ":" and "." indicate conservatively substituted aminoacids shared between the protein pair. The three structural functional domains identified by the Pfam database are highlighted as follows: DNA damage-inducible (DinB) (light blue), formylglycine-generating sulfatase (FGE-sulfatase) (magenta), and S-adenosylmethionine (SAM) methyltransferase (green).

Table 1. OvoA in marine arthropods. The list includes the organisms for which a single OvoA transcript was found as result of the in silico transcriptome mining that included a reciprocal blast and structural domain analysis. For each organism, phylum, subphylum, subclass, and order are listed. For each sequence, detailed information on the mined database and National Center for Biotechnology Information (NCBI) accession number are provided in Table S1.

Phylum	Subphylum	Subclass	Order	Organism
Arthropoda	Crustacea	Copepoda	Calanoida	Neocalanus flemingeri
				Calanus finmarchicus
				Calanus helgolandicus
				Labidocera madurae
				Eurytemora affinis
				Temora longicornis
				Pseudodiaptomus annandalei
				Rhincalanus gigas
				Pleuromamma xiphias
				Hemidiaptomus amblyodon
				Metridia pacifica
			Cyclopoida	Eucyclops serrulatus
				Apocyclops royi
				Paracyclopina nana
			Harpacticoida	Tigriopus californicus
				Tigriopus japonicus
				Tisbe furcata
			Siphonostomatoida	Caligus rogercresseyi
				Lepeophtheirus salmonis
		Malacostraca	Amphipoda	Gammarus fossarum
				Gammarus pulex
			Decapoda	Paralithodes camtschaticus
				Halocaridinides trigonophthalma
				Scylla paramamosain
				Eriocheir sinensis
				Callinectes sapidus
				Gecarcinus lateralis
				Homarus americanus

2.2. Phylogenetic Analysis of OvoA Transcripts from Marine Metazoans

Phylogenetic analysis of OvoA sequences deduced in this study for marine arthropods was used to support their annotation and to investigate their relationship to each other and to those from other marine metazoans. The analysis generated a consensus tree with several clades representing the different phyla. Consistent with what has been previously reported for marine metazoans, OvoA sequences from Mollusca, Echinodermata, Cnidaria, and Chordata phylum cluster separately and in individual clades (Figure 3). The OvoA sequences identified in this study for marine arthropods separated into two clades (Figure 3). The first clade, highly separated from all other metazoans, is closely related to OvoA from Placozoa and from two Porifera (Figure 3). This clade included 15 OvoA sequences, including 12 sequences from copepods and three from decapods (Figure 3). The second clade, with a total of 13 OvoA sequences, included seven copepods, four decapods and two amphipods. The seven copepods included five OvoA sequences from Calanoida and two sequences from Cyclopoida (Figure 3).

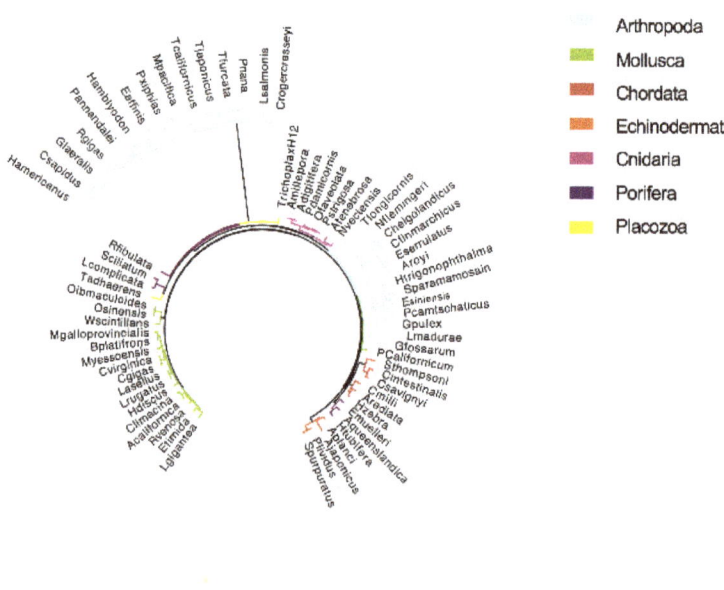

Figure 3. Phylogenetic tree for OvoA gene in marine metazoans. The unrooted tree shows the relationships between OvoA identified in this study for marine arthropods and OvoA from selected marine metazoans. Amino acid sequences were aligned using ClustalW, and FASTTREE was used to build a maximum-likelihood phylogenetic tree (Galaxy v. 2.1.10+ galaxy1) using the protein evolution model JTT+ CAT. Color coding refers to the different phylum: light blue = Arthropoda (sequences identified in this study), green = Mollusca, red = Chordata, orange = Echinodermata, pink = Cnidaria, purple = Porifera, yellow = Placozoa. Scale bar indicates the number of amino acid substitution per site.

2.3. Ovo A Expression in Calanus finmarchicus and C. helgolandicus

The expression of OvoA was examined in the copepods *C. finmarchicus* and *C. helgolandicus* using previous RNA-Seq data for these copepods feeding on toxic algal species [28,29].

In *C. finmarchicus*, exposure to the saxitoxin producing dinoflagellate *Alexandrium fundyense* induced changes in the expression of OvoA (Figure 4A). The increase in expression of OvoA did not depend on the dose of the toxic algae but was time affected (Figure 4A). Specifically, at two days, OvoA was found up-regulated in females fed with toxic algae at low (LD) and high (HD) doses (LD = 5.1 ± 0.11 Log2 [RPKM + 1], HD = 5.03 ± 0.5 Log2 [RPKM + 1]) compared with females on the control diet *Rhodomonas* sp. (Figure 4A). In contrast, a longer exposure to the dinoflagellate had no significant effect; at five days, the expression of OvoA was similar between diets and not significantly different compared with females on the control diet (Figure 4A).

In *C. helgolandicus* exposure to a toxic diet did not affect the expression of OvoA. In females exposed for 5 days to the toxic diatom *Skeletonema marinoi*, OvoA expression was not significantly different from the expression of females feeding on the control diet *P. minimum* (TOXIC = 9.97 ± 1.35, Log2 [RPKM + 1]; CONTROL = 9.80 ± 0.36, Log2 [RPKM + 1]). The reported lack of OvoA differential expression after 5 days on the toxic algae is similar to that reported for *C. finmarchicus* (Figure 4A).

Changes in the expression of OvoA were also examined in *C. finmarchicus* through development. Using previously published RNA-Seq expression data, we examined the expression of OvoA in different stages including embryos (E), early nauplii (EN), early copepodites (CI), late copepodites (CIV and CV), and adult females (F). Compared with all other stages, the lowest and significantly different expression of OvoA was found in embryos (0.2 Log2 [RPKM + 1]) (Figure 4B). The OvoA expression significantly increased across development reaching its peak in the first copepodite stage (CI) (6.2 ± 0.19 Log2 [RPKM + 1]). A high expression was also maintained through the pre-adult stage (CV) (5.7 ± 0.19 Log2 [RPKM + 1]) but it decreased in the adult stage (Figure 4B).

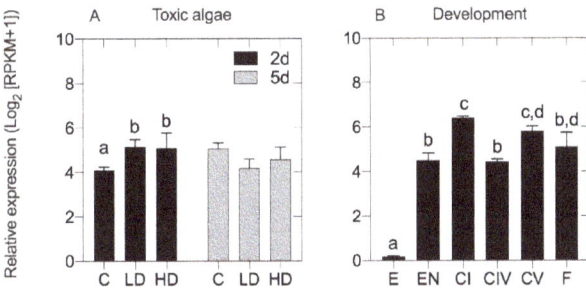

Figure 4. OvoA expression in *Calanus finmarchicus*. In both graphs, relative expression was normalized by length RPKM (Log2) adding pseudocounts of 1. (**A**) Expression of OvoA in adult females exposed for 2 days (2d) and 5 days (5d) to a control diet *Rhodomonas* sp. (C), and low (LD) and high doses (HD) of the toxic dinoflagellate *Alexandrium fundyense* [29]. Bar graphs indicate mean with standard deviation (SD) of the three replicates in each diet; (**B**) Expression of OvoA across development: embryos [E], early nauplii (NII-NIII) [EN], early copepodites [CI], late copepodites (preadult CIV and CV) [CIV] [CV], females [F]. Bar graphs indicate 2-way ANOVA of the three replicates in each sample (exception CI and CIV with two replicates). Significant differences ($p < 0.05$; 2-way ANOVA followed by post-hoc Tukey's test) among stages are indicated by small letters over the bars.

3. Discussion

Ovothiols are small sulfur-containing natural metabolites playing a key role in protecting the organisms against oxidative stress. For its chemical properties and low molecular weight, Ovothiol A is one of the strongest antioxidants reacting with ROS and radicals significantly faster than other natural thiols. Ovothiols are biosynthesized in a two-way step with OvoA, 5-histidylcysteine sulfoxide synthase, being the key regulator. The OvoA gene is highly conserved and found in almost all marine metazoans including Porifera, Cnidaria, Hemicordata, and Echinoderamata [15]. Interestingly, some organisms such as insects and fish, are unable to produce those secondary compounds. This seems to be related to the two gene loss event that occurred through evolution for the ancestral Ecdysozoa (nematodes and arthropods) and the ancestor of Osteichthyes fish. Although fish lack the OvoA to biosynthesize the compounds, ovothiols have been found in different tissues of freshwater fish suggesting that those organisms acquire the metabolite through their nutrition [15]. For arthropods, there was no evidence of OvoA gene and no reports on the presence of ovothiols. In our study, we present the results for the mining of the publicly available transcriptomic resources on the National Center for Biotechnology Information (NCBI) database (TSA) limiting the results to the marine arthropods, mostly represented by the Crustacea subphylum. However, during our searches, OvoA hits resulted also for terrestrial species. For the completeness of our mining (data are not shown) we further examined those sequences with reciprocal blast and structural domain analysis as part of our workflow. This resulted in the identification of OvoA transcripts from eight insects (6 Hemiptera and 2 Diptera). Considering that the focus of the study is on marine organisms, we did not expand the investigation on the terrestrial arthropods. However, our preliminary results might suggest that more investigations are needed in order to clarify also the presence of this gene in terrestrial species.

Marine arthropods are among the most distributed living organism in aquatic environment; copepods, the insects of the sea, dominate the zooplankton. Zooplanktonic organisms have a key role in the energy transfer to higher trophic levels. Through their lifecycle, copepods are commonly exposed to abiotic and biotic stressors that disturb their cellular homeostasis with negative effects on their fitness and in extreme conditions their survival. To cope with the stress, organisms typically activate a cellular stress response (CSR) [30]. This response has the goal to repair and prevent macromolecular damage, to activate cell cycle checkpoints, to reallocate energy resources, and in extreme cases to activate a programmed cell death [30]. The critical part of the CSR is the antioxidant system, a set of enzymes acting against the oxidative protein damage induced by elevated concentration of reactive oxygen species (ROS). Antioxidant proteins, commonly used as biomarkers of oxidative stress, include thioredoxin/thioredoxin reductase, glutaredoxin/glutathione/glutathione reductases, metallothioneins, and cytochrome P450 proteins.

The increase of new transcriptomic resources for marine arthropods, mostly for organism from the copepoda order, has provided the opportunity to expand targeted gene discovery in these organisms. A better understanding of the complexity of gene families of interest, in particular those associated with response to stress, opens new opportunities to discover new biomarkers that could be used for functional studies. For its antioxidant properties, OvoA could be a new biomarker to evaluate antioxidant stress responses in marine organisms. Here we focused on the target identification in marine arthropods of the transcripts encoding for the OvoA enzyme. Our study describes the ovothiol gene distribution in many marine arthropods providing the first report of OvoA gene in the Arthropoda phylum. For mining transcriptomic resources for marine organisms, which included 19 copepods and nine malacrostacans, we found in each organism a single OvoA transcript encoding protein. Seventy percent of the proteins deduced from the predicted OvoA transcript appear to be full-length and showed the expected structural hallmark. Phylogenetic analysis was used to support the annotation and also to evaluate the relationship of OvoA from marine arthropods with other marine metazoans. Based on our results we found that the OvoA sequences from marine arthropods are significantly different from the other metazoans by clustering in independent clades. However, to our surprise, the OvoA sequences separated in two clades that included both copepods and malacrostacans with no distinction between copepod orders. The separation of two clades might suggest that through evolution the OvoA has diverged, however more studies are needed.

In many marine organisms, ovothiols are known for their role in the oxidative response against environmental stressors. In sea urchins, ovothiols are significantly over-expressed in response to metals and toxic algae [2]. In the starlet sea anemone *Nematostella vectensis* OvoA has been suggested as protector against environmental pollutants [31]. A significant high expression of OvoA was found in organisms exposed to dispersant and/or sweet crude oil exposure alone or combined with ultraviolet radiation (UV) [31]. Here, to support a possible role of OvoA as antioxidant in copepods, we used previously generated RNA-Seq data for two calanoid copepods exposed to harmful microalgae to examine the expression of OvoA. In the previously published study, the physiological response of *C. finmarchicus* females exposed to the neurotoxin-producing dinoflagellate *Alexandrium fundyense* was investigated after two- and five-days exposure [28]. The authors reported that at 2 days, *C. finmarchicus* activates a cellular stress response that involves differential expression of many genes associated with molecular chaperoning, apoptosis, cell cycle checkpoint, intracellular signaling, and protein turnover [28]. Although detoxification was not the major component of the response, up-regulated with the diet there were also some antioxidant biomarkers such as glutathione S-transferase (GST), sulfotransferase, and thioredoxin. Here, we found that the expression of OvoA was significantly high in *C. finmarchicus* exposed to the toxic diet compared with individuals on a control diet. The differential regulation of OvoA at 2 days reported here, is consistent with a role of OvoA as antioxidant as part of the CSR previously reported [28]. Furthermore, the lack of significant difference in the expression between the two toxic diets (low and high doses) agrees with the findings that the *C. finmarchicus* response to the toxic algae is not dose dependent. At 5 days, we did not report differences in the expression of OvoA between individuals on the toxic diets (both doses) and the control. This agrees with the fact that at 5 days the *C. finmarchicus* CSR became a cellular homeostatic response, characterized by fewer differentially expressed genes [28]. A homeostatic response is activated when the organism physiologically adapts to new conditions and starts to re-establish homeostasis by counteracting the stress in a specific way [30].

Consistent with *C. finmarchicus*, we also observed no significant differences in OvoA expression when the congener *C. helgolandicus* was fed for 5 days on the oxylipin-producing diatom *S. marinoi*, with respect to the control diet. Oxylipins are lipid-derived info chemicals that regulate the structure and functioning of natural phytoplankton communities [25], and also act as defensive compounds against consumer copepods, by inducing offspring abnormalities, thereby reducing population recruitment at sea [25,32]. Interestingly, the same *C. helgolandicus* females for which we examined the expression of OvoA, showed strong up regulation of genes involved in stress response and xenobiotic detoxification, such as GST and cytochrome P450 [29]. Hence, it is possible that these *C. helgolandicus* individuals were activating a detoxification system based on other antioxidants than ovothiols, that protected the adult copepod from the direct ingestion of the harmful diet. Although we did not have information on OvoA expression in *C. helgolandicus* females feeding for 2 days on *S. marinoi*, a previous study showed that these copepods activated a CSR by over-expressing genes encoding for cellular chaperons, as well as for proteins involved in signal transduction pathways and cell cycle [33]. Given the similar cellular response of the two copepod species when exposed for short feeding times to harmful algal diets, we could speculate that ovothiols may play a role in the antioxidant defensive system of *C. helgolandicus*, as well. However, further studies are needed to confirm this hypothesis.

In addition to their role in response to stressor, ovothiols play a role also during development [2]. In the sea urchin *P. lividus*, a significant high expression of the OvoA gene was found not only in the post-fertilized eggs but also in the pluteus stage during larval development. At the pluteus stage, the organism undergoes a series of morphological changes leading to the final metamorphosis. Alteration of the redox homeostasis is common through development as a consequence of oxygen radicals or reactive oxygen species (ROS) that act as primary or secondary messengers to promote cell growth [34]. The periods associated with morphological changes are characterized by an increase of metabolic activity and apoptosis that leads to elevated concentration of ROS. Thus, it is not strange that OvoA transcript is highly expressed in those stages of development due to its role in ROS scavenging. Copepods have a molt cycle with six nauplier and five copepodite stages [35]. A significant high expression of OvoA was found here in *C. finmarchicus* in the first and the last copepodite stages. Those two stages are key through development. Between the six nauplier and the first copepodite stage the organism undergoes morphological rearrangements while the 5th copepodite stage is when the organism sexually differentiates [35]. Although copepods have a molt cycle that does not involve a pupal stage as in sea urchin (with final metamorphosis), the high expression at those two key stages is like the sea urchin findings, with OvoA playing a key role during late development. Taken together, the pattern of expression reported for OvoA transcript in *C. finmarchicus* fed on the toxic diet suggests that the production of ovothiols is a possible adaptive strategy to cope with environmental stressors. A differential expression through development could be associated either with an antioxidant response to the byproducts that are generated during metamorphosis or to a specific signaling role that these metabolites can have through development.

In addition to its role as antioxidant, ovothiols have also been reported to have antiproliferative and anti-inflammatory activities [2,10]. Our results provide the first evidence that OvoA is present in copepods, decapods, and amphipods, opening new questions on its distribution also among other zooplanktonic species. The high expression of OvoA in *C. finmarchicus* in response to a toxic diet as well as during the key transition stages of the molt cycle, might suggest that ovothiol A has an antioxidant role also in copepods. In the recent years, drug discovery has focused on marine planktonic organisms, rather than macroorganisms because of their advantage of easy culturing in closed controlled systems and to obtain huge biomass [36,37]. Both phytoplanktonic and zooplanktonic species, have been shown to have the capability of producing several antioxidant, anti-inflammatory, anti-diabetes, anticancer, and other bioactivities compounds useful for the prevention and treatment of human pathologies [38–42]. Thus, the findings that ovothiol A might be produced by zooplankters can have interesting possible future biotechnological applications and can stimulate further studies on planktonic metabolites for pharmaceutical, nutraceutical, and cosmeceutical applications.

4. Materials and Methods

4.1. In Silico Mining, Reciprocal Blast, and Protein Structural Analysis

In silico search for putative OvoA encoding transcript was performed using a well-established vetting protocol that involves a mining, a reciprocal BLAST, and a structural motif analysis [43,44]. The transcriptome shotgun assembly (TSA) database on the National Center for Biotechnology Information (NCBI) was searched (October 2021) using the OvoA sequence from *Paracentrotus lividus* (AMM72581) as query (tblastn algorithm) limiting the results to Arthropoda (taxid: 6656). Among the hits, we focused on the marine organisms, mostly represented by crustacean including the Copepoda and Malacrostaca subphyla. For completeness, we also mined the Crustybase [45] to search additional available transcriptomes for other marine arthropods. Using *P. lividus* OvoA protein sequence we mined (tblastn algorithm) transcriptomes for the decapods *Eriocheir sinensis, Litopenaeus vannamei, Callinectes sapidus, Gecarcinus lateralis, Homarus americanus* whose references were not available on NCBI (Table S1). The transcripts encoding sequences OvoA for all the newly identified arthropods are provided in Supplementary File S3.

Reciprocal blast was used to confirm the identity of the putative OvoA transcripts by blasting each transcript against the non-redundant (nr) protein database. Briefly, each putative OvoA transcript was fully translated using ExPASy [46] and then the deduced protein was used to query the NCBI non-redundant (nr) protein database (blastp algorithm). Protein sequences were further inspected by searching the Pfam database for structural domains [47]. Specifically, we searched for the three expected conserved domains: the DinB-like domain, the FGE-sulfatase domain, and the methyltransferase 11 domain pertaining to the SAM-dependent methyl-transferase homologous superfamily. OvoA sequences from the calanoid *C. finmarchicus* and *C. helgolandicus* were aligned using ClustalW software (Galaxy version 2.1 [48]).

4.2. Phylogenetic Analysis

Phylogenetic analysis was used to support the assignment of the predicted OvoA sequences from marine arthropods, to establish their relationship to each other and to those from other metazoans. An unrooted phylogenetic tree was generated using OvoA amino acid sequences deduced from this study and from known marine metazoans [1]. The selected sequences included organisms from Mollusca, Chordata, Hemichordata, Echinodermata, Placozoa, and Porifera phylum (Table S2). An unrooted phylogenetic tree was generated using amino acid sequences that were aligned using ClustalW software (Galaxy version 2.1 [48]). FASTTREE was used to build a maximum-likelihood phylogenetic tree (Galaxy Version 2.1.10+ galaxy1) using the protein evolution model JTT+ CAT [49].

4.3. Expression of OvoA in Calanus finmarchicus and C. helgolandicus

Expression of OvoA transcript was examined in the copepods *Calanus finmarchicus* and *Calanus helgolandicus* exposed to stress conditions and in *C. finmarchicus* across development using previously published data [28,29]. The datasets were searched for the OvoA sequences identified in this study for *C. finmarchicus* and *C. helgolandicus*. The expression data for OvoA obtained from the three datasets was normalized using the Reads Per Kilobase per Million mapped reads RPKM method. A 2-way ANOVA ($p < 0.05$) followed by post-hoc Tukey's test which was used to assess statistical significance in each study. A brief description of the datasets mined for the expression data is presented below.

The *C. finmarchicus* RNA-Seq dataset included expression data for females incubated for two and five days under three experimental diets: control (*Rhodomonas* sp.) and two doses (low and high) of the toxic dinoflagellate *Alexandrium fundyense* [24,50]. The toxic concentrations used for the dinoflagellate (LD = 50,000 cells L^{-1}; HD = 200,000 cells L^{-1}) were comparable with low and high bloom conditions reported in the Gulf of Maine [28]. Detailed methods for copepod collection, algal-incubation, RNA extraction and RNA-Seq processing are described in Roncalli et al. [28]. Briefly, females were exposed to the three diets for a total of 7 days with samples being harvested for RNA-Seq at day 2 and day 5 (three replicates/treatment). Expression was quantified by mapping each RNA-Seq library against the *C. finmarchicus* reference transcriptome (NCBI: PRJNA236528) using bowtie software (v.2.0.6). The second *C. finmarchicus* RNA-Seq dataset included expression data for six developmental stages: embryos, early nauplii (NII-NIII), early copepodites (CI), late copepodites (CIV), pre-adults (CV), and females (F) [50–52]. For each stage three samples were processed for RNA-Seq (exception CI and CIV with two replicates) and expression rate was measured by mapping each RNA-Seq library against the *C. finmarchicus* reference transcriptome (NCBI: PRJNA236528) using bowtie software (v.2.0.6).

Lastly, the *C. helgolandicus* dataset consisted of RNA-Seq data for laboratory-incubated females feeding for five days on the oxylipin-producing diatom *Skeletonema marinoi* and the control diet *Prorocentrum minimum*. Detailed methods for copepod collection, algal-incubation experiments, transcriptome sequencing, de novo assembly and annotation, are described in [29]. In brief, *C. helgolandicus* females collected in the Gulf of Naples (Mediterranean Sea) were fed for five days with either *S. marinoi* or *P. minimum* at 1 mg C L^{-1} (three replicates each). RNA-Seq libraries were pooled to generate a de novo assembly (NCBI: PRJNA640515) that was used to quantify expression levels by self-mapping using bowtie. Reads were normalized by length using the RPKM methods Reads Per Kilobase per Million mapped reads (RPKM).

5. Conclusions

This study reports for the first time the presence of the OvoA gene, a key player of the ovothiol biosynthetic pathway, in arthropods. By mining the new transcriptomic resources for marine arthropods, we report a single OvoA gene in copepods, decapods, and amphipods. Phylogenetic analysis places all the marine arthropod sequences in two separate branches, suggesting possible events through evolution. Changes in expression of the OvoA gene across development and under stress conditions, suggest that ovothiol may play a role as a defensive compound in *C. finmarchicus*, thus proposing this gene as a new biomarker of stress in holozooplanktonic species. The finding that many copepods have the OvoA gene and are thus capable of producing bioactive compounds opens up further possibilities for both new drug discovery as well as in the marine biotechnology field.

Supplementary Materials: The following are available online at https://www.mdpi.com/article/10.3390/md19110647/s1, Table S1: List of in publicly available marine arthropod datasets mined for OvoA using the query from *P. lividus*. For each dataset, information on Genus, Species, Phylum, class, and Order are provided. Accession number of the mined transcriptome (TSA database) and the Bioproject are listed. For *Eurytemora affinis* and *Tigriopus californicus* the protein sequence database was mined (blastp algoritm). For *Lepeophtheirus salmonis* the TSA accession number was not provided. For three decapods, transcriptomes were mined using CrustyBase repository. Table S2: List of OvoA protein sequences used for the phylogenetic analysis. The list includes sequences identified in this study (light blue) and sequences publicly available for selected marine metazoan [1]. For each sequence, information on Genus, Species, Phylum, class, and Order are provided. Supplementary File S3: FASTA file of OvoA transcript encoding protein identified in this study for marine arthropods.

Author Contributions: Conceptualization, V.R., C.L. and Y.C.; methodology, V.R.; writing—original draft preparation, V.R., C.L. and Y.C.; writing—review and editing, V.R., C.L. and Y.C. All authors have read and agreed to the published version of the manuscript.

Funding: This research received no external funding.

Institutional Review Board Statement: Not applicable.

Informed Consent Statement: Not applicable.

Data Availability Statement: Bioproject and transcriptome shotgun assembly (TSA) numbers of the National Center for Biotechnology Information (NCBI) database for the datasets examined in the present study are indicated in Supplementary Table S1. In Supplementary File S3, the OvoA transcript encoding protein identified in this study for marine arthropods is indicated.

Acknowledgments: We would like to thank P. Lenz from the University of Hawai'i at Manoa and A. Ianora from Stazione Zoologica A. Dohrn for their intellectual contributions.

Conflicts of Interest: The authors declare no conflict of interest.

References

1. Gerdol, M.; Sollitto, M.; Pallavicini, A.; Castellano, I. The complex evolutionary history of sulfoxide synthase in ovothiol biosynthesis. *Proc. R. Soc. B* **2019**, *286*, 20191812. [CrossRef]
2. Castellano, I.; Migliaccio, O.; D'Aniello, S.; Merlino, A.; Napolitano, A.; Palumbo, A. Shedding light on ovothiol biosynthesis in marine metazoans. *Sci. Rep.* **2016**, *6*, 1–11. [CrossRef]
3. Diaz de Cerio, O.; Reina, L.; Squatrito, V.; Etxebarria, N.; Gonzalez-Gaya, B.; Cancio, I. Gametogenesis-Related Fluctuations in Ovothiol Levels in the Mantle of Mussels from Different Estuaries: Fighting Oxidative Stress for Spawning in Polluted Waters. *Biomolecules* **2020**, *10*, 373. [CrossRef]
4. Krauth-Siegel, R.L.; Leroux, A.E. Low-molecular-mass antioxidants in parasites. *Antioxid. Redox Signal.* **2012**, *17*, 583–607. [CrossRef] [PubMed]
5. Ariyanayagam, M.R.; Fairlamb, A.H. Ovothiol and trypanothione as antioxidants in trypanosomatids. *Mol. Biochem. Parasitol.* **2001**, *115*, 189–198. [CrossRef]
6. Gonçalves, C.; Costa, P.M. Histochemical detection of free thiols in glandular cells and tissues of different marine Polychaeta. *Histochem. Cell Biol.* **2020**, *154*, 315–325. [CrossRef]
7. O'neill, E.C.; Trick, M.; Hill, L.; Rejzek, M.; Dusi, R.G.; Hamilton, C.J.; Zimba, P.V.; Henrissat, B.; Field, R.A. The transcriptome of *Euglena gracilis* reveals unexpected metabolic capabilities for carbohydrate and natural product biochemistry. *Mol. BioSyst.* **2015**, *11*, 2808–2820. [CrossRef]
8. Milito, A.; Orefice, I.; Smerilli, A.; Castellano, I.; Napolitano, A.; Brunet, C.; Palumbo, A. Insights into the Light Response of *Skeletonema marinoi*: Involvement of Ovothiol. *Mar. Drugs* **2020**, *18*, 477. [CrossRef] [PubMed]
9. Torres, J.P.; Lin, Z.; Watkins, M.; Salcedo, P.F.; Baskin, R.P.; Elhabian, S.; Safavi-Hemami, H.; Taylor, D.; Tun, J.; Concepcion, G.P. Small-molecule mimicry hunting strategy in the imperial cone snail, *Conus imperialis*. *Sci. Adv.* **2021**, *7*, eabf2704. [CrossRef]
10. Russo, G.L.; Russo, M.; Castellano, I.; Napolitano, A.; Palumbo, A. Ovothiol isolated from sea urchin oocytes induces autophagy in the Hep-G2 cell line. *Mar. Drugs* **2014**, *12*, 4069–4085. [CrossRef] [PubMed]
11. Castellano, I.; Di Tomo, P.; Di Pietro, N.; Mandatori, D.; Pipino, C.; Formoso, G.; Napolitano, A.; Palumbo, A.; Pandolfi, A. Anti-inflammatory activity of marine ovothiol A in an in vitro model of endothelial dysfunction induced by hyperglycemia. *Oxidative Med. Cell. Longev.* **2018**, *2018*, 2087373. [CrossRef]
12. Brancaccio, M.; D'Argenio, G.; Lembo, V.; Palumbo, A.; Castellano, I. Antifibrotic effect of marine ovothiol in an in vivo model of liver fibrosis. *Oxidative Med. Cell. Longev.* **2018**, *2018*, 5045734. [CrossRef]
13. Palumbo, A.; Castellano, I.; Napolitano, A. Ovothiol: A potent natural antioxidant from marine organisms. *Blue Biotechnol. Prod. Use Mar. Mol.* **2018**, *2*, 583–610. [CrossRef]
14. Braunshausen, A.; Seebeck, F.P. Identification and characterization of the first ovothiol biosynthetic enzyme. *J. Am. Chem. Soc.* **2011**, *133*, 1757–1759. [CrossRef]
15. Castellano, I.; Seebeck, F.P. On ovothiol biosynthesis and biological roles: From life in the ocean to therapeutic potential. *Nat. Prod. Rep.* **2018**, *35*, 1241–1250. [CrossRef] [PubMed]
16. Yanshole, V.V.; Yanshole, L.V.; Zelentsova, E.A.; Tsentalovich, Y.P. Ovothiol A is the main antioxidant in fish lens. *Metabolites* **2019**, *9*, 95. [CrossRef]
17. Tsentalovich, Y.P.; Zelentsova, E.A.; Yanshole, L.V.; Yanshole, V.V.; Odud, I.M. Most abundant metabolites in tissues of freshwater fish pike-perch (*Sander lucioperca*). *Sci. Rep.* **2020**, *10*, 1–12. [CrossRef]
18. Brancaccio, M.; Tangherlini, M.; Danovaro, R.; Castellano, I. Metabolic adaptations to marine environments: Molecular diversity and evolution of ovothiol biosynthesis in Bacteria. *Genome Biol. Evol.* **2021**, *13*, evab169. [CrossRef] [PubMed]
19. Migliaccio, O.; Castellano, I.; Romano, G.; Palumbo, A. Stress response to cadmium and manganese in *Paracentrotus lividus* developing embryos is mediated by nitric oxide. *Aquat. Toxicol.* **2014**, *156*, 125–134. [CrossRef] [PubMed]

20. Sommer, U.; Stibor, H. Copepoda–Cladocera–Tunicata: The role of three major mesozooplankton groups in pelagic food webs. *Ecol. Res.* **2002**, *17*, 161–174. [CrossRef]
21. Steinberg, D.K.; Landry, M.R. Zooplankton and the ocean carbon cycle. *Annu. Rev. Mar. Sci.* **2017**, *9*, 413–444. [CrossRef] [PubMed]
22. Turner, J.T. Zooplankton fecal pellets, marine snow, phytodetritus and the ocean's biological pump. *Prog. Oceanogr.* **2015**, *130*, 205–248. [CrossRef]
23. Lauritano, C.; Romano, G.; Roncalli, V.; Amoresano, A.; Fontanarosa, C.; Bastianini, M.; Braga, F.; Carotenuto, Y.; Ianora, A. New oxylipins produced at the end of a diatom bloom and their effects on copepod reproductive success and gene expression levels. *Harmful Algae* **2016**, *55*, 221–229. [CrossRef]
24. Roncalli, V.; Turner, J.T.; Kulis, D.; Anderson, D.M.; Lenz, P.H. The effect of the toxic dinoflagellate *Alexandrium fundyense* on the fitness of the calanoid copepod *Calanus finmarchicus*. *Harmful Algae* **2016**, *51*, 56–66. [CrossRef] [PubMed]
25. Russo, E.; Lauritano, C.; d'Ippolito, G.; Fontana, A.; Sarno, D.; von Elert, E.; Ianora, A.; Carotenuto, Y. RNA-Seq and differential gene expression analysis in *Temora stylifera* copepod females with contrasting non-feeding nauplii survival rates: An environmental transcriptomics study. *BMC Genom.* **2020**, *21*, 1–22. [CrossRef]
26. Carotenuto, Y.; Vitiello, V.; Gallo, A.; Libralato, G.; Trifuoggi, M.; Toscanesi, M.; Lofrano, G.; Esposito, F.; Buttino, I. Assessment of the relative sensitivity of the copepods *Acartia tonsa* and *Acartia clausi* exposed to sediment-derived elutriates from the Bagnoli-Coroglio industrial area. *Mar. Environ. Res.* **2020**, *155*, 104878. [CrossRef] [PubMed]
27. Bai, Z.; Wang, N.; Wang, M. Effects of microplastics on marine copepods. *Ecotoxicol. Environ. Saf.* **2021**, *217*, 112243. [CrossRef] [PubMed]
28. Roncalli, V.; Cieslak, M.C.; Lenz, P.H. Transcriptomic responses of the calanoid copepod *Calanus finmarchicus* to the saxitoxin producing dinoflagellate *Alexandrium fundyense*. *Sci. Rep.* **2016**, *6*, 25708. [CrossRef] [PubMed]
29. Asai, S.; Sanges, R.; Lauritano, C.; Lindeque, P.K.; Esposito, F.; Ianora, A.; Carotenuto, Y. De novo transcriptome assembly and gene expression profiling of the copepod *Calanus helgolandicus* feeding on the PUA-producing diatom *Skeletonema marinoi*. *Mar. Drugs* **2020**, *18*, 392. [CrossRef]
30. Kültz, D. Defining biological stress and stress responses based on principles of physics. *J. Exp. Zool. Part A Ecol. Integr. Physiol.* **2020**, *333*, 350–358. [CrossRef]
31. Tarrant, A.M.; Payton, S.L.; Reitzel, A.M.; Porter, D.T.; Jenny, M.J. Ultraviolet radiation significantly enhances the molecular response to dispersant and sweet crude oil exposure in *Nematostella vectensis*. *Mar. Environ. Res.* **2018**, *134*, 96–108. [CrossRef]
32. Ianora, A.; Miralto, A.; Poulet, S.A.; Carotenuto, Y.; Buttino, I.; Romano, G.; Casotti, R.; Pohnert, G.; Wichard, T.; Colucci-D'Amato, L. Aldehyde suppression of copepod recruitment in blooms of a ubiquitous planktonic diatom. *Nature* **2004**, *429*, 403–407. [CrossRef] [PubMed]
33. Carotenuto, Y.; Dattolo, E.; Lauritano, C.; Pisano, F.; Sanges, R.; Miralto, A.; Procaccini, G.; Ianora, A. Insights into the transcriptome of the marine copepod *Calanus helgolandicus* feeding on the oxylipin-producing diatom *Skeletonema marinoi*. *Harmful Algae* **2014**, *31*, 153–162. [CrossRef] [PubMed]
34. Dennery, P.A. Effects of oxidative stress on embryonic development. *Birth Defects Res. Part C Embryo Today: Rev.* **2007**, *81*, 155–162. [CrossRef]
35. Mauchline, J. *Adv. Mar. Biol. 33: The Biology of Calanoid Copepods*; Academic Press: Cambridge, MA, USA, 1998.
36. Saide, A.; Martínez, K.A.; Ianora, A.; Lauritano, C. Unlocking the Health Potential of Microalgae as Sustainable Sources of Bioactive Compounds. *Int. J. Mol. Sci.* **2021**, *22*, 4383. [CrossRef]
37. Carotenuto, Y.; Esposito, F.; Pisano, F.; Lauritano, C.; Perna, M.; Miralto, A.; Ianora, A. Multi-generation cultivation of the copepod *Calanus helgolandicus* in a re-circulating system. *J. Exp. Mar. Biol. Ecol.* **2012**, *418*, 46–58. [CrossRef]
38. Riccio, G.; Ruocco, N.; Mutalipassi, M.; Costantini, M.; Zupo, V.; Coppola, D.; de Pascale, D.; Lauritano, C. Ten-Year Research Update Review: Antiviral Activities from Marine Organisms. *Biomolecules* **2020**, *10*, 1007. [CrossRef] [PubMed]
39. Brillatz, T.; Lauritano, C.; Jacmin, M.; Khamma, S.; Marcourt, L.; Righi, D.; Romano, G.; Esposito, F.; Ianora, A.; Queiroz, E.F. Zebrafish-based identification of the antiseizure nucleoside inosine from the marine diatom *Skeletonema marinoi*. *PLoS ONE* **2018**, *13*, e0196195. [CrossRef] [PubMed]
40. Gasmi, A.; Mujawdiya, P.K.; Shanaida, M.; Ongenae, A.; Lysiuk, R.; Doşa, M.D.; Tsal, O.; Piscopo, S.; Chirumbolo, S.; Bjørklund, G. *Calanus* oil in the treatment of obesity-related low-grade inflammation, insulin resistance, and atherosclerosis. *Appl. Microbiol. Biotechnol.* **2020**, *104*, 967–979. [CrossRef]
41. Vingiani, G.M.; De Luca, P.; Ianora, A.; Dobson, A.D.; Lauritano, C. Microalgal enzymes with biotechnological applications. *Mar. Drugs* **2019**, *17*, 459. [CrossRef] [PubMed]
42. Lauritano, C.; Helland, K.; Riccio, G.; Andersen, J.H.; Ianora, A.; Hansen, E.H. Lysophosphatidylcholines and chlorophyll-derived molecules from the diatom *Cylindrotheca closterium* with anti-inflammatory activity. *Mar. Drugs* **2020**, *18*, 166. [CrossRef] [PubMed]
43. Roncalli, V.; Cieslak, M.C.; Passamaneck, Y.; Christie, A.E.; Lenz, P.H. Glutathione S-transferase (GST) gene diversity in the crustacean *Calanus finmarchicus*– contributors to cellular detoxification. *PLoS ONE* **2015**, *10*, e0123322. [CrossRef]
44. Christie, A.E.; Roncalli, V.; Lenz, P.H. Diversity of insulin-like peptide signaling system proteins in *Calanus finmarchicus* (Crustacea; Copepoda)—Possible contributors to seasonal pre-adult diapause. *Gen. Comp. Endocrinol.* **2016**, *236*, 157–173. [CrossRef] [PubMed]

45. Hyde, C.J.; Fitzgibbon, Q.P.; Elizur, A.; Smith, G.G.; Ventura, T. CrustyBase: An interactive online database for crustacean transcriptomes. *BMC Genom.* **2020**, *21*, 1–10. [CrossRef]
46. Gasteiger, E.; Gattiker, A.; Hoogland, C.; Ivanyi, I.; Appel, R.D.; Bairoch, A. ExPASy: The proteomics server for in-depth protein knowledge and analysis. *Nucleic Acids Res.* **2003**, *31*, 3784–3788. [CrossRef]
47. Finn, R.D.; Bateman, A.; Clements, J.; Coggill, P.; Eberhardt, R.Y.; Eddy, S.R.; Heger, A.; Hetherington, K.; Holm, L.; Mistry, J. Pfam: The protein Families database. *Nucleic Acids Res.* **2014**, *42*, D222–D230. [CrossRef] [PubMed]
48. Larkin, M.A.; Blackshields, G.; Brown, N.P.; Chenna, R.; McGettigan, P.A.; McWilliam, H.; Valentin, F.; Wallace, I.M.; Wilm, A.; Lopez, R.; et al. Clustal W and Clustal X version 2.0. *Bioinformatics* **2007**, *23*, 2947–2948. [CrossRef]
49. Price, M.N.; Dehal, P.S.; Arkin, A.P. FastTree 2–approximately maximum-likelihood trees for large alignments. *PLoS ONE* **2010**, *5*, e9490. [CrossRef]
50. Christie, A.E.; Fontanilla, T.M.; Nesbit, K.T.; Lenz, P.H. Prediction of the protein components of a putative Calanus finmarchicus (Crustacea, Copepoda) circadian signaling systems using a de novo assembled transcriptome. *Comp. Biochem. Physiol. D Genom. Proteom.* **2013**, *8*, 165–193. [CrossRef] [PubMed]
51. Cieslak, M.C.; Castelfranco, A.M.; Roncalli, V.; Lenz, P.H.; Hartline, D.K. t-Distributed Stochastic Neighbor Embedding (t-SNE): A tool for eco-physiological transcriptomic analysis. *Mar. Genom.* **2020**, *51*, 100723. [CrossRef]
52. Lenz, P.H.; Roncalli, V.; Hassett, R.P.; Wu, L.S.; Cieslak, M.C.; Hartline, D.K.; Christie, A.E. *De novo* assembly of a transcriptome for *Calanus finmarchicus* (Crustacea, Copepoda)-the dominant zooplankter of the North Atlantic Ocean. *PLoS ONE* **2014**, *9*, e88589. [CrossRef] [PubMed]

MDPI
St. Alban-Anlage 66
4052 Basel
Switzerland
Tel. +41 61 683 77 34
Fax +41 61 302 89 18
www.mdpi.com

Marine Drugs Editorial Office
E-mail: marinedrugs@mdpi.com
www.mdpi.com/journal/marinedrugs

www.ingramcontent.com/pod-product-compliance
Lightning Source LLC
LaVergne TN
LVHW070638100526
838202LV00012B/832